SURGICAL RECALL
3rd edition

"In the operating room we can save more lives, cure more cancer, restore more function, and relieve more suffering than anywhere else in the hospital."

—R. Scott Jones, M.D.

SURGICAL RECALL
3rd edition

RECALL SERIES EDITOR AND SENIOR EDITOR

LORNE H. BLACKBOURNE, M.D., F.A.C.S.
Fellow, Trauma/Critical Care
Department of Surgery
University of Miami
Jackson Memorial Hospital
Miami, Florida
MEDSTUD.com

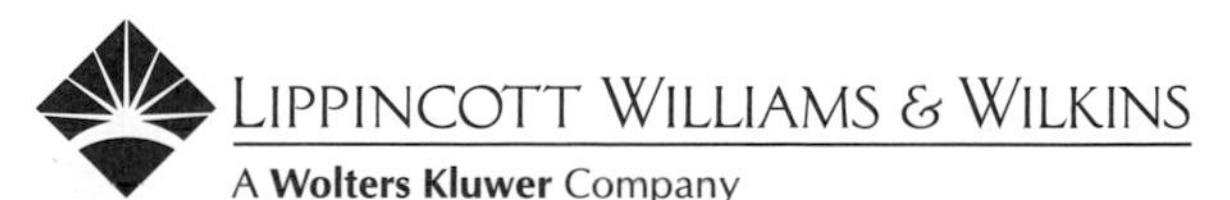

A **Wolters Kluwer** Company
Philadelphia • Baltimore • New York • London
Buenos Aires • Hong Kong • Sydney • Tokyo

Editor: Neil Marquardt
Managing Editor: Emilie Linkins
Marketing Manager: Scott Lavine
Senior Production Editor: Karen M. Ruppert
Designer: Risa Clow
Compositor: Peirce Graphic Services
Printer: RRD-Crawfordsville

351 West Camden Street
Baltimore, MD 21201
530 Walnut St.
Philadelphia, PA 19106

Printed in the United States of America

First Edition, 1994
Second Edition, 1998

Library of Congress Cataloging-in-Publication Data

Surgical recall / editor, Lorne H. Blackbourne.—3rd ed.
p. cm.
Includes index.
ISBN 0-7817-2973-4 (alk. paper)
1. Surgery—Examinations, questions, etc. I. Blackbourne, Lorne H.

RD37.2 .S9748 2002
617′.0076—dc21

2002023582

To purchase additional copies of this book, call our customer service department at **(800) 638-3030** or fax orders to **(301) 824-7390.** International customers should call **(301) 714-2324.**

Visit Lippincott Williams & Wilkins on the Internet: http://www.LWW.com. Lippincott Williams & Wilkins customer service representatives are available from 8:30 am to 6:00 pm, EST.

02 03 04 05 06
1 2 3 4 5 6 7 8 9 10

Dedication

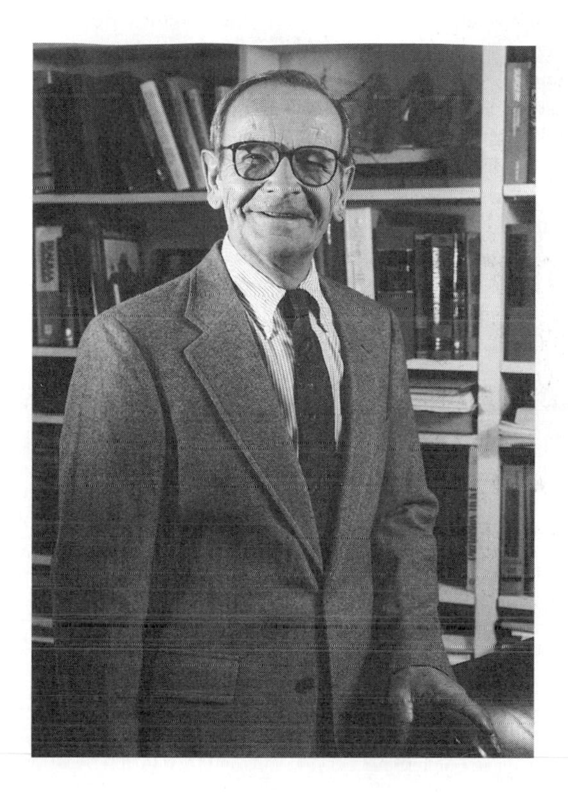

This manual is dedicated to the memory of Leslie E. Rudolf, Professor of Surgery and Vice Chairman of the Department of Surgery at the University of Virginia. Dr. Rudolf was born on November 12, 1927 in New Rochelle, New York. He served in the U.S. Army Counter-intelligence Corps in Europe after World War II.

He graduated from Union College in 1951 and attended Cornell Medical College, from which he graduated in 1955. He then entered his surgical residency at Peter Brigham Hospital in Boston, Massachusetts and completed his residency there serving as Chief Resident Surgeon in 1961.

Dr. Rudolf came to Charlottesville, Virginia as an Assistant Professor of Surgery in 1963. He rapidly rose through the ranks, becoming Professor of Surgery and Vice Chairman of the Department in 1974 and a Markle Scholar in Academic Medicine from 1966 until 1971. His research interests included organ and tissue transplantation and preservation. Dr. Rudolf was instrumental in initiating the Kidney Transplant Program at the University of Virginia Health Sciences Center. His active involvement in service to the Charlottesville community is particularly exemplified by his early work with the Charlottesville/Albemarle Rescue Squad, and he received the Governor's Citation for the Commonwealth of Virginia Emergency Medical Services in 1980.

His colleagues at the University of Virginia Health Sciences Center, including faculty and residents, recognized his keen interests in teaching medical students, evaluating and teaching residents, and helping the young surgical faculty. He took a serious interest in medical student education, and he would have strongly approved of this teaching manual, affectionately known as the "Rudolf" guide, as an extension of ward rounds and textbook reading.

In addition to his distinguished academic accomplishments, Dr. Rudolf was a talented person with many diverse scholarly pursuits and hobbies. His advice and counsel on topics ranging from Chinese cooking to orchid raising were sought by a wide spectrum of friends and admirers.

This manual is a logical extension of Dr. Rudolf's interests in teaching. No one book, operation, or set of rounds can begin to answer all questions of surgical disease processes; however, in a constellation of learning endeavors, this effort would certainly have pleased him.

John B. Hanks, M.D.
Professor of Surgery
University of Virginia
Charlottesville, Virginia

EDITORS:

Anikar Chhabra, M.D.
Resident in Orthopaedic Surgery
University of Virginia
Charlottesville, Virginia

Mark I.E. Cockburn, M.D.
Fellow in Surgical Critical Care/Trauma
Department of General Surgery
University of Miami—Jackson Memorial Hospital
Miami, Florida

Robert L. Hannan, M.D.
Senior Staff Surgeon
Cardiovascular Surgery
Miami Children's Hospital
Miami, Florida

ASSOCIATE EDITORS:

Joseph J. Dubois
Medical Student
University of Virginia
Charlottesville, Virginia

Dennis Kim, M.P.H.
Albany Medical College
New York, New York

Oliver A.R. Binns, M.D.
Resident in Thoracic Surgery
University of Virginia Health Sciences Center
Charlottesville, Virginia

Jared Antevil, M.D.
General Surgeon
San Diego, California

INTERNATIONAL EDITORS:

Mohammad Azfar, MBBS, F.R.C.S.
General Surgeon
Kuwait City, Kuwait

Stephen Washington, MBChB
Department of Surgery
University of Manchester
Manchester, United Kingdom

Elizabeth Cheshire MBBS (Hons), LLB(Hons)
Hampshire, United Kingdom

ADVISOR:

Curtis G. Tribble, M.D. FACS
Professor of Surgery
University of Virginia

Contributors

The following contributed to the third edition of this book:

Suzanne Clements
Medical Student
University of Manchester
Manchester, United Kingdom

Adam C. Crowl, M.D.
Resident in Orthopaedic Surgery
University of Virginia
Charlottesville, Virginia

Joseph J. DuBois, M.D.
Medical Student
University of Virginia
Charlottesville, Virginia

Johnathan A. Engh, M.D.
Medical Student
University of Virginia Health Sciences Center
Charlottesville, Virginia

Johann Farley, M.D.
Medical College of Wisconsin
Racine Family Practice
Racine, Wisconsin

Mark G. Freeman, M.D.
Medical Student
University of Virginia School of Medicine
Charlottesville, Virginia
Resident in Orthopaedic Surgery
Chattanooga, Tennessee

Michael H. Handy, M.D.
Resident in Orthopaedic Surgery
University of Virginia Health Sciences Center
Charlottesville, Virginia

Clara M. Holt
Columbia University
New York, New York

Steven A. Koziol, M.D.
Department of Surgery
Wilford Hall Air Force Base
University of Texas
San Antonio, Texas

Dr. P. Moradi, M.D.
Senior House Officer
Ophthalmology
Salisbury NHS Trust
Salisbury, United Kingdom

Brett Odum, M.D.
Resident in Neurosurgery
Medical College of Virginia
Richmond, Virginia

Kornelis A. Poelstra, M.D., PhD
Resident in Orthopaedic Surgery
University of Virginia
Charlottesville, Virginia

Derek B. Purcell, M.D.
Medical Student
University of Virginia
Charlottesville, Virginia

Clifton C. Reade, M.D.
Resident in General Surgery
East Carolina University
Greenville, North Carolina

Joshua R. Simmons
Medical Student
University of Virginia
Charlottesville, Virginia

Angelique M. Reitsma, M.D.
Resident in Family Medicine
University of Virginia
Charlottesville, Virginia

Brian P. Struyk, M.D.
Transitional Intern
Naval Medical Center
San Diego, California

Francis Shen, M.D.
Resident in Orthopaedic Surgery
University of Virginia
Charlottesville, Virginia

L. Erik Westerlund, M.D.
Resident in Orthopaedic Surgery
University of Virginia
Charlottesville, Virginia

The following people contributed to previous editions of this book:

Lorne H. Blackbourne, M.D.
Kirk J. Fleischer, M.D.
Colt Peyton, M.D.
Oliver A.R. Binns, M.D.
Christopher Bogaev, M.D.
R. Bradford Bowles III, M.D.
James A. Burns, M.D.
David deHoll, M.D.
Hong J. Kim, M.D.
Carolyn Lederman, M.D.
L. Carr McClain, M.D.
Gregory Paine, M.D.
Richard S. Polin, M.D.
Henry M. Prillaman, M.D.
Donald Schmidt, M.D.
Walter Scott, M.D.
Nathan E. Simmons, M.D.
Owen B. Tabor, M.D.
Anne Whitworth, M.D.
Linda C. Ahn, M.D.
Robert A. Buckmire, M.D.
David C. Cassada, M.D.
John W. Davis, M.D.
Nicolisa DeSouza, M.D.
Barbara M. Fried, M.D.
W. Glover Garner, M.D.
Christopher Hogan, M.D.
Nancy A. Huff, M.D.
Stephen S. Kim, M.D.
Timothy Kwiatkowski, M.D.
J. Pieter Noordzij, M.D.
David M. Powell, M.D.
G. Bino Rucker, M.D.
Julius P. Smith III, M.D.
Mehrdad Soroush, M.D.
John Sperling, M.D.
Sandeep S. Teja, M.D.
Eric E. Walk, M.D.
T. Lisle Whitman, M.D.
William J. Wirostko, M.D.
David Bentrem, M.D.
Paul Shin, M.D.
Jennifer Deblasi, M.D.
Jonas R. Rudziki, M.D.
Albert Weed, B.A.
Joseph Wells, M.D.
Jeffry Claridge, M.D.
John Sperling, M.D.
Jonas Sheehan, M.D.
David Graham, M.D.
Charles Hobson, M.D.
Christopher Hogan, M.D.
Bradley Kesser, M.D.
John Jane, M.D.
Scott Langenburg, M.D.
Christopher Moore, M.D.
Paul Mosca, M.D.

Foreword

Surgical Recall represents the culmination of several years' effort by Lorne Blackbourne and his friends, who began the project when they were third-year medical students. Lorne, who completed his residency in General Surgery at the University of Virginia, has involved other surgical residents and medical students to provide annual updates and revisions to this text.

This book reflects the interest, enthusiasm, and true dedication to learning and teaching that permeates the medical school classes and surgical residencies in our institution. It is an honor, privilege, and a continuing stimulus to work in the midst of this group of dedicated young people. I congratulate all the students and residents involved in this project and also acknowledge the leadership of the surgical faculty. The professor's ultimate satisfaction occurs when all the learners assume ownership of learning and teaching.

This book encompasses the essential information in general surgery and surgical specialties usually imparted to students in our surgical clerkship and reviewed and developed further in electives. Developed from the learner's standpoint, the text includes fundamental information such as a description of the diseases, signs, symptoms, essentials of pathophysiology, treatments, and possible outcomes. The unique format of this study guide uses the Socratic method by employing a list of questions or problems posed along the left side of the page with answers and responses on the right. In addition, the guide includes numerous practical tips for students and junior residents to facilitate comprehensive and effective management of patients. This material is essential for students in the core course of surgery and for those taking senior electives.

In this third edition of *Surgical Recall*, the authors have added several new chapters and have expanded the existing chapters for a fuller and more complete coverage of all subjects, including the new subjects. We hope you find this expanded version of this work stimulating and easy to use.

R. Scott Jones, M.D.
Professor and Chairman
Department of Surgery
University of Virginia
Charlottesville, Virginia

Preface

Surgical Recall began as a source of surgical facts during my Surgery Clerkship when I was a third-year medical student at the University of Virginia. My goal has been to provide concise information that every third-year surgical student should know, placed in a "rapid fire" two-column format.

The format of *Surgical Recall* is conducive to the recall of basic surgical facts because it relies upon repetition and positive feedback. As one repeats the question-and-answer format, one gains success.

This new third edition includes updated information, new acronyms and mnemonics, new illustrations, and more streamlined rapid-fire answers.

We have dedicated our work to the living memory of Professor Leslie Rudolf. It is our hope that those who knew Dr. Rudolf will remember him and those who did not will ask.

Lorne H. Blackbourne, M.D., F.A.C.S
Fellow, Trauma/Critical Care
Department of Surgery
University of Miami
Miami, Florida

P.S. We would like to hear from you if you have any corrections, acronyms, classic ward or operating room questions (all contributors will be credited). You can reach me via email in care of Lippincott Williams & Wilkins at book_comments@lww.com.

Contents

Section I

Overview and Background Surgical Information

1 Introduction

PREPARING FOR THE SURGERY CLERKSHIP

USING THE STUDY GUIDE

This study guide was written to accompany the surgical clerkship. It has evolved over the years through student feedback and continued updating. In this regard, we welcome any feedback (both positive and negative) or suggestions for improvement. The objective of the guide is to provide a rapid overview of common surgical topics, but keep in mind that **it is NOT written as an all-encompassing source. You will have to consult major textbooks to round out the information in this guide.** The guide is organized in a self-study/quiz format. By covering the information/answers on the right with the bookmark, you can attempt to answer the questions on the left to assess your understanding of the information. Keep the guide with you at all times, and when you have even a few spare minutes (e.g., between cases) hammer out a page or at least a few questions. Many students read this book as a primer before the clerkship even begins!

Your study objectives in surgery should include the following four points:

1. OR question-and-answer periods
2. Ward questioning
3. Oral exam
4. Written exam

The optimal plan of action would include daily reading in a text, such as McKenney, Mangonon, and Moylan's *Understanding Surgical Disease*, anatomy review prior to each OR case, and *Surgical Recall.* But remember, this guide helps you recall basic facts about surgical topics. Reading should be done daily! The average general surgery clerkship is 6 weeks, or 42 days. If you read 10 pages a day, that is 420 pages, or the entire text of McKenney, Mangonon, and Moylan's *Understanding Surgical Disease!* As you read the text, take notes.

To facilitate learning a surgical topic, first break down each topic into the following categories and, in turn, master each category:

1. What is it?
2. Incidence
3. Risk factors
4. Signs and symptoms

5. Laboratory and radiologic tests
6. Diagnostic criteria
7. Differential diagnoses
8. Medical and surgical treatment
9. Postoperative care
10. Complications
11. Stages and prognosis

Granted, it is hard to read after a full day in the OR. For a change, go to sleep right away and wake up a few hours early the next day and read **before** going to the hospital. It sounds crazy, but it does work.

APPEARANCE

Why is your appearance so important?

The patient sees only the wound dressing, the skin closure, and you. You can wear whatever you want, **but you best look clean. Do not wear religious or political buttons as this is not fair to your patients.**

WHAT THE PERFECT SURGICAL STUDENT CARRIES IN HER COAT

Stethoscope
Penlight
Scissors
Minibook on medications (e.g., trade names, doses)
Tape/4 × 4s
Sutures to practice tying
Pen/notepad/small notebook to write down pearls
Notebook or clipboard with patient's data (always write down chores with a box next to them so you can check off the box when the chore is completed)
Small calculator
List of commonly used telephone numbers (e.g., radiology)

THE PERFECT PREPARATION FOR ROUNDS

Interview your patient (e.g., problems, pain, wishes).
Talk with your patient's nurse (e.g. "Were there any events during the last shift?").
Examine patient (e.g., cor/pulm/abd/**wound**).
Record vital signs (e.g., T_{max}).
Record input (e.g., IVF, PO).
Record output (e.g., urine, drains).
Check labs.
Check microbiology (e.g., culture reports, Gram stains).
Check x-rays.
Check pathology reports.

Check allied health updates (e.g., PT, OT).
Read chart.
Check medication (don't forget H_2 blocker in the hyperalimentation).
Check nutrition.
Always check with the intern for chores, updates, insider information, **before** rounds.

PRESENTING ON ROUNDS

Your presentation on rounds should be like an iceberg. State important points about your patient (the tip of the iceberg visible above the ocean), but know **everything** else about your patient that your chief might ask about (that part of the iceberg under the ocean). Always include:
Name
Postoperative day s/p-procedure
A concise overall assessment of how the patient is doing
Vital signs/temp status/antibiotics day
Input/output-urine, drains, po intake, IVF
Change in physical examination
Any complaints (not yours—the patient's)
Plan

Your presentation should be concise, with good eye contact (you should not simply read from a clipboard). The intangible element of confidence cannot be overemphasized; if you do not know the answer to a question about a patient, however, the correct response should be "I do not know, but I will find out." Never lie or hedge on an answer because it will only serve to make the remainder of your surgical rotation less than desirable. Furthermore, do your best to be enthusiastic and motivated. **Never, ever whine.** And remember to be a **team player.** Never make your fellow students look bad! Residents pick up on this immediately and will slam you.

THE PERFECT SURGERY STUDENT

Never whines
Never pimps his residents or fellow students (or attendings)
Never complains
Is never hungry, thirsty, or tired
Is always enthusiastic
Loves to do scut work and can never get enough
Never makes a fellow student look bad
Is always clean (a patient sees only you and the wound dressing)
Is never late
Smiles a lot and has a good sense of humor
Makes things happen
Is not a "know it all"
Never corrects anyone **during** rounds unless it will affect patient care
Makes the intern/resident/chief look good at all times, if at all possible

Knows more about her patients than anyone else
Loves the OR
Never wants to leave the hospital
Takes correction, direction, and instruction very well
Says "Sir" and "Ma'am" to the scrub nurses (and to the attending, unless corrected)
Never asks questions he can look up for himself
Knows the patient's disease, surgery, indication for surgery, and the anatomy before going to the OR
Is the first one to arrive at clinic and the last one to leave
Always places x-rays up in the OR
Reads from a surgery text **every day**
Is a team player
Asks for feedback
Never has a chip on her shoulder
Loves to suture
Is honest and always admits fault and errors
Knows when his patient is going to the OR (e.g., by calling)
Is confident but **not** cocky
Has a **"Can Do"** attitude and can figure out things on her own
Is not afraid to get help when needed
Never says **"No"** or **"Maybe"** to involvement in patient care
Treats everyone (e.g., nurses, fellow students) with respect
Follows the chain of command
Never wears scrubs to conference
Praises others when appropriate
Checks with the intern beforehand for information for rounds (test results/ surprises)
RUNS for materials, lab values, test results, etc., during rounds before any house officer
Gives credit where credit is due
Dresses and undresses wounds on rounds
Has a steel bladder, a cast-iron stomach, and a heart of gold
Always writes the op note without question
Always checks with the intern after rounds for chores
Always makes sure there is a medical student in every case
Always follows the patient to the recovery room
In the OR, always asks permission to ask a question
Always reviews anatomy prior to going to the OR
Does what the intern asks (i.e., the chief will get feedback from the intern)
Is a high-speed, low-drag, hardcore **HAMMERHEAD**

Define HAMMERHEAD	A hammerhead is an individual who places his head to the ground and **hammers** through any and all obstacles to get a job done and then asks for more work. One who gives 110% and never complains. One who **desires** work.

OPERATING ROOM

Your job in the OR will be to retract (water-skiing) and answer questions posed by the attending physicians and residents. Retracting is basically idiot-proof. Many students emphasize anticipating the surgeon's next move, but stick to following the surgeon's request. More than 75% of the questions asked in the OR deal with anatomy; therefore, read about the anatomy and pathophysiology of the case, which will reduce the "I don't knows."

Never argue with the scrub nurses—they are always right. They are the selfless warriors of the operating suite's sterile field, and arguing with one will only **make matters worse.**

Never touch or take instruments from the Mayo tray (tray with instruments on it over the patient's feet) unless given explicit permission to do so. Every day when you approach the OR suite door **STOP** and ask yourself if you have on scrubs, shoe covers, a cap, and a mask to avoid the embarrassing situation of being yelled at by the OR staff (a.k.a. the 3 strikes test: strike 1 = no mask, strike 2 = no headcover, strike 3 = no shoe covers. . . . . any strikes and you are outta here—place a mental stop sign outside of the OR with the 3 strikes rule on it)! When entering the OR, first introduce yourself to the scrub nurse and ask if you can get your gloves or gown. If you have questions in the OR, first **ask** if you can ask a question because it may be a bad time and this way it will not appear as though you are pimping the resident/attending.

Other thoughts on the OR:

When scrubbed, if you need to sneeze, step straight back and do not turn your head. If you feel faint, ask if you can sit down (try to eat prior to going to the OR). If your feet swell in the OR, try wearing support hose socks. If your back hurts, try taking some ibuprofen (with a meal) **prior** to the case. Also, sit-ups or abdominal crunches help to relieve back pain by strengthening the abdominal muscles. At the end of the case, ask the scrub nurse for some leftover ties (clean ones) to practice tying knots with and, if there is time, start writing your OP Note.

Why always wipe the Betadine (povidone-iodine) off your patient at the end of the procedure?	The Betadine can become very irritating and itchy.

SURGICAL NOTES

HISTORY AND PHYSICAL REPORT

The history and physical examination report, better known as the H & P, can make the difference between life and death. You should take this responsibility very **seriously.** Fatal errors can be made in the H & P, including the incorrect diagnosis, the wrong medications, the wrong allergies, and the wrong past surgical history. Operative reports of the patient's past surgical procedures are invaluable! The surgical H & P needs to be both accurate and **concise.** To save space, use − for a negative sign/symptom and + for a positive sign/symptom.

What are the words most commonly misspelled in a surgical history note?

1. guaiac
2. abscess

Example H & P (very brief—for illustrative purposes only—see below or next section for abbreviation key):

Mr. Smith is a 22-year-old white man who was in his normal state of excellent health until he noted the onset of periumbilical pain 1 day prior to admission. This pain was followed approximately 4 hours later by pain in his right lower quadrant that any movement exacerbated. + vomiting, anorexia. − fever, urinary tract symptoms, change in bowel habits, constipation, BRBPR, hematemesis, or diarrhea.
Medications: Ibuprofen prn headaches
Allergies: NKDA (no known drug allergies)
PMH: none
PSH: none
SH: ETOH, tobacco
FH: − CA
ROS: − resp disease, − cardiac disease, − renal disease
PE:
HEENT ncat, tms clear
cor nsr, − m,r,g
pulm clear b/l
abd nondistended, + bs, + tender RLQ, + rebound RLQ
rectal guaiac − nl tone, − mass
ext nt, − c,c,e
neuro wnl
LABS: urinalysis (ua) normal. chem 7, PT/PTT, CBC pending
X-RAYS: none
ASSESSMENT: 22 y.o. wm with hx and physical findings of right lower quadrant peritoneal signs consistent with (c/w) appendicitis.
Plan:
Consent
IVF with Lactated Ringer's
IV cefoxitin
To OR for appendectomy
Wilson Tyler cc III/

PMH = past medical history; PSH = past surgical history; SH = social history; FH = family history; ROS = review of systems, ncat = normocephalic atraumatic; tms = tympanic membranes; cor = heart; m, r, g = murmur, rub, gallop; NSR = normal sinus rhythm; b/l = both lungs; bs = bowel sounds; cc III = clinical clerk, third year; ext = extremity; nt = nontender; c, c, e = cyanosis, clubbing, or erythema; wnl = within normal limits

PREOP NOTE

The preop note is written in the progress notes the day before the operation.

Example:

Preop Dx:	Colon CA
Labs:	CBC, chem 7, PT/PTT
CXR:	- infiltrate
Blood:	T & C × 2 units
ECG:	NSR, wnl
Anesthesia:	Pre-op completed
Consent:	Signed and on front of chart

Orders:

1. Void OCTOR (on call to OR)
2. 1 gm cefoxitin OCTOR
3. Hibiclens scrub this p.m.
4. Bowel prep today
5. NPO p midnight (MN)

p=after

OP NOTE

The op note is written in the OR before the patient is in the PACU (or recovery room) in the progress note section of the chart.

Example:

Preop Dx:	Acute appendicitis
Postop Dx:	Same
Procedure:	Appendectomy
Surgeon:	Halsted
Assistants:	Harvey Cushing, Curt Tribble, Joebob Dubose cc III
Op findings:	No perforation
Anesthesia:	GET
*I/O:	1000 mL LR/ uo 600 ml
*EBL:	50 mL
Specimen:	Appendix to pathology
Drains:	None
Complications:	None (if there are complications ask what you should write)

To PACU in stable condition

cc III = clinical clerk, third year; EBL = estimated blood loss; GET = general endotracheal; I/O = ins and outs; PACU = postanesthesia care unit

*Ask the anesthesiologist or Certified Registered Nurse Anesthetist (CRNA) for this information.

How do I remember what is in the OP note when I am in the OR?	Bring the *Surgical Recall* BOOKMARK with you to the OR, or remember the acronym PPP SAFE DISC:

P	Pre op dx
P	Post op dx
P	Procedure
S	Surgeon (and assistants)
A	Anesthesia
F	Fluids
E	Estimated blood loss (EBL)
D	Drains
I	IV Fluids
S	Specimen
C	Complications

POSTOP NOTE

The postop note is written on the day of the operation in the progress notes.
Example:

Procedure:	Appendectomy
Neuro:	A and O × 3
V/S:	Stable/afebrile
I/O:	1 L LR/ uo 600 ml (urine output)
Labs:	post-op Hct: 36
PE:	cor RRR
	pulm CTA
	abd drsg dry & intact
Drains:	JP 30 ml serosanguinous fluid
Assess:	Stable postop

Plan:

1. IV hydration
2. 1 g cefoxitin q 8 hr

V/S = vital signs; Hct = hematocrit; RRR = regular rhythm and rate; JP = Jackson-Pratt; A and O × 3 = alert and oriented times 3

ADMISSION ORDERS

The admission orders are written in the physician orders section of the patient's chart on admission, transfer, or postop.
Example:

Admit to 5E Dr. DeBakey

Dx:	AAA
Condition:	Stable

V/S:	q 4 hr or q shift; if post-op, q 15 min × 2 hr, then q 1 hr × 4, then q 4 hr
Activity:	Bedrest or OOB to chair
Nursing:	Daily wgt; I/O; change drsg q shift; call
HO for:	
	L = Temp > 38.5
	UO < 30 ml/hr
	SBP > 180 < 90
	DBP > 100
	HR < 60 > 110
Diet:	NPO
IVF:	D5 1/2 NS c̄ 20 KCL
Drugs:	ANCEF
Labs:	CBC

HO = House Officer; I/O = ins and outs; OOB = out of bed; SBP = systolic blood pressure; DBP = diastolic blood pressure, HR = heart rate; KCL = potassium chloride

ADMISSION ORDERS/POSTOP ORDERS

AC/DC AVA PAIN DUD

A = Admit to 5E
C = Care Provider
D = Diagnosis
C = Condition

A = Allergies
V = Vitals
A = Activity

P = Pain meds
A = Antibiotics
I = IVF/Incentive Spirometry
N = Nursing (Drains, Etc.)

D = DVT prophylaxis
U = Ulcer prophylaxis
D = Diet

DAILY NOTE—PROGRESS NOTE

Basically a SOAP note, but it is not necessary to write out SOAP. For many reasons, make your notes very OBJECTIVE and, as a student, do not mention discharge because this leads to confusion.

Example:
10/1/90 Blue Surgery
POD #4 s/p appendectomy
Day #5 cefoxitin
Pt without c/o
V/S: 120/80 76 12 afebrile (Tmax 38)
I/O: 1000/600
Drains: JP #1 60 last shift (JP = Jackson-Pratt drain)
PE: cor RRR-no m,g,r
pulm CTA
abd +BS, +flatus, -rigidity
ext nt, -cyanosis, -erythema
(nt = nontender)
ASSESS: Stable POD #4 on IV antibiotics
PLAN:
1. Increase PO intake.
2. Increase ambulation.
3. Follow cultures.
Grayson Stuart, cc III/
** Always sign your notes and leave the room for them to be cosigned!
POD = Postop day (The day after operation is POD 1. The day of operation is the operative day. **But note: antibiotic day #1 is the day the antibiotics were started.)
The acronym for what should be checked on your patient daily before rounding with the surgical team: AVOID WTE
A Appearance—any subjective complaints
V Vital signs
O Output-urine/drains
I Intake—IV/PO
D Drains—# of/output/character
W Wound/dressing/weight
T Temperature
E Exam—cor, pulm, abd, etc.

INTENSIVE CARE NOTE

The note is by systems:
Neurologic (GCS, MAE)
Pulmonary (vent settings, etc.)
CVS (pressors, swann numbers, etc.)
Heme (CBC)
F.E.N. (Chem 10, nutrition, etc.)
Renal (urine output, bun, cr, etc.)
I.D. (Tmax, WBC, antibiotics, etc.)
Assessment
Plan
(CVS = current vital signs; F.E.N. = fluids, electrolytes, nutrition; BUN = blood urea nitrogen; Cr = creatinine; I.D. = incision and drainage). PE, labs,

radiology studies, etc. are included in each section. This is also an excellent way to write progress notes for the very complicated floor patient.

CLINIC NOTE

Often the clinic note is a letter to the referring doctor. It should always include:
1. Patient name, history #, date
2. Brief hx, current complaints/symptoms
3. PE, labs, x-rays
4. Assessment
5. Plan

How is a medication prescription written?	Tylenol® 500 mg tablet Disp (dispense): 100 tablets *sig:* 1–2 P.O. q 4 hrs PRN pain

COMMON ABBREVIATIONS YOU SHOULD KNOW

ā	Before
AAA	Abdominal aortic aneurysm, "triple A"
ABD	Army battle dressing
ABG	Arterial blood gas
ABI	Ankle to brachial index
AKA	Above the knee amputation
A.K.A.	Also known as
Ao	Aorta
APR	Abdominoperineal resection
ARDS	Adult respiratory distress syndrome
ASA	Aspirin
AXR	Abdominal x-ray
B1	Billroth 1 gastroduodenostomy
B2	Billroth 2 gastrojejunostomy
BCP	Birth control pill

BE	Barium enema
BIH	Bilateral inguinal hernia
BKA	Below the knee amputation
BRBPR	Bright red blood per rectum
BS	Bowel sounds, breath sounds, blood sugar
BSE	Breast self-examination
c̄	With
CA	Cancer
CABG	Coronary artery bypass graft ("CABBAGE")
CBC	Complete blood cell count
CBD	Common bile duct
C/O	Complains of
COPD	Chronic obstructive pulmonary disease
CP	Chest pain
CTA	Clear to auscultation
CVA	Cerebral vascular accident, costovertebral angle
CVP	Central venous pressure
CXR	Chest x-ray
Dx	Diagnosis
DDx	Differential diagnosis
DI	Diabetes insipidus
DP	Dorsalis pedalis
DPL	Diagnostic peritoneal lavage

DPC	Delayed primary closure
DT	Delirium tremens
DVT	Deep venous thrombosis
EBL	Estimated blood loss
ECG	Electrocardiogram (also EKG)
ECMO	Extracorporeal membrane oxygenation
EGD	Esophagogastroduodenoscopy (UGI scope)
EOMI	Extraocular muscles intact
ERCP	Endoscopic retrograde cholangio-pancreatography
ETOH	Alcohol
EUA	Exam under anesthesia
FAP	Familial adenomatous polyposis
FAST	Focused abdominal sonogram for trauma
FEN	Fluids, electrolytes, nutrition
FNA	Fine needle aspiration
FOBT	Fecal occult blood test
GCS	Glasgow Coma Scale
GERD	Gastroesophageal reflux disease
GET(A)	General endotracheal (anesthesia)
GU	Genitourinary
HCT	Hematocrit
HEENT	Head, Eyes, Ears, Nose, and Throat
HO	House officer

IABP	Intra-aortic balloon pump
IBD	Inflammatory bowel disease
ICU	Intensive care unit
I& D	Incision and drainage
I& O	Ins and outs, in and out
IMV	Intermittent mandatory ventilation
IVC	Inferior vena cava
IVF	Intravenous fluids
IVP	Intravenous pyelography
IVPB	Intravenous piggyback
JVD	Jugular venous distention
Ⓛ	Left
LAP APPY	Laparoscopic appendectomy
LAP CHOLE	Laparoscopic cholecystectomy
LE	Lower extremity
LES	Lower esophageal sphincter
LIH	Left inguinal hernia
LLQ	Left lower quadrant
LR	Lactated Ringer's
LUQ	Left upper quadrant
MAE	Moving all extremities
MAST	Military antishock trousers
MEN	Multiple endocrine neoplasia
MI	Myocardial infarction

MSO4	Morphine sulfate
NGT	Nasogastric tube
NPO	Nothing per os
NS	Normal saline
OBR	Ortho bowel routine
OCTOR	On call to OR
OOB	Out of bed
ORIF	Open reduction internal fixation
p̄	After
PCWP	Pulmonary capillary wedge pressure
PE	Pulmonary embolism, Physical examination
PEEP	Positive end-expiratory pressure
PEG	Percutaneous endoscopic gastrostomy (via EGD and skin incision)
PERRL	Pupils equal and react to light
PFT	Pulmonary function tests
PICC	Peripherally inserted central catheter
PGV	Proximal gastric vagotomy (i.e., leaves fibers to pylorus intact to preserve emptying)
PID	Pelvic inflammatory disease
PO	Per os (by mouth)
POD	Postoperative day
PT	Physical therapy, Patient, Posterior tibial
PR	Per rectum

PRN	As needed: literally "pro re nata"
PTC	Percutaneous transhepatic cholangiogram (dye injected via a catheter through skin and into dilated intrahepatic bile duct)
PTCA	Percutaneous transluminal coronary angioplasty
PTX	pneumothorax
q̄	Every
QD	Every day
QOD	Every other day
Ⓡ	Right
RIH	Right inguinal hernia
RLQ	Right lower quadrant
Rx	Treatment
RTC	Return to clinic
SBO	Small bowel obstruction
SCD	Sequential compression device
SIADH	Syndrome of inappropriate antidiuretic hormone
SICU	Surgical intensive care unit
SOAP	Subjective, objective, assessment, and plan
STSG	Split thickness skin graft
SVC	Superior vena cava
s̄	Without
Sx	Symptoms
TEE	Transesophageal echocardiography

T & C	Type and cross
T & S	Type and screen
Tmax	Maximal temperature
TPN	Total parenteral nutrition
TURP	Transurethral resection of the prostate
UE	Upper extremity
UGI	Upper gastrointestinal
UO	Urine output
US	Ultrasound
UTI	Urinary tract infection
VAD	Ventricular assist device
VOCTOR	Void on call to OR
W→D	Wet-to-dry dressing
XRT	X-ray therapy
ZE	Zollinger-Ellison syndrome
−	No, negative
+	Yes, positive
↑	Increase, more
↓	Decrease, less
<	Less than
>	Greater than

GLOSSARY OF SURGICAL TERMS YOU SHOULD KNOW

Abscess — Localized collection of pus anywhere in the body, surrounded and walled off by damaged and inflamed tissues

Achlorhydria	Absence of hydrochloric acid in the stomach
Acholic stool	Light-colored stool as a result of decreased bile content
Adeno-	Prefix denoting gland or glands
Adhesion	Union of two normally separate surfaces
Adnexa	Adjoining parts; usually means ovary/fallopian tube
Adventitia	Outer coat of the wall of a vein or artery (composed of loose connective tissue)
Afferent	Toward
-algia	Suffix denoting pain
Amaurosis fugax	Transient visual loss in one eye
Ampulla	Enlarged or dilated ending of a tube or canal
Analgesic	Drug that prevents pain
Anastomosis	Connection between two tubular organs or parts
Anergy	Lack of response to a specific antigen
Angio-	Prefix denoting blood or lymph vessels
Anomaly	Any deviation from the normal (i.e., congenital or developmental defect)
Apnea	Cessation of breathing
Atelectasis	Collapse of alveoli
Bariatric	Weight reduction; bariatric surgery is performed on morbidly obese patients to effect weight loss
Beta	β-HCG (pregnancy test)

Bifurcation	Point at which division into two branches occurs
Bile salts	Alkaline salts of bile necessary for the emulsification of fats
Bili-	Prefix denoting bile
Boil	Tender inflamed area of the skin containing pus
Bovie	Electrocautery
Cachexia	Abnormally low weight associated with chronic disease
Calculus	Stone
Carbuncle	A collection of boils (furuncle) with multiple drainage channels (CARbuncle = car = big)
Caudal	Relating to the lower part or tail of the body
Cauterization	Destruction of tissue by direct application of heat
Celiotomy	Surgical incision into the peritoneal cavity (laparotomy = celiotomy)
Cephal-	Prefix denoting the head
Chole-	Prefix denoting bile
Cholecyst-	Prefix denoting gallbladder
Choledocho-	Prefix denoting the common bile duct
Chyme	Semiliquid mass of food that passes from the stomach to the duodenum
Cicatrix	Scar
Cleido-	Prefix denoting the clavicle

Colic — Intermittent abdominal pain usually indicating pathology in a tubular organ (e.g., small bowel)

Colloid — Serum proteins, albumin

Colonoscopy — Endoscopic examination of the colon

Colostomy — Surgical operation in which part of the colon is brought through the abdominal wall

Constipation — Infrequent or difficult passage of stool

Cor pulmonale — Enlargement of the right ventricle caused by lung disease and resultant pulmonary hypertension

Curettage — Scraping of the internal surface of an organ or body cavity by means of a spoon-shaped instrument

Cyst — Abnormal sac or closed cavity lined with epithelium and filled with fluid or semisolid material

Direct bilirubin — Conjugated bilirubin (indirect = unconjugated)

Dolor — Pain, one of the classic signs of inflammation

-dynia — Suffix denoting pain

Dys- — Prefix: difficult/painful/abnormal

Dyspareunia — Painful sexual intercourse

Dysphagia — Difficulty in swallowing

Ecchymosis — Bruise

-ectomy — Suffix denoting the surgical removal of a part or all of an organ (e.g., gastrectomy)

Efferent — Away from

Endarterectomy — Surgical removal of an atheroma and the inner part of the vessel wall to relieve an obstruction (carotid endarterectomy = CEA)

Enteritis — Inflammation of the small intestine, usually causing diarrhea

Enterolysis — Lysis of peritoneal adhesions; not to be confused with enteroclysis, which is a contrast study of the small bowel

Eschar — Scab produced by the action of heat or a corrosive substance on the skin

Excisional biopsy — Biopsy with removal of entire tumor (think, Excisional = Entire removal)

Fascia — Sheet of strong connective tissue

Fistula — Abnormal communication between two hollow, epithelialized organs or between a hollow organ and the exterior (skin)

Foley — Bladder catheter

Frequency — Abnormally increased frequency (e.g., urinary frequency)

Furuncle — Boil, small subcutaneous staphylococcal infection of follicle (think furuncle = follicle < car = carbuncle)

Gastropexy — Surgical attachment of the stomach to the abdominal wall

Hemangioma — Benign tumor of blood vessels

Hematemesis — Vomiting of blood

Hematoma — Accumulation of blood within the tissues, which clots to form a solid swelling

Hemoptysis — Coughing up blood

Hemothorax — Blood in the pleural cavity

Hepato- — Prefix denoting the liver

Herniorrhaphy	Surgical repair of a hernia
Hesitancy	Difficulty in initiating urination
Hiatus	Opening or aperture
Hidradenitis	Inflammation of the apocrine glands, usually caused by blockage of the glands
Icterus	Jaundice
Ileostomy	Surgical connection between the lumen of the ileum and the skin of the abdominal wall
Ileus	Abnormal intestinal motility (usually paralytic)
Incisional biopsy	Biopsy with only a "slice" of tumor removed
Induration	Abnormal hardening of a tissue or organ
Inspissated	Hard
Intussusception	Telescoping of one part of the bowel into another
-itis	Suffix denoting inflammation of an organ, tissue, etc. (e.g., gastritis)
Lap appy	Appendectomy via laparoscopy
Laparoscopy	Visualization of the peritoneal cavity via a laparoscope
Laparotomy	Surgical incision into the abdominal cavity (laparotomy = celiotomy)
Lap chole	Cholecystectomy via laparoscopy
Leiomyoma	Benign tumor of smooth muscle
Leiomyosarcoma	Malignant tumor of smooth muscle
Melena	Black tarry stool (melenic, not melanotic stools)

Necrotic	Dead
Obstipation	Failure to pass flatus or stool
Odynophagia	Painful swallowing
-orraphy	Surgical repair (e.g., herniorrhaphy)
-ostomy	General term referring to any operation in which an artificial opening is created between two hollow organs or between one viscera and the abdominal wall for drainage purposes (e.g., colostomy) or for feeding (e.g., gastrostomy)
-otomy	Suffix denoting surgical incision into an organ
Percutaneous	Performed through the skin
-pexy	Suffix denoting fixation
Phleb-	Prefix denoting vein or relating to veins
Phlebolith	Calcification in a vein— a vein stone
Phlegmon	Diffuse inflammation of soft tissue, resulting in a swollen mass of tissue (most commonly seen with pancreatic tissue)
Plica	Fold or ridge
Plicae semilunares	Folds (semicircular) into lumen of the large intestine
Plicae circulares	Circular (complete circles) folds in the lumen of the small intestine (A.K.A. valvulae conniventes)
Pneumaturia	Passage of urine containing air
Pneumothorax	Collapse of lung with air in pleural space
Pseudocyst	Fluid-filled cavity resembling a true cyst, but not lined with epithelium

Pus	Liquid product of inflammation, consisting of dying leukocytes and other fluids from the inflammatory response
Rostral	Referring to the upper body/head region (toward the beak)
Rubor	Redness; a classic sign of inflammation
Steatorrhea	Fatty stools as a result of decreased fat absorption
Stenosis	Abnormal narrowing of a passage or opening
Sterile field	Area covered by sterile drapes or prepped in sterile fashion using antiseptics (e.g., Betadine)
Succus	Fluid (e.g., succus entericus is fluid from the bowel lumen)
Tenesmus	Urge to defecate with ineffectual (and often painful) straining
Thoracotomy	Surgical opening of the chest cavity
Transect	To divide transversely (to cut in half)
Trendelenburg	Patient posture with pelvis higher than the head, inclined about 45° (A.K.A. "Headdownenburg")
Urgency	Sudden strong urge to urinate; often seen with a UTI
Wet-to-dry dressing	Damp gauze dressing placed on a wound and removed after the dressing dries to the wound, providing microdébridement

SURGERY SIGNS, TRIADS, ETC. YOU SHOULD KNOW

What are the A, B, C, Ds of melanoma?

Signs of melanoma:
- A—Asymmetric
- B—Border irregularities
- C—Color variation
- D—Diameter > 0.6 cm **and** Dark black color

What is the Allen's test?

Test for patency of ulnar artery prior to placing a radial arterial line or performing an ABG. Simply stated, occlude both ulnar and radial arteries with the examiner's fingers with the patient's hand in a fist; open fist and release ulnar artery occlusion and assess blood flow to hand

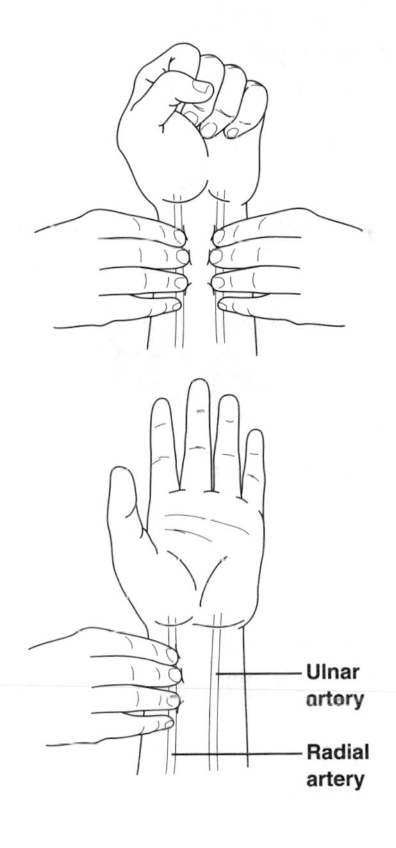

Define the following terms:

Ballance's sign

Dullness to percussion in the left flank/LUQ and resonance to percussion in the right flank seen with splenic rupture/hematoma

Barrett's esophagus

Columnar metaplasia of the distal esophagus (GERD related)

Battle's sign

Ecchymosis over the mastoid process in patients with basilar skull fractures

Beck's triad

Seen in patients with cardiac tamponade:
1. JVD
2. Decreased or muffled heart sounds
3. Decreased blood pressure

Bergman's triad

Seen with fat emboli syndrome:
1. Mental status changes
2. Petechiae (often in the axilla/thorax)
3. Dyspnea

Blumer's shelf

Metastatic disease to the rectouterine (pouch of Douglas) or rectovesical pouch creating a "shelf" that is palpable on rectal examination

Boas's sign

Right subscapular pain resulting from cholelithiasis

Carcinoid triad

Seen with carcinoid syndrome:
1. Flushing
2. Diarrhea
3. Right-sided heart failure (FDR)

Charcot's triad

Seen with cholangitis:
1. Fever (chills)
2. Jaundice
3. Right upper quadrant pain

(Pronounced "char-cows")

Chvostek's sign

Twitching of facial muscles upon tapping the facial nerve in patients with hypocalcemia

Courvoisier's law

An enlarged nontender gallbladder seen with obstruction of the common bile duct, most commonly with pancreatic cancer
Note: not seen with acute cholecystitis because the gallbladder is scarred secondary to chronic cholelithiasis (pronounced "koor-vwah-ze-ay")

Cullen's sign

Bluish discoloration of the periumbilical area due to retroperitoneal hemorrhage tracking around to the anterior abdominal wall through fascial planes (e.g., acute hemorrhagic pancreatitis)

Cushing's triad	Signs of increased intracranial pressure: 1. Hypertension 2. Bradycardia 3. Irregular respirations
Dance's sign	Empty right lower quadrant in children with ileocecal intussusception
Fothergill's sign	Used to differentiate an intra-abdominal mass from one in the abdominal wall; if mass is felt while there is tension on the musculature, then it is in the wall (i.e., sitting halfway upright)
Fox's sign	Ecchymosis of inguinal ligament seen with retroperitoneal bleeding
Goodsall's rule	Anal fistulae course in a straight path anteriorly and take a curved path posteriorly (think of a dog with a straight anterior nose and a curved posterior tail)
Grey Turner's sign	Ecchymosis or discoloration of the flank in patients with retroperitoneal hemorrhage as a result of dissecting blood from the retroperitoneum (think: turn side to-side = flank)
Hamman's sign/crunch	Crunching sound on auscultation of the heart resulting from emphysematous mediastinum, seen with Boerhaave's syndrome, pneumomediastinum, etc.
Homans' sign	Calf pain on forced dorsiflexion of the foot in patients with DVT
Howship-Romberg sign	Pain along the inner aspect of the thigh; seen with an obturator hernia as the result of nerve compression
Kehr's sign	Severe left shoulder pain in patients with splenic rupture (as a result of referred pain from diaphragmatic irritation)
Krukenberg tumor	Metastatic tumor to the ovary (classically from gastric cancer)

Kelly's sign	Visible peristalsis of the ureter in response to squeezing or retraction; used to identify the ureter during surgery
Laplace's law	Wall tension = pressure × radius (thus, the colon perforates preferentially at the cecum because of the increased radius and resultant increased wall tension)
McBurney's point	One-third the distance from the anterior iliac spine to the umbilicus on a line connecting the two
McBurney's sign	Tenderness at McBurney's point in patients with appendicitis
Meckel's diverticulum rule of 2s	Two percent of the population have a Meckel's diverticulum, 2% of those are symptomatic, and they occur within approximately 2 feet of the ileocecal valve
Mittelschmerz	Lower quadrant pain due to ovulation
Murphy's sign	Cessation of inspiration while palpating under the right costal margin; the patient cannot continue to inspire deeply because it brings an inflamed gallbladder under pressure (seen in acute cholecystitis)
Obturator sign	Pain upon internal rotation of the leg with the hip and knee flexed; seen in patients with appendicitis/pelvic abscess

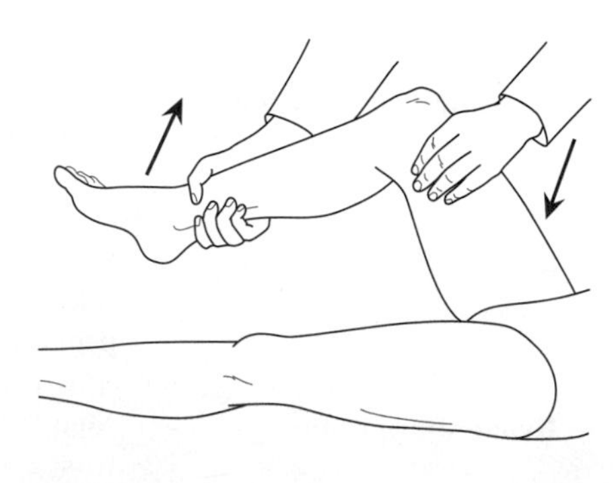

Psoas

Pain elicited by extending the hip with the knee in full extension, seen with appendicitis and psoas inflammation

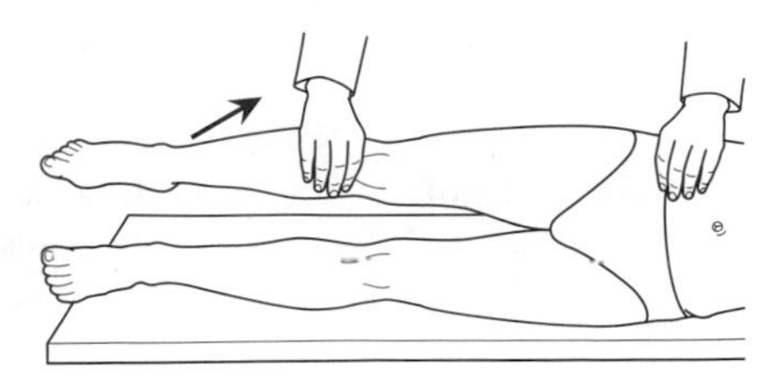

Pheochromocytoma SYMPTOMS triad

Think of the first three letters in the word pheochromocytoma—P-H-E:
1. **P**alpitations
2. **H**eadache
3. **E**pisodic diaphoresis

Pheochromocytoma rule of 10s

10% bilateral, 10% malignant, 10% in children, 10% extra-adrenal, 10% have multiple tumors

Raccoon eyes

Bilateral black eyes as a result of basilar skull fracture

Reynold's pentad

1. Fever
2. Jaundice
3. Right upper quadrant pain
4. Mental status changes
5. Shock/sepsis

Thus, Charcot's triad plus # 4 and # 5; seen in patients with suppurative cholangitis

Rovsing's sign

Palpation of the left lower quadrant resulting in pain in the right lower quadrant; seen in appendicitis

Saint's triad

1. Cholelithiasis
2. Hiatal hernia
3. Diverticular disease

Silk glove sign

Indirect hernia sac in the pediatric patient; the sac feels like a finger of a silk glove when rolled under the examining finger

Sister Mary Joseph's sign (A.K.A. Sister Mary Joseph's node)	Metastatic tumor to umbilical lymph node(s)
Virchow's node	Metastatic tumor to left supraclavicular node (classically due to gastric cancer)
Virchow's triad	Risk factors for thrombosis: 1. Stasis 2. Abnormal endothelium 3. Hypercoagulability
Trousseau's sign	Carpal spasm after occlusion of blood to the forearm with a BP cuff in patients with hypocalcemia
Valentino's sign	Right lower quadrant pain from a perforated peptic ulcer due to succus/pus draining into the RLQ
Westermark's sign	Decreased pulmonary vascular markings on CXR in a patient with pulmonary embolus
Whipple's triad	Evidence for insulinoma: 1. Hypoglycemia (< 50) 2. CNS and vasomotor symptoms (e.g., syncope, diaphoresis) 3. Relief of symptoms with administration of glucose

2 Surgical Syndromes

What is Leriche's syndrome?

Claudication of buttocks **I**mpotence **A**trophy of buttocks (seen with iliac occlusive disease) (Think: **CIA**)

What is RED reaction syndrome?

Syndrome of rapid vancomycin infusion, resulting in skin erythema

What is Ogilvie's syndrome?

Massive **nonobstructive** colonic dilatation

What is Gardner's syndrome?

GI polyps and associated findings of **S**ebaceous cysts, **O**steomas, and **D**esmoid tumors (**SOD**); polyps have high malignancy potential (think: a Gardner plants **SOD**)

What is Peutz-Jeghers syndrome?

Benign GI polyps and buccal pigmentation (think: **P**eutz = **P**igmentation)

What is Fitz-Hugh-Curtis syndrome?

Perihepatic gonorrhea infection

What is SIADH?

Syndrome of inappropriate antidiuretic hormone (think: **I**nappropriately **I**ncreased ADH)

What is toxic shock syndrome?

Staphylococcus aureus toxin induced syndrome marked by fever, hypotension, organ failure, and **rash** (desquamation—especially palms and soles)

What is Tietze's syndrome?

Costochondritis of rib cartilage; aseptic (treat with NSAIDs)

What is Plummer-Vinson syndrome?

Syndrome of:
1. Esophageal web
2. Iron-deficiency anemia

3. Dysphagia
4. Spoon-shaped nails
5. Atrophic oral and tongue mucosa

Usually occurs in elderly women; 10% develop squamous cell carcinoma

What is carcinoid syndrome?

Syndrome of **B FDR:**
Bronchospasm
Flushing
Diarrhea
Right-sided heart failure (caused by factors released by carcinoid tumor)

What does ARDS stand for?

Acute respiratory distress syndrome (poor oxygenation caused by leaky capillaries)

What is dumping syndrome?

Delivery of a large amount of hyperosmolar chyme into the small bowel, usually after vagotomy and a gastric drainage procedure (pyloroplasty/gastrojejunostomy); results in autonomic instability, abdominal pain, and diarrhea

What is afferent loop syndrome?

Obstruction of the afferent loop of a Billroth II gastrojejunostomy

What is short-gut syndrome?

Malnutrition resulting from less than 100 cm of viable small bowel

What is blind loop syndrome?

Bacterial overgrowth of intestine caused by stasis

What is Cushing's syndrome?

Excessive cortisol production

What is Rendu-Osler-Weber (ROW) syndrome?

Syndrome of GI tract Telangiectasia/A-V malformations

What is Boerhaave's syndrome?

Esophageal perforation

What is thoracic outlet syndrome?

Compression of the structures exiting from the thoracic outlet

What is Munchausen syndrome?

Self-induced illness

What is superior vena cava (SVC) syndrome?	Obstruction of the SVC (e.g., by tumor, thrombosis)
What is another name for Sipple's syndrome?	MEN II
What is another name for Wermer's syndrome?	MEN I
What is Trousseau's syndrome?	Syndrome of deep venous thrombosis (DVT) associated with carcinoma
What is Mirrizzi's syndrome?	Extrinsic obstruction of the common hepatic bile duct from a cystic duct gallstone
What is refeeding syndrome?	Hypokalemia, hypomagnesemia, and hypophosphatemia after refeeding a starved patient
What is compartment syndrome?	Compartmental hypertension caused by edema, resulting in muscle necrosis of the lower extremity, seen in the calf; patient may have a distal pulse
What is HITT syndrome?	Heparin-induced thrombocytopenic thrombosis (HITT) syndrome: Heparin-induced platelet antibodies cause platelets to thrombose vessels, often resulting in loss of limb or life (also known as "white clot syndrome").
What is Budd-Chiari syndrome?	Thrombosis of hepatic veins
What is Mendelson's syndrome?	Chemical pneumonitis after aspiration of gastric contents
What is Zollinger-Ellison syndrome?	Gastrinoma and PUD

3

Surgical Most Commons

What is the most common:	
Indication for surgery with Crohn's disease?	Small bowel obstruction (SBO)
Type of melanoma?	Superficial spreading
Type of breast cancer?	Infiltrating ductal
Site of breast cancer?	Upper outer quadrant
Vessel involved with a bleeding duodenal ulcer?	Gastroduodenal artery
Cause of common bile duct obstruction?	Choledocholithiasis
Cause of cholangitis?	Bile duct obstruction resulting from choledocholithiasis
Cause of pancreatitis?	ETOH
Bacteria in stool?	*Bacteroides fragilis* ("B. frag")
Cause of SBO in adults in the United States?	Adhesions
Cause of SBO in children?	Hernias
Cause of emergency abdominal surgery in the United States?	Acute appendicitis
Site of GI carcinoids?	Appendix
Abdominal x-ray (AXR) finding with SBO?	Air-fluid levels

Cause of large bowel obstruction?	Colon cancer
Type of colonic volvulus?	Sigmoid volvulus
Cause of fever < 48 post-operative hours?	Atelectasis
Bacterial cause of urinary tract infection (UTI)?	*Escherichia coli*
Chest x-ray (CXR) finding with traumatic thoracic aortic injury?	Widened mediastinum
Abdominal organ injured in blunt abdominal trauma?	Spleen
Abdominal organ injured in penetrating abdominal trauma?	Small bowel
Benign tumor of the liver?	Hemangioma
Malignancy of the liver?	Mets
Pneumonia in the ICU?	Gram-negative bacteria
Cause of epidural hematoma?	Middle meningeal artery injury
Cause of lower GI bleeding?	Upper GI bleeding
Hernia?	Inguinal hernia (right>left)

4 Surgical Percentages

What percentage of people in the United States will develop acute appendicitis?

Approximately 7%

What is the acceptable percentage of normal appendices removed with the preoperative diagnosis of appendicitis?

Up to 20%; it is better to remove some normal appendices than to miss a case of acute appendicitis, which could result in a ruptured appendix

In what percentage of cases can ultrasound diagnose cholelithiasis?

98%

In what percentage of cases does a thoracic aortogram to rule out a torn thoracic aorta after blunt trauma yield a positive study?

Approximately 10%

In what percentage of cases does a lower GI bleed stop spontaneously?

Approximately 90%

In what percentage of cases does a UGI bleed stop spontaneously?

Approximately 80%

What percentage of patients undergoing laparotomy develop a postoperative small bowel obstruction at some time later?

Approximately 5%

What percentage of American women develop breast cancer?	10%
What percentage of patients with acute appendicitis will have a radiopaque fecalith on abdominal x-ray (AXR)?	Only about 5%
What percentage of patients with gallstones will have radiopaque gallstones on AXR?	Approximately 10%
What percentage of kidney stones are radiopaque on AXR?	Approximately 90%
At 6 weeks, wounds have achieved what percentage of their total tensile strength?	Approximately 90%
What percentage of patients with ARDS will die?	Approximately 50%
What percentage of the population has a Meckel's diverticulum?	2%
What is the risk of appendiceal rupture 24 hours after the onset of symptoms?	Approximately 25%
What percentage of colonic villous adenomas contain cancer?	Approximately 40% (think: VILLous = VILLain)

5 Surgical History

Identify the following:	
First to use antiseptic (carbolic acid)?	Lister (British surgeon)
First to advocate surgical gloves?	Halsted (made by GOODYEAR®)
Father of antiseptic surgery?	Lister (1827–1912)
Father of American neurosurgery?	Harvey Cushing
Developer of vascular grafts?	DeBakey (his wife hand sewed them!)
Developed electrocautery for surgery with Dr. Cushing?	Bovie (1928)
The Mayo Brother's scrub nurse?	Sister Joseph (of St. Mary's hospital)
Developed the cardiopulmonary bypass?	Gibbon
Identify the year the following procedures were first performed and the physician who performed them:	
Renal transplant	1954; Murray
CABG	1962; Sabiston
CEA	1953; DeBakey

Heart transplant	1967; Barnard
Artificial heart valve	1960; Starr
Liver transplant	1963; Starzl
Total parenteral nutrition (TPN)	1968; Rhoades
Vascular anastomosis	1902; Carrel
Lung transplant	1964; Hardy
Pancreatic transplant	1966; Najarian
Heart-lung transplant	1982; Reitz
AAA rx	1951; Dubost
1st lap chole?	1987; Mouret and Dubois in France
First appendectomy?	1848; Hancock
First gastric resection?	1881; Billroth
First lap appy?	1983; Semm (GYN DOCTOR!)

Who was the only surgeon to win the Pulitzer Prize?

Cushing (for his biography on Osler)

Which surgeons have won the Nobel Prize?

Kocher 1909 (thyroid surgery)
Gullstrand 1911 (ophthalmology)
Carrel 1912 (transplantation/vascular anastomosis)
Bárány 1914 (inner ear disease-vestibular disease)
Banting 1922 (insulin)
Hess 1949 (brain physiology)
Forssman 1956 (cardiac catheterization)
Huggins 1966 (oncology)
Murray 1990 (kidney transplant)

6 Surgical Instruments

How should a pair of scissors/needle-driver/ clamp be held?

With the thumb and **fourth** finger, using the index finger to steady

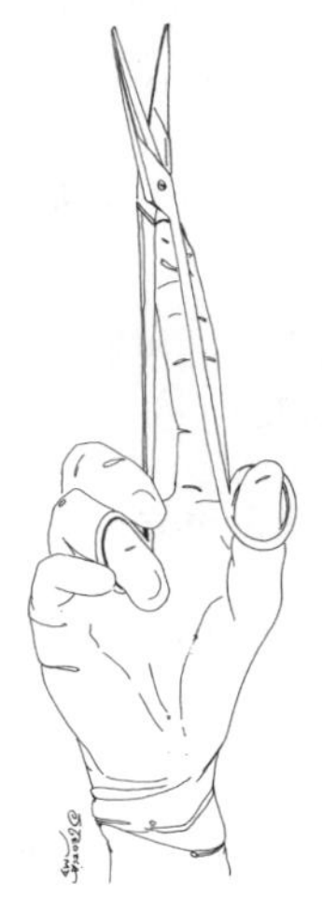

Is it better to hold the skin with a DeBakey or an Adson or toothed forcep?

Better to use an Adson or toothed pickup as it is better to cut the skin rather than crush it!

What helps steady the scissor- or Bovie-hand?

Resting it on the opposite hand

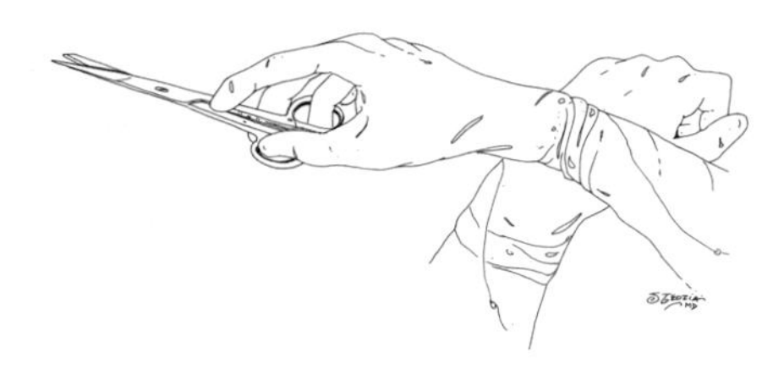

What can be done to guarantee that you do not cut the knot when cutting sutures?

Slide the scissors down to the knot then turn the scissors at a 45° angle and cut

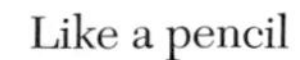

How should a pair of forceps be held?

Like a pencil

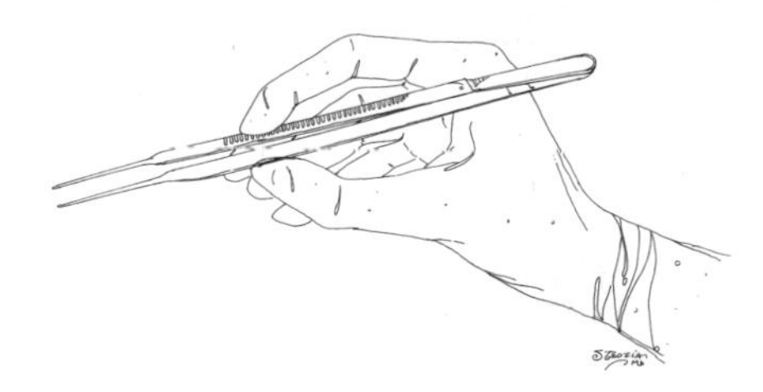

What are forceps also known as?

"Pickups"

Identify the following instruments:

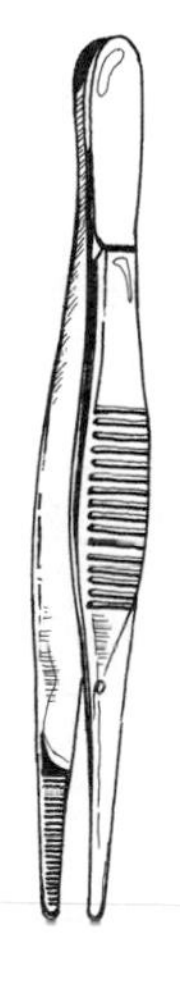

Forcep

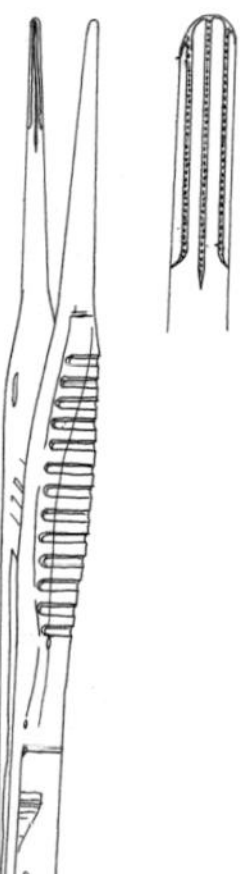

DeBakey pickup

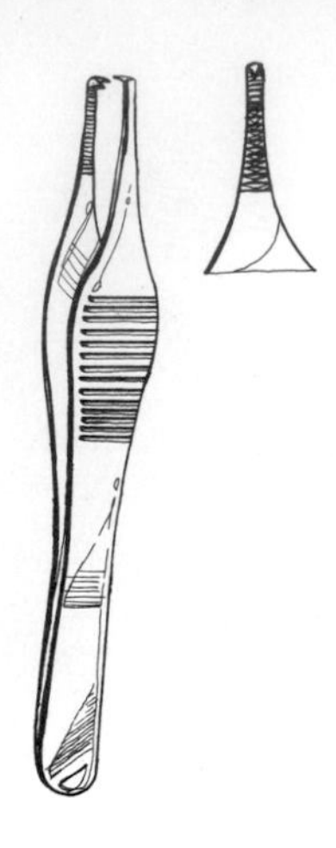

Adson pickup

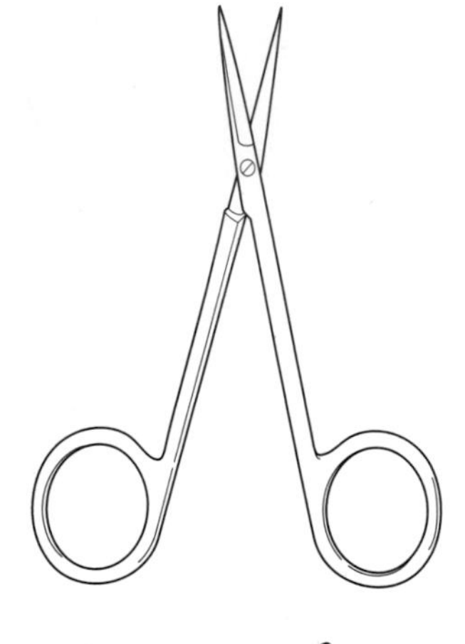

Iris scissors

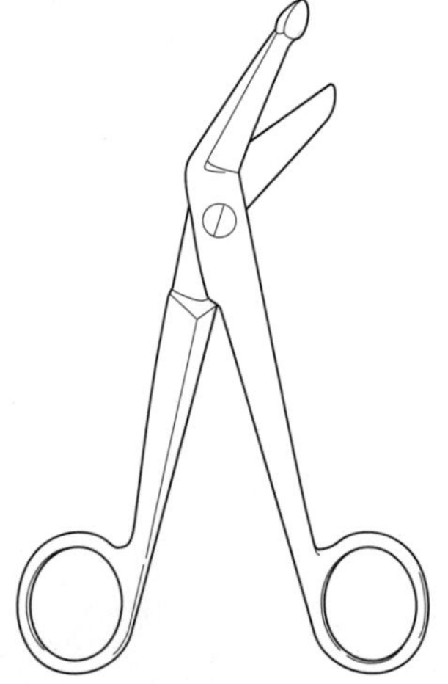

Bandage scissors

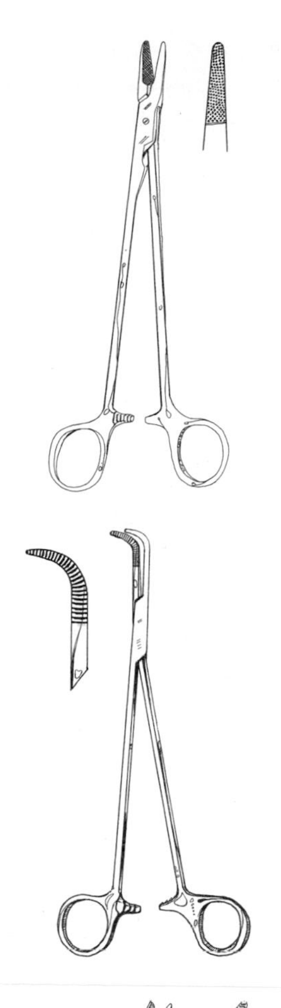

Needle-driver

Right-angle clamp

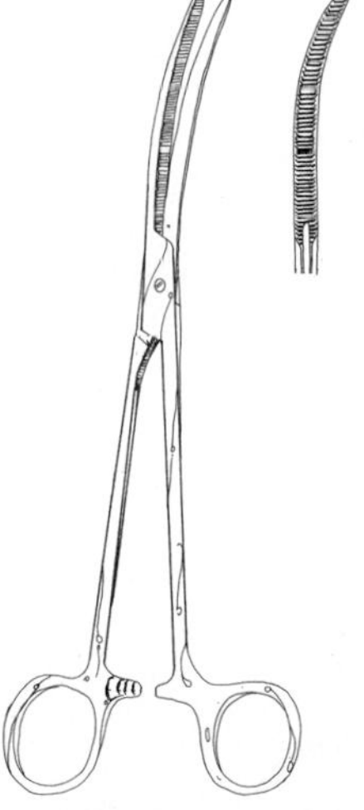

Kelly clamp

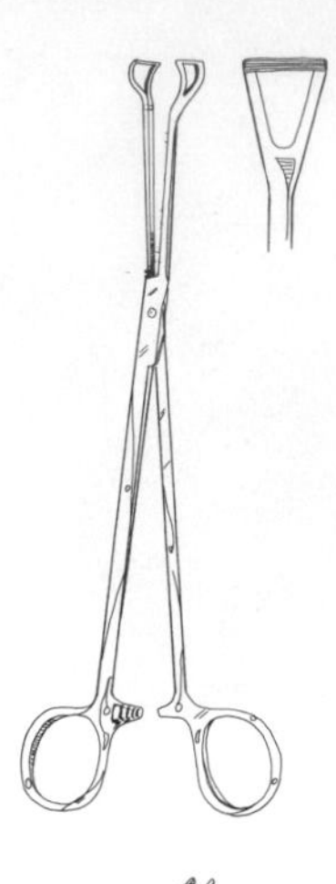

Babcock clamp

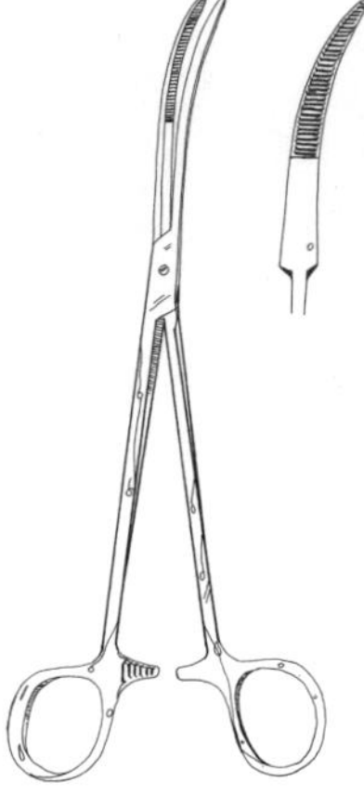

Tonsil clamp

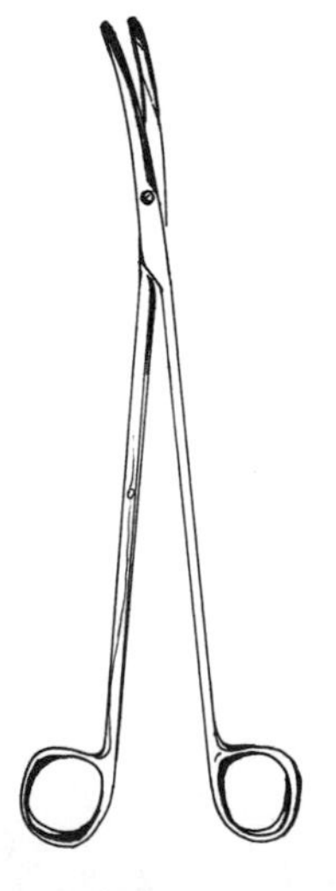

Metzenbaum scissors

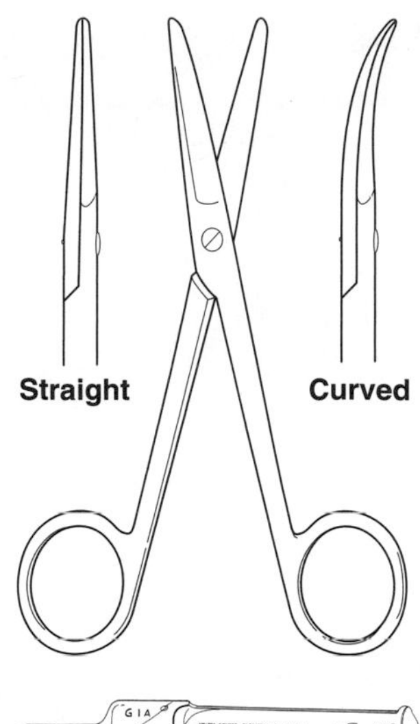

Mayo scissors (heavy scissors)

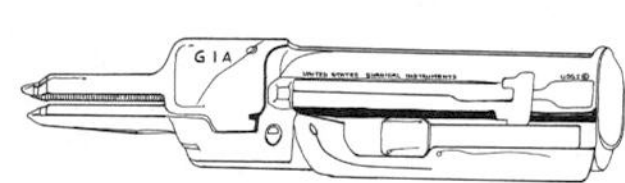

GIA stapler

What does "GIA" stand for? **G**astro **I**ntestinal **A**nastomosis

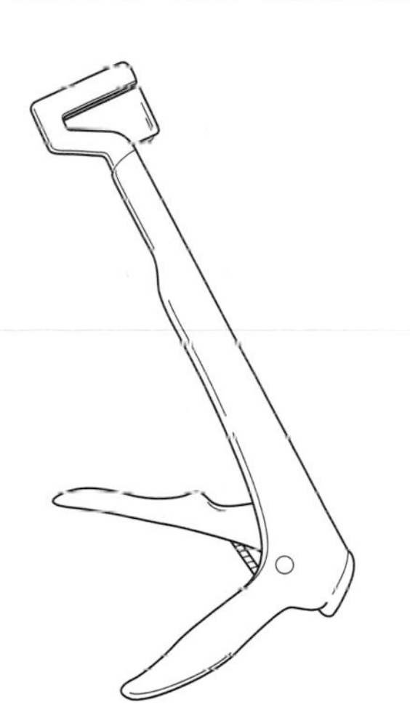

TA stapler

What does "TA" stand for? **T**horaco **A**bdominal

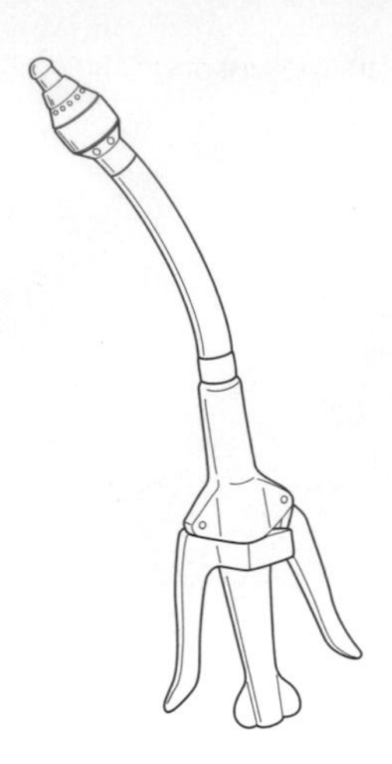

EEA stapler

What does "EEA" stand for? **E**nd-to-**e**nd **a**nastomosis

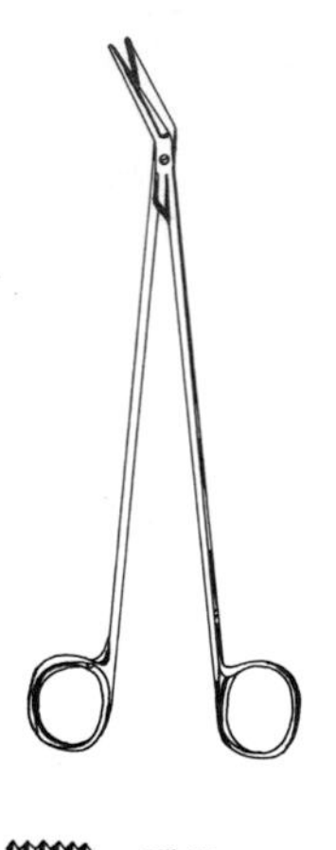

Pott's scissors

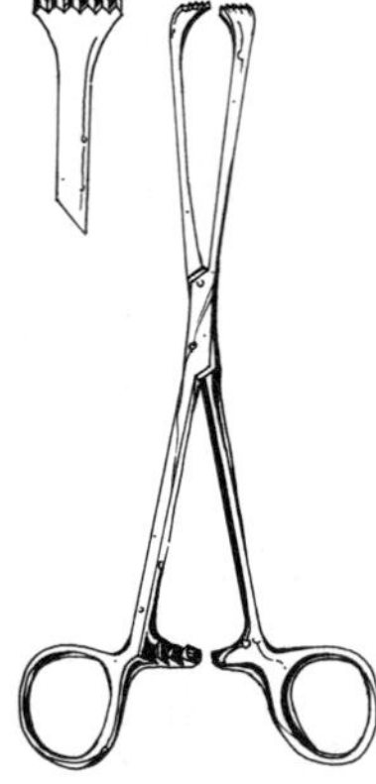

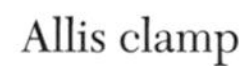

Allis clamp

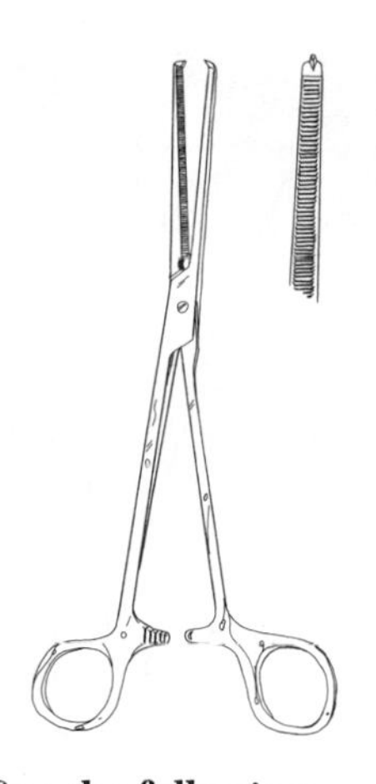

Kocher clamp, for very thick tissue (e.g., fascia)

Define the following scalpel blades:

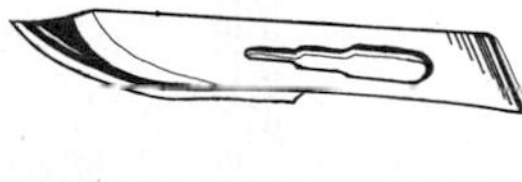

Number 10

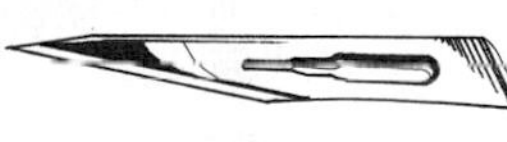

Number 11

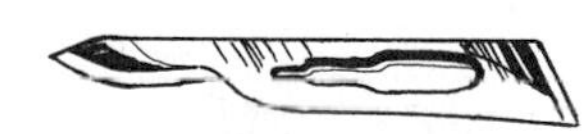

Number 15

Bovie electrocautery

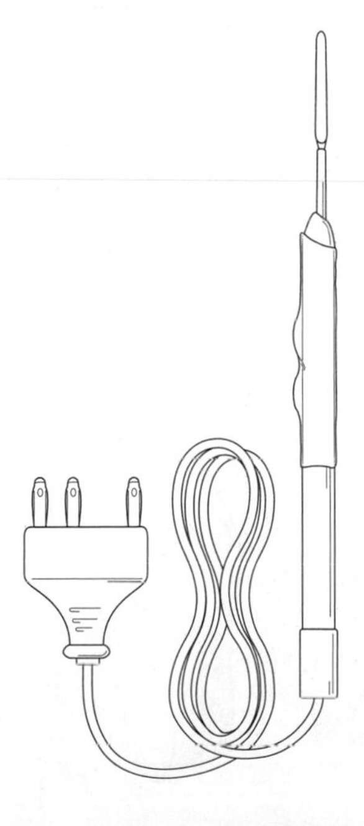

Yankauer suction (sucker)

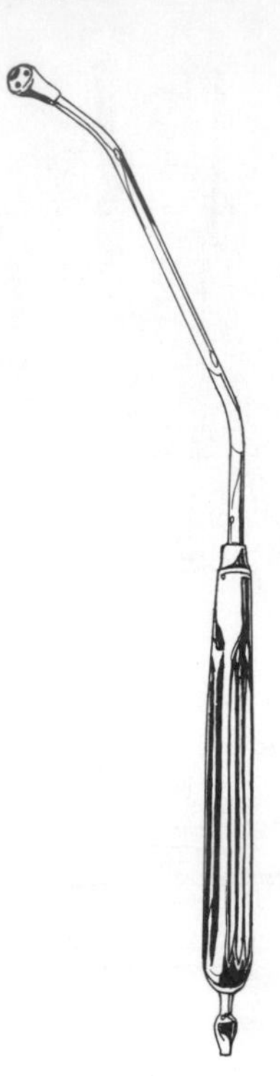

RETRACTORS (YOU WILL GET TO KNOW THEM WELL!)

What does it mean to "toe in" the retractor?

To angle the tip of the retractor in by angling the retractor handle up

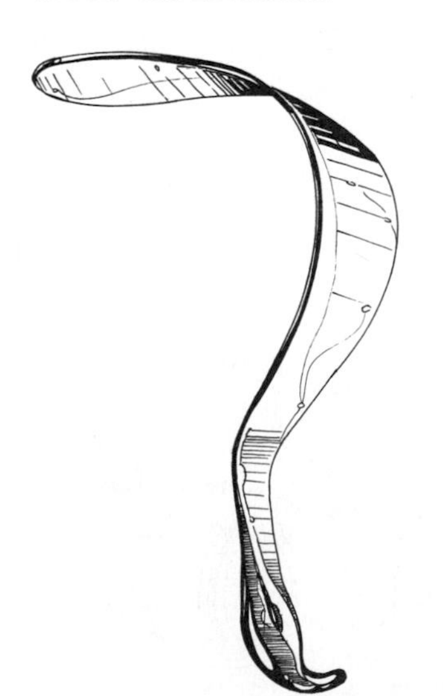

Deaver retractor

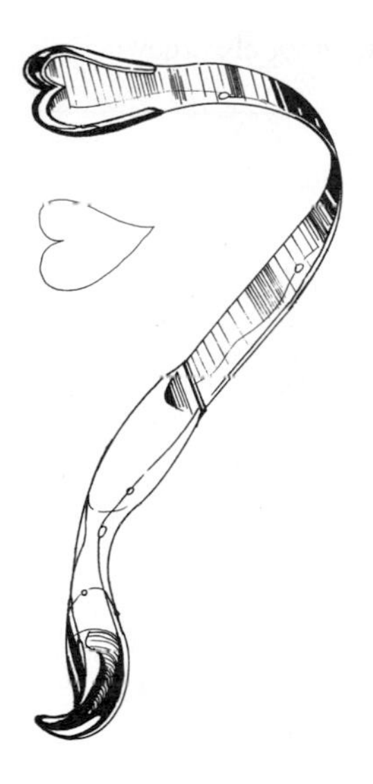

Sweetheart retractor (Harrington)

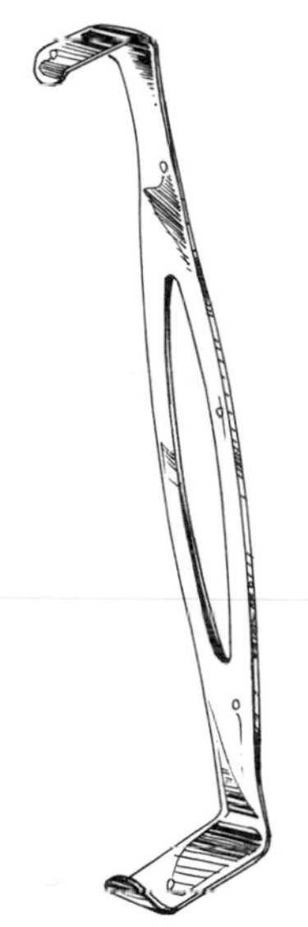

Army–Navy retractor

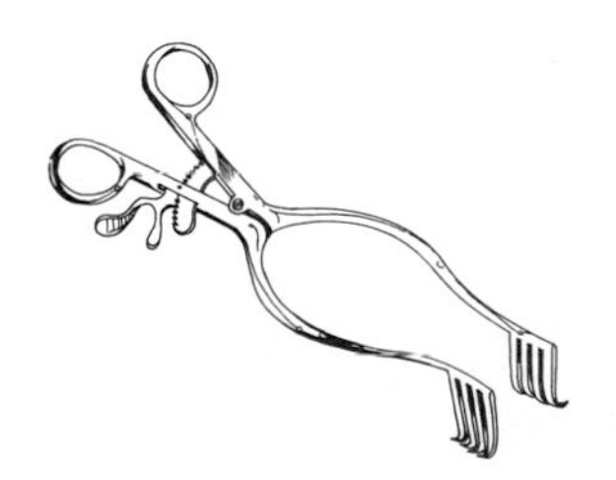

Weitlaner retractor also known as a "WHEATY" (self-retaining retractor; sorry, operates without a student!)

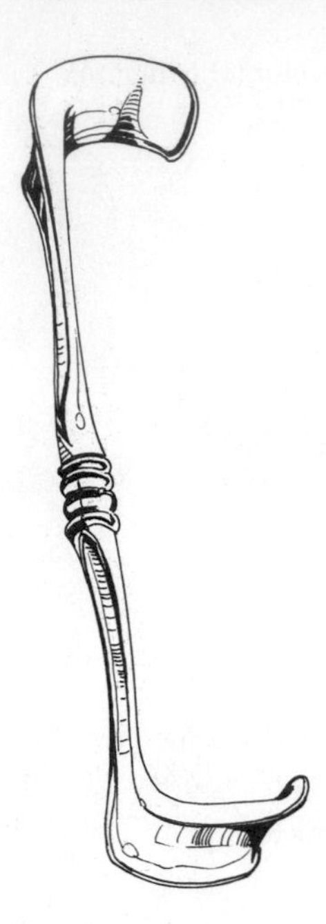

Richardson retractor also known as a "RICH"

What is a "malleable" retractor?

A metal retractor that can be bent to customize to the situation at hand

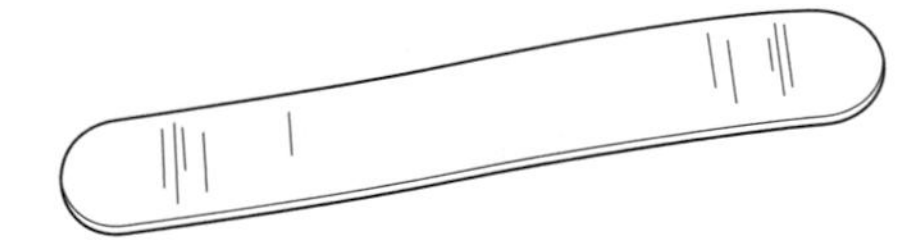

7 Sutures and Stitches

SUTURE MATERIALS

GENERAL INFORMATION

What is a suture?
Any strand of material used to ligate blood vessels or to approximate tissues

How are sutures sized?
By diameter; stated as a number of O's: the higher the number of O's, the smaller the diameter (e.g., 2-O suture has a larger diameter than 5-O suture)

Which is thicker, 1-O suture or 3-O suture?
1-O suture (pronounced one oh")

CLASSIFICATION

What are the two most basic suture types?
Absorbable and nonabsorbable

What is an absorbable suture?
The suture is completely broken down by the body (dissolving suture).

What is a nonabsorbable suture?
The suture is not broken down (permanent suture).

SUTURES

Catgut

What are "catgut" sutures made of?
Purified collagen fibers from the intestines of healthy cows or sheep (sorry, no cats)

What are the two types of gut sutures?
Plain and chromic

What is the difference between plain and chromic gut?

Chromic gut is treated with chromium salts (chromium trioxide), which results in more collagen crosslinks, making the suture more resistant to breakdown by the body.

Vicryl® Suture

What is it?

Absorbable, braided, multifilamentous copolymer of lactide and glycoside

How long does it retain its strength?

60% at 2 weeks, 8% at 4 weeks

PDS®

What is it?

Absorbable, monofilament polymer of polydioxanone (absorbable fishing line)

How long does it maintain its tensile strength?

70% to 74% at 2 weeks, 50% to 58% at 4 weeks, 25% to 41% at 6 weeks

How long does it take to complete absorption?

180 days (6 months)

What is silk?

Braided protein filaments spun by the silkworm larva; known as a nonabsorbable suture

What is Prolene?

Nonabsorbable suture (used for vascular anastomoses, hernias, abdominal fascial closure)

What is nylon?

Nonabsorbable "fishing line"

WOUND CLOSURE

GENERAL INFORMATION

What is the purpose of a suture closure?

To approximate divided tissues to enhance wound healing

What are the three types of wound healing?

1. Primary closure (intention)
2. Secondary intention
3. Tertiary intention (**d**elayed **p**rimary **c**losure = DPC)

What is primary intention?

When the edges of a clean wound are closed in some manner immediately (e.g., suture, Steri-Strips®, staples)

What is secondary intention?

When a wound is allowed to remain open and heal by granulation, epithelization, and contraction—used for dirty wounds, otherwise an abscess can form

What is tertiary intention?

When a wound is allowed to remain open for a time and then closed, allowing for debridement and other wound care to reduce bacterial counts prior to closure (i.e., delayed primary closure)

What is another term for tertiary intention?

DPC = delayed primary closure

Classic time to wait before closing an open abdominal wound by DPC?

5 days

What rule is constantly told to medical students about wound closure?

"Approximate, don't strangulate!" Translation: If sutures are pulled too tight, then the tissue becomes ischemic as the blood supply is decreased, resulting in necrosis, infection, or both

SUTURE TECHNIQUES

What is a taper-point needle?

Round body, leaves a round hole in tissue (spreads without cutting tissue)

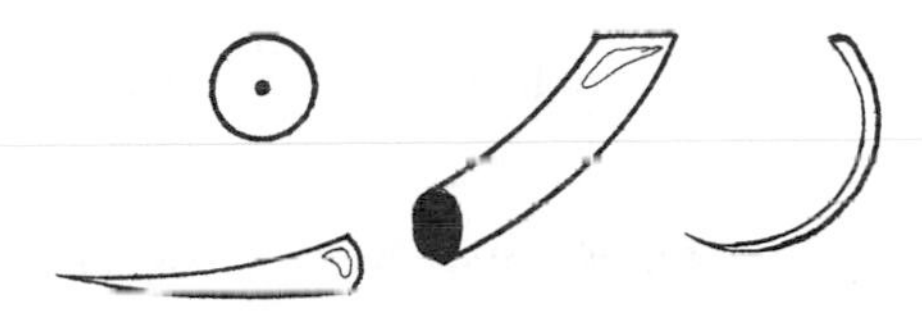

What is it used for?

Suturing of soft tissues other than skin (e.g., GI tract, muscle, nerve, peritoneum, fascia)

What is a conventional cutting needle?

Triangular body with the sharp edge toward the inner circumference; leaves a triangular hole in tissue

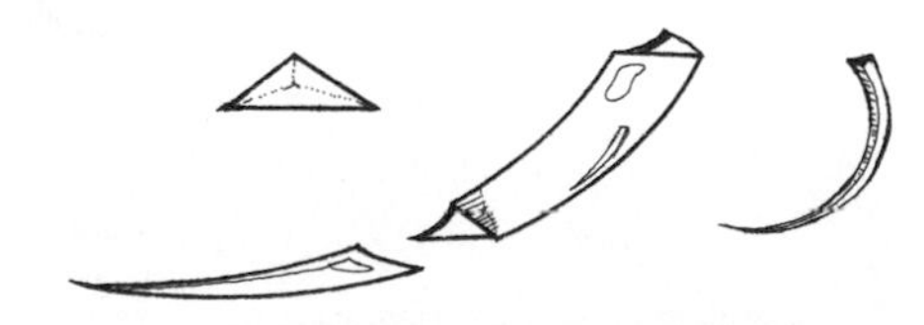

What are its uses? Suturing of **skin**

What is a simple interrupted stitch?

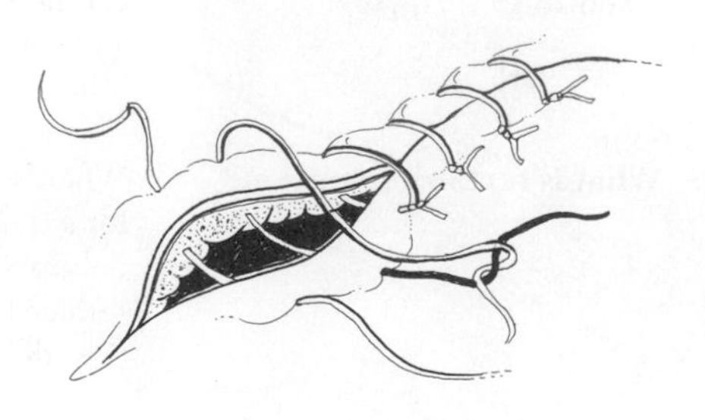

What is a vertical mattress stitch? A simple stitch is made, the needle is reversed, and a small bite is taken from each wound edge; the knot ends up on one side of the wound.

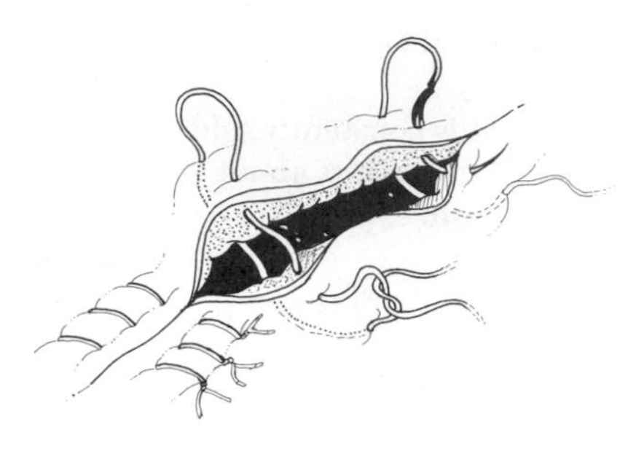

What is the vertical mattress stitch also known as? Far-far, near-near stitch—oriented perpendicular to wound

What is it used for? Difficult-to-approximate skin edges; everts tissue well

What is a horizontal mattress stitch? A simple stitch is made, the needle is reversed, and the same size bite is taken again—oriented parallel to wound

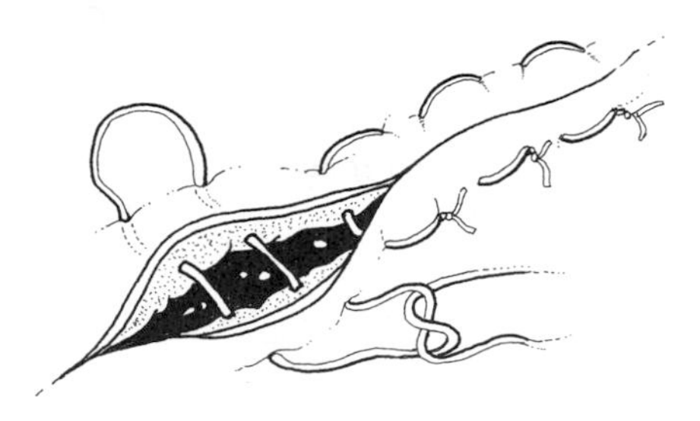

What is a simple running (continuous) stitch?

Stitches made in succession without knotting each stitch

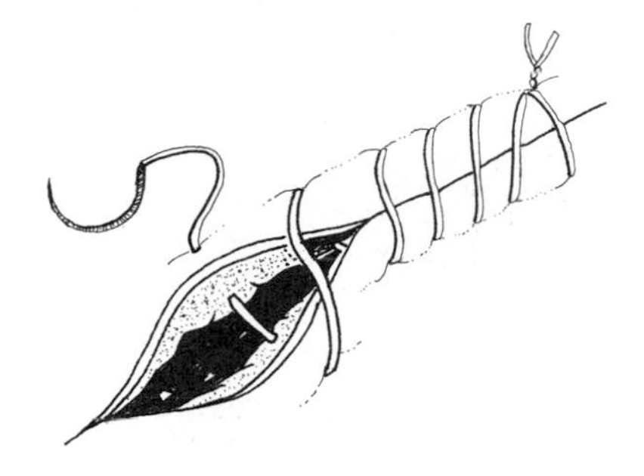

What is a subcuticular stitch?

A stitch (usually running) placed just underneath the epidermis, can be either absorbable or nonabsorbable (e.g., pull-out stitch if nonabsorbable)

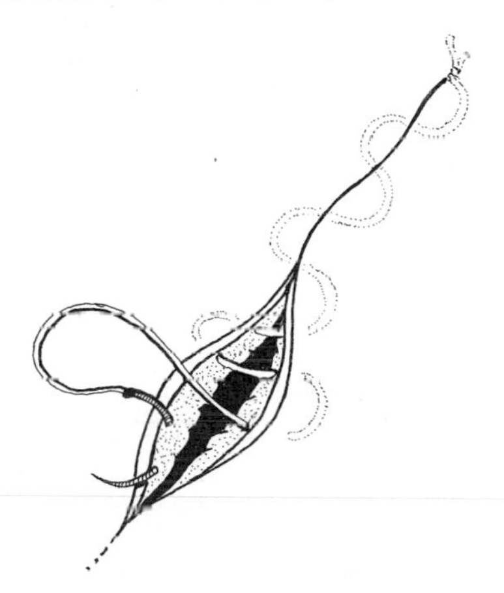

What is a pursestring suture?

A stitch that encircles a tube perforating a hollow viscus (e.g., gastrostomy tube), allowing the hole to be drawn tight and thus preventing leakage

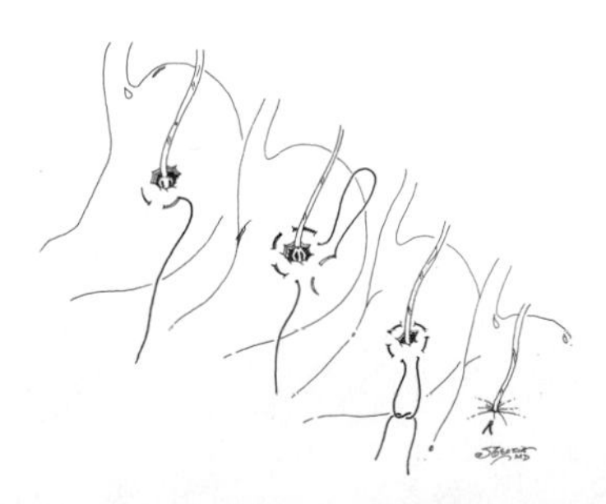

What are metallic skin staples?

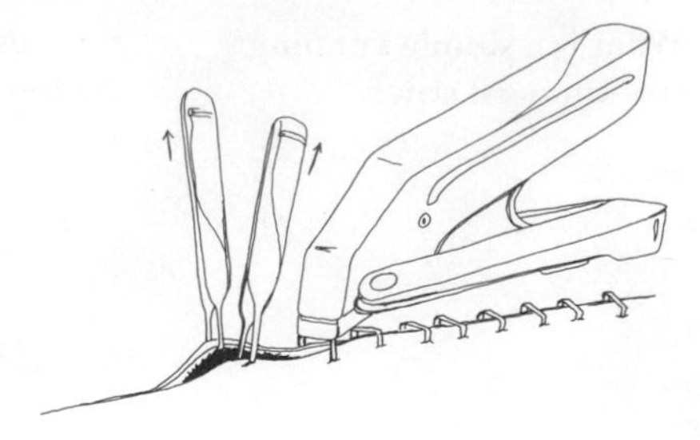

What is a staple removal device?

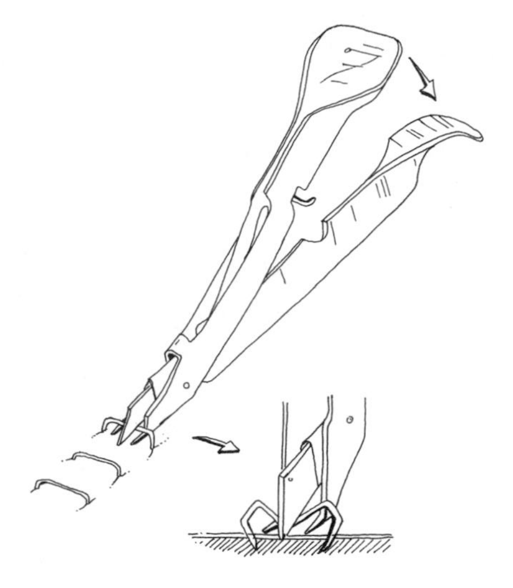

What is a gastrointestinal anastomosis (GIA) device?

A stapling device that lays two rows of small staples in a hemostatic row and **automatically cuts** in between them

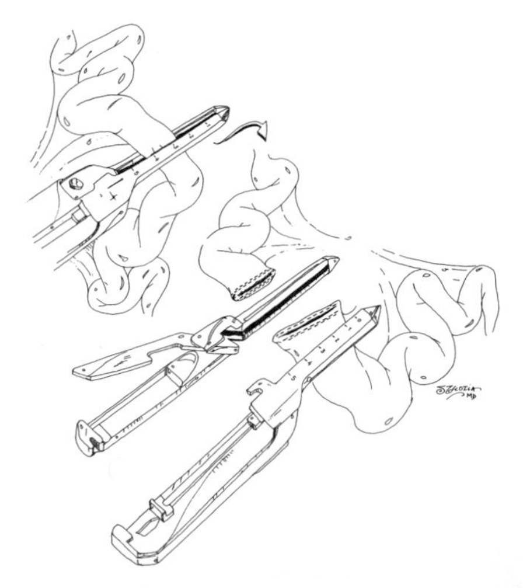

What is a suture ligature (A.K.A. stick tie)?

The suture is anchored by passing it through the vessel **on a needle** before wrapping it around and occluding the vessel; it prevents slippage of knot-use on larger vessels.

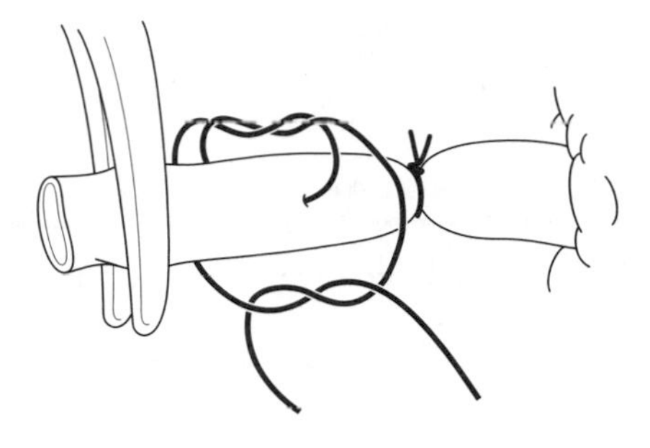

What is a retention suture?

A large suture (No. 2) that is full thickness through the entire abdominal wall except the peritoneum. To buttress an abdominal wound at risk for dehiscence

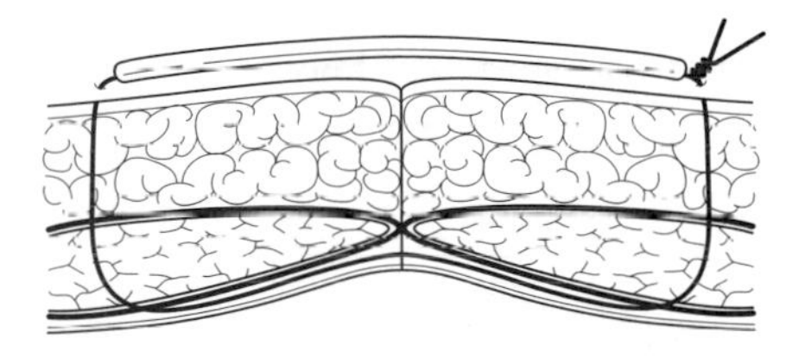

What is a pop-off suture?

A suture that is not permanently swaged to the needle, allowing the surgeon to "pop" off the needle from the suture without cutting the suture

8 Surgical Knot Tying

KNOTS AND EARS

What is the basic surgical knot?

The square knot

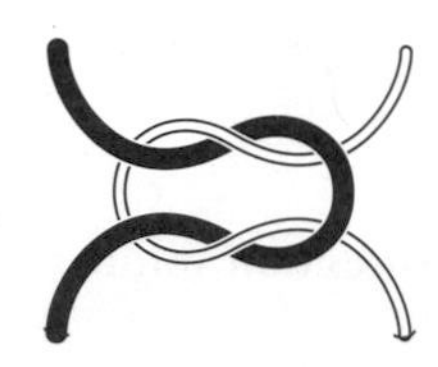

What is the first knot that should be mastered?

Instrument knot

What is a "surgeon's knot"?

A double-wrap throw

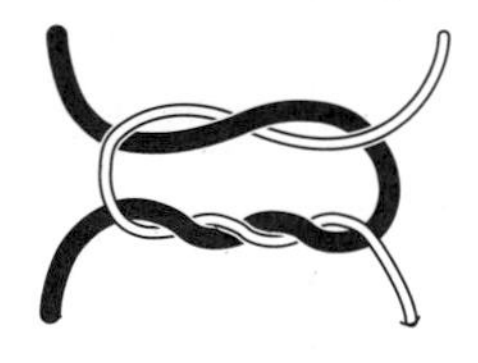

How many (correct) throws are necessary to ensure that your knots do not slip?

As many as the attending surgeon wants

What are the guidelines for the number of throws needed?

Depends on the suture material
Silk—3
Gut—4
Vicryl®, Dexon®, other braided synthetics—4
Nylon, polyester, polypropylene, PDS, Maxon—6

How long should the ears of the knot be cut?

To the length requested by the attending surgeon
Some guidelines are:
Silk vessel ties—1 to 2 mm
Abdominal fascia closure—5 mm
Skin sutures, drain sutures—5 to 10 mm (makes them easier to find and remove)

When should skin sutures be removed?

As soon as the wound has healed enough to withstand expected mechanical trauma
Any stitch left in more than approximately 10 days will leave a scar guidelines are:
Face:—3 to 5 days
Extremities—10 days
Joints—10–14 days
Back—14 days
Abdomen—7 days

How can strength be added to an incision during and after suture removal?

With Steri-Strips®

In general, in which group of patients should skin sutures be left in longer than normal?

Patients on steroids

How should the sutures be cut?

Use the tips of the scissors to avoid cutting other tissues
Try to remove the cut ends (less foreign material decreases risk of infection)
Rest the scissor-hand on the non-scissor-hand to steady

How is an instrument knot tied?

Always start with a double wrap, known as a "surgeon's knot" and then use a single wrap, pulling the suture in the opposite directions after every "throw"

Does a student need to know a one-hand tie?

No! Master the two-hand tie and the instrument tie.

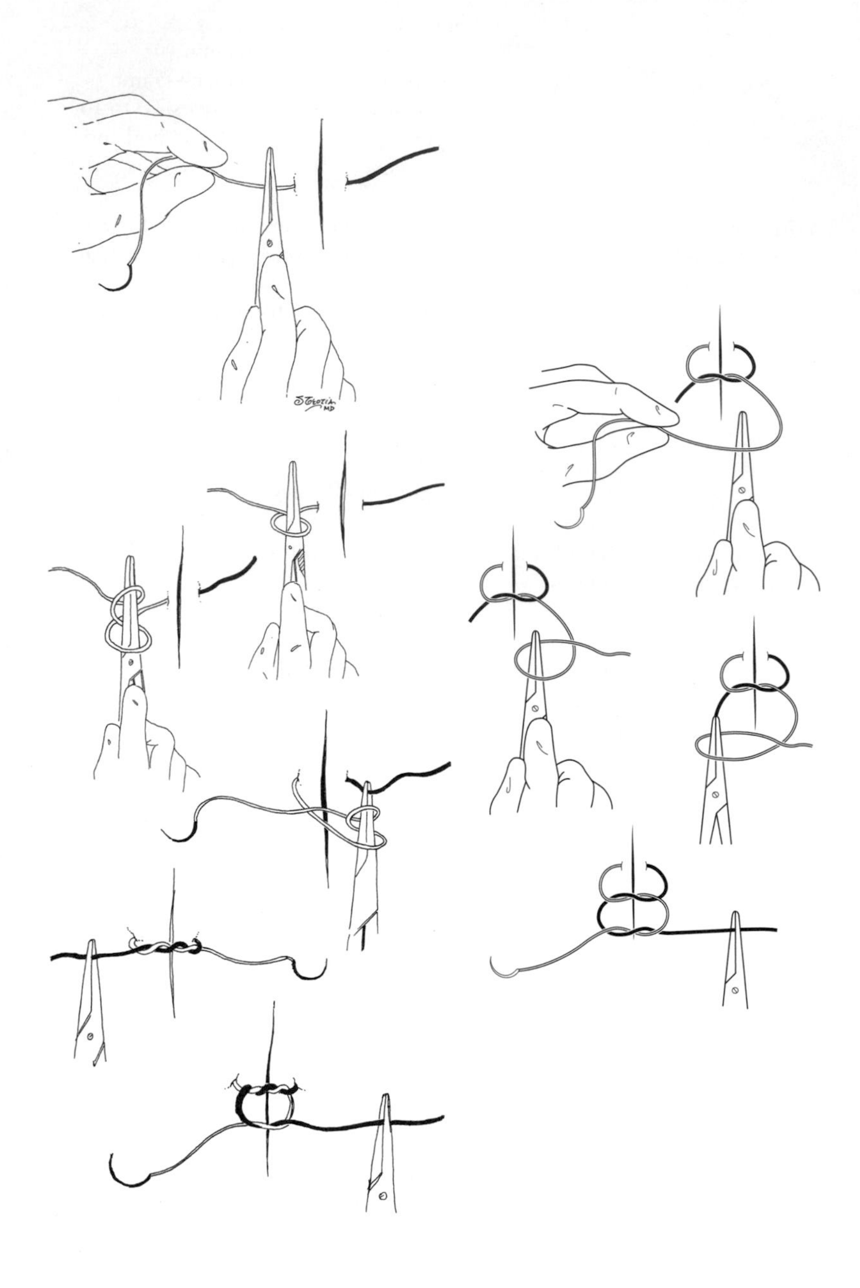

TWO-HAND TIE

What is the basic position for the two-hand tie?

The "C" position, formed by the thumb and index finger; the suture will **alternate** over the thumb and then the index finger for each throw

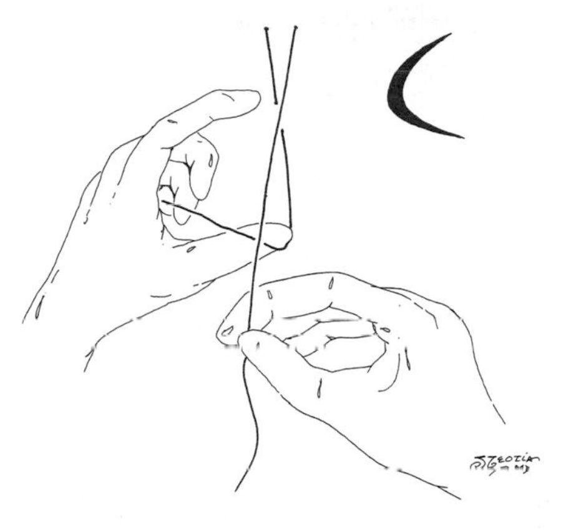

How is a two-hand knot tied?

First, use the index to lead.

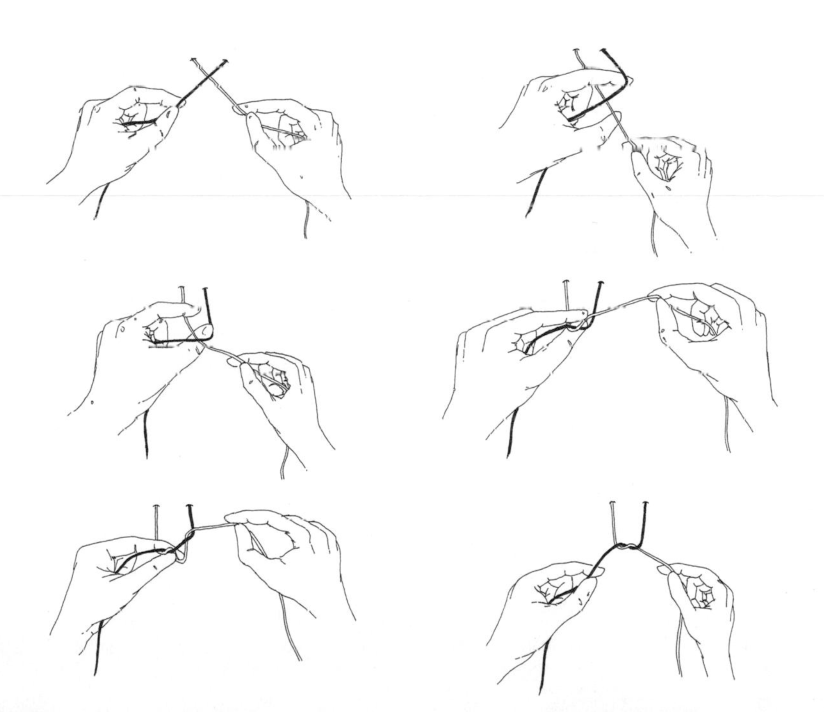

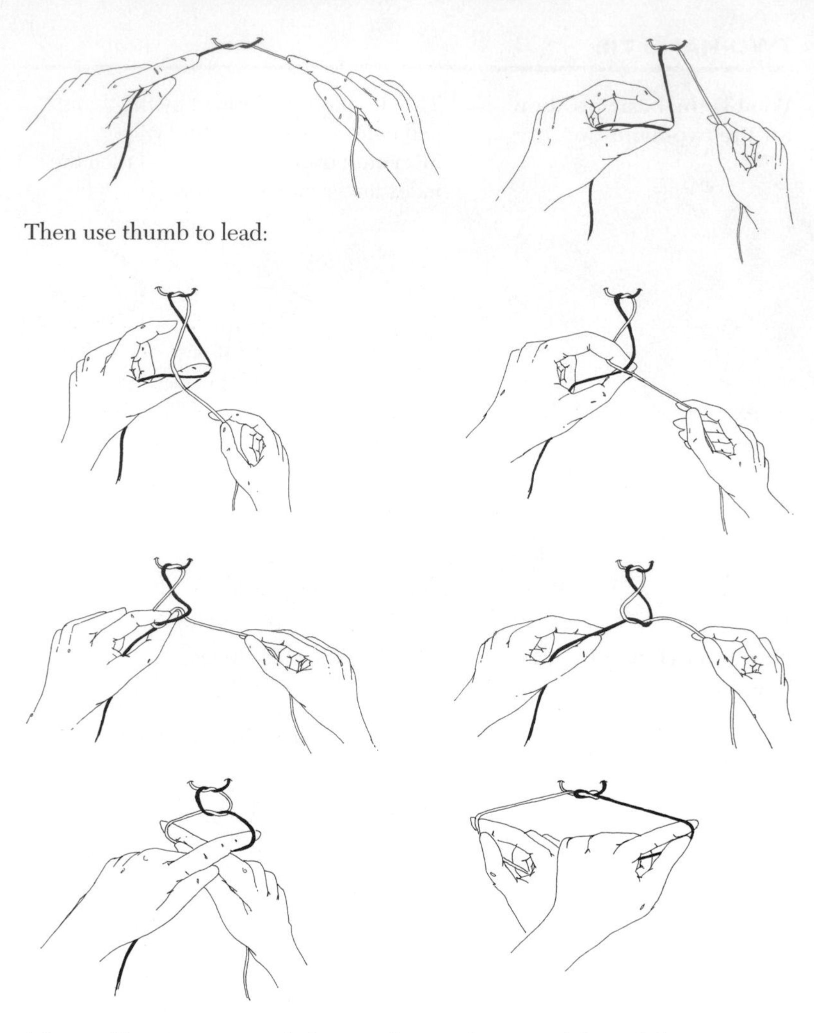

Then use thumb to lead:

Ask a resident or intern to help you after you have tried for awhile.

9 Incisions

If a patient has an old incision, is it best to make a subsequent incision next to or through the old incision?

Through the old incision, or excise the old incision, because it has scar tissue that limits the amount of collaterals that would be needed to heal an incision placed next to it

What is used to incise the epidermis?

Scalpel blade

What is used to incise the dermis?

Scalpel or electrocautery

Describe the following incisions:

Kocher

Right subcostal incision for open cholecystectomy

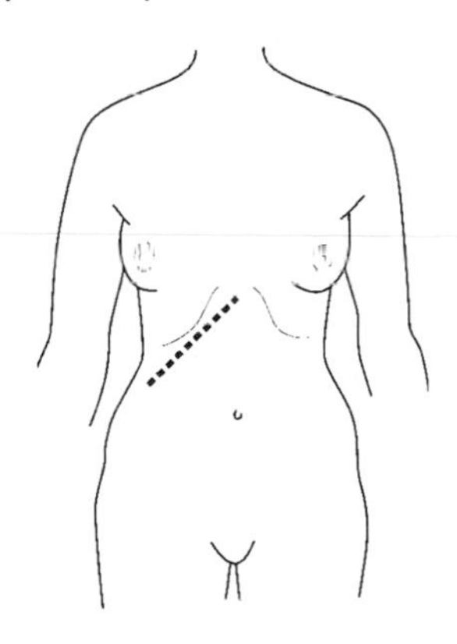

Midline laparotomy

Incision down the middle of abdomen along and through the linea alba

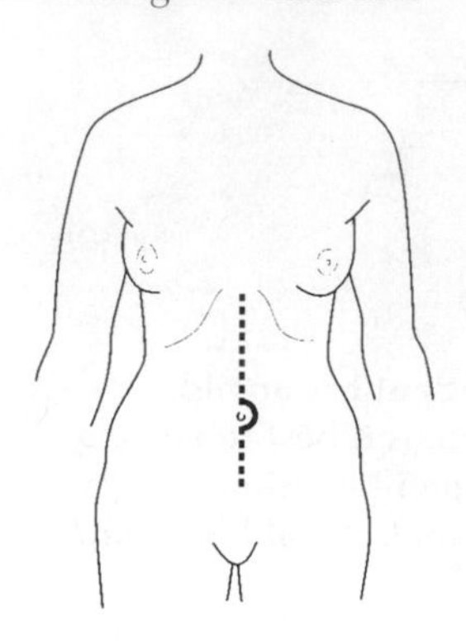

McBurney's

Small oblique right lower quadrant incision for an appendectomy through McBurney's point (one-third from the anterior superior iliac spine to the umbilicus)

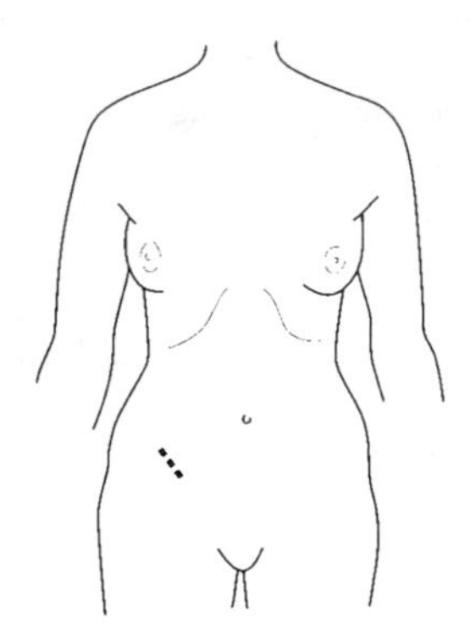

Rocky-Davis

Like a McBurney's incision except transverse (straight across)

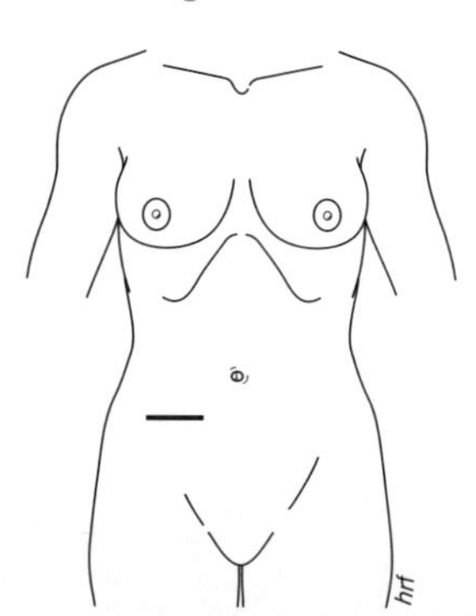

Paramedian

Incision that is longitudinal, but lateral to the linea alba (rarely used)

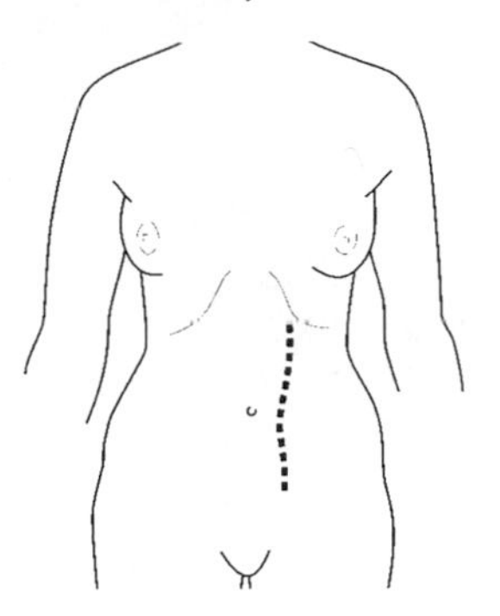

Pfannenstiel

Low transverse abdominal incision with retraction of the rectus muscles laterally; most often used for gynecologic procedures

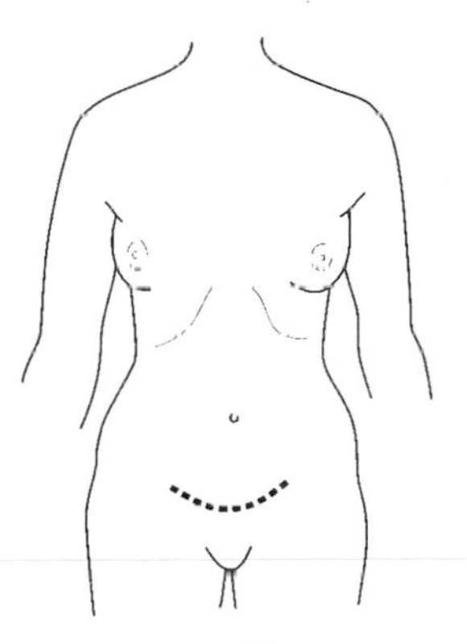

Kidney transplant

Lower quadrant; kidney placed extraperitoneally

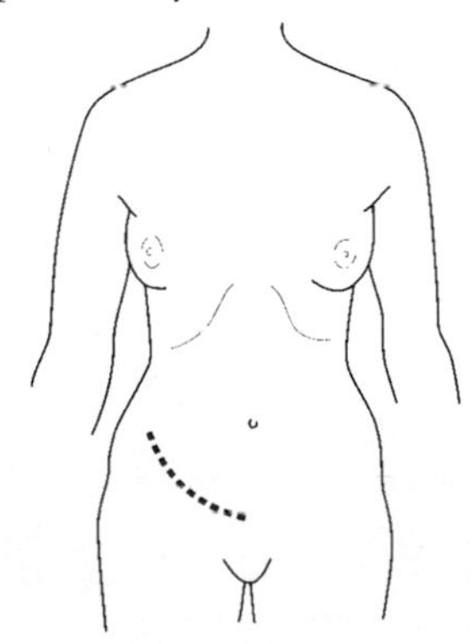

Liver transplant

Chevron or Mercedes-Benz® incision in the upper abdomen

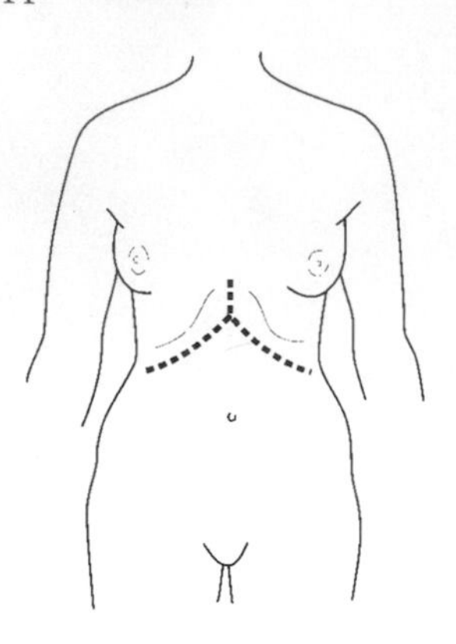

Transverse abdominal

Used mainly in infants and children (or for hemicolectomy in adults)

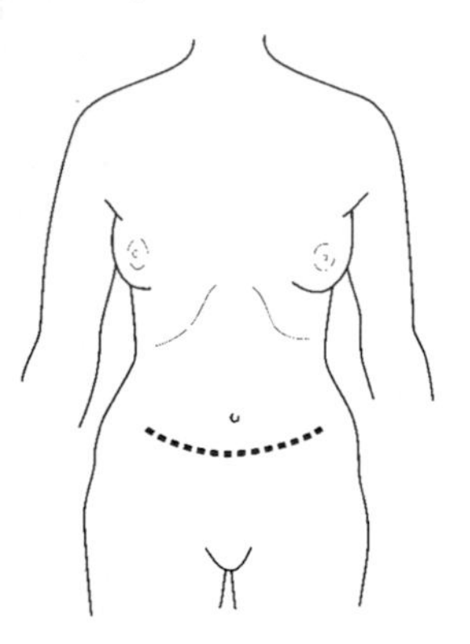

Median sternotomy

Midline sternotomy incision for heart procedures; less painful than a lateral thoracotomy

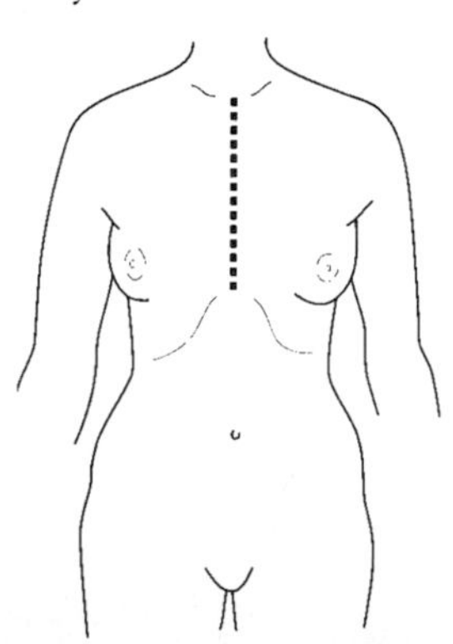

Thoracotomy

Usually through the fourth or fifth intercostal space; may be anterior or posterior lateral incisions

Very painful, but many are performed with muscle sparing (muscle retraction and not muscle transection)

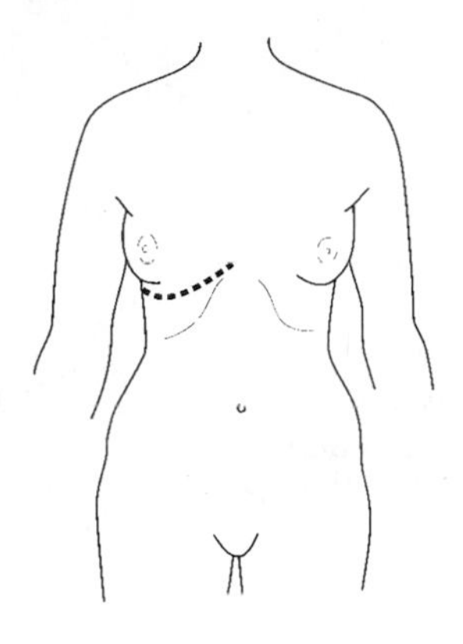

CEA (carotid endarterectomy)

Incision down anterior border of the sternocleidomastoid muscle to expose the carotid

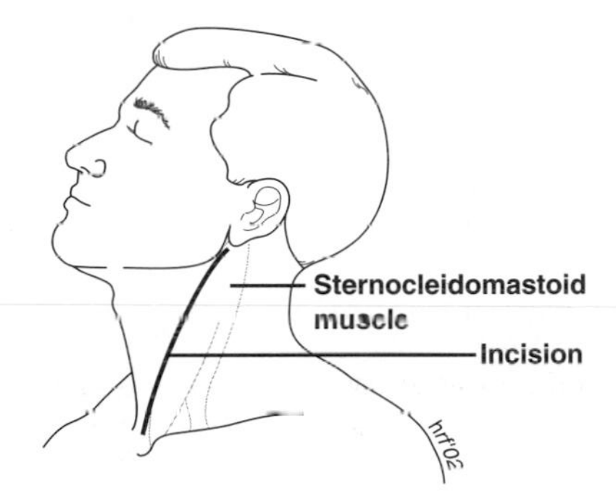

Inguinal hernia repair (open)

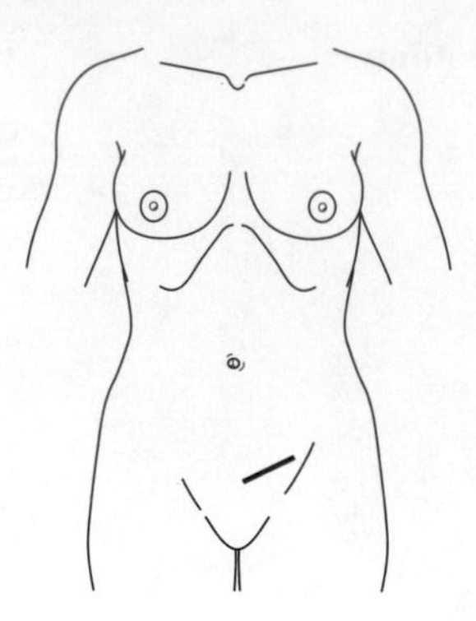

Laparoscopic cholecystectomy

Four trocar incisions

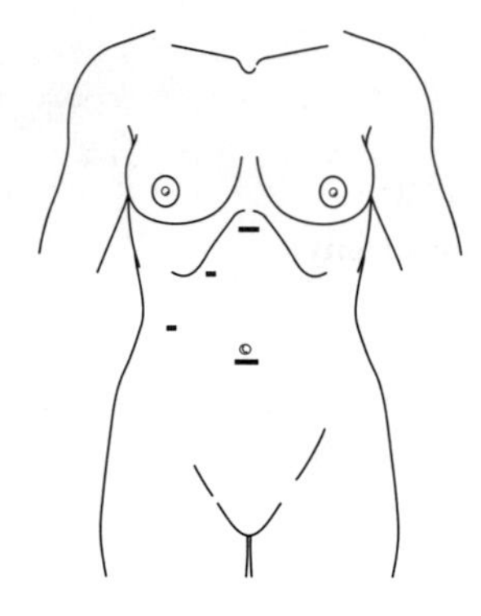

10 Surgical Positions

Define the following positions:

Supine	Patient lying flat on his back
Prone	Patient lying flat, face down
Left lateral decubitus	Patient lying down on her left side (think, "left lateral decubitus = left side down")
Right lateral decubitus	Patient lying down on his right side (think, "right lateral decubitus = right side down")
Lithotomy	Patient lying supine with legs spread

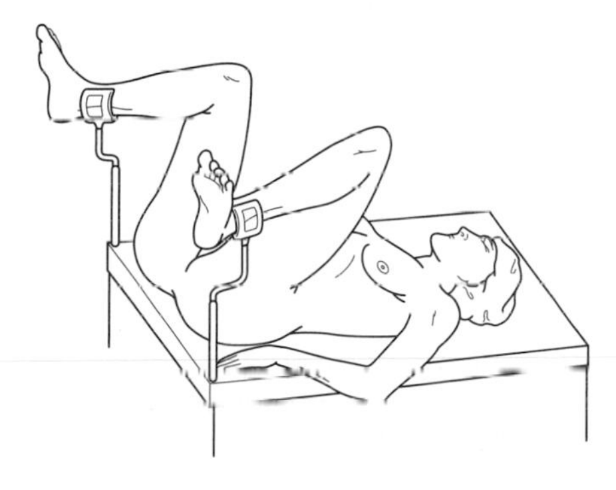

Trendelenburg	Patient supine with head lowered (A.K.A. "headdownenburg"—used during placement of a subclavian vein catheter as the veins distend with blood from gravity flow)

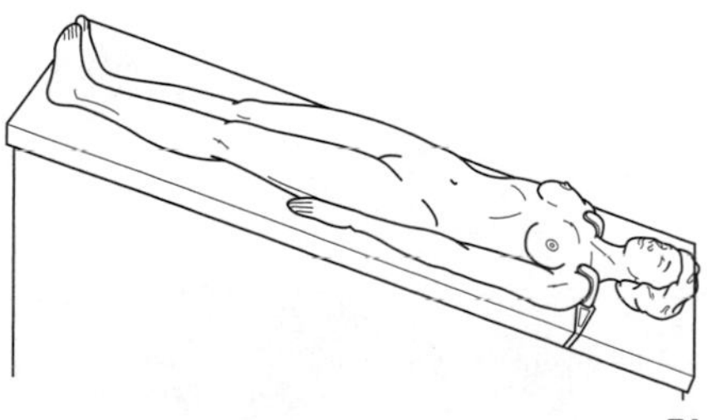

Reverse Trendelenburg	Patient supine with head elevated (usual position for laparoscopic cholecystectomy to make the intestines fall away from the operative field)

11 Surgical Speak

The language of surgery is quite simple if you master a few suffixes.

Define the suffix:

-ectomy	To surgically **remove** part of or an entire structure/organ
-orraphy	Surgical **repair**
-otomy	Surgical **incision into** an organ
-ostomy	Surgically created **opening** between two organs or organ and skin
-plasty	Surgical “shaping” or formation

Now test your knowledge of surgical speak:

Word for the surgical repair of a hernia	Herniorrhaphy
Word for the surgical removal of the stomach	Gastrectomy
Word for the surgical creation of an opening between the colon and the skin	Colostomy
Word for the surgical formation of a “new” pylorus	Pyloroplasty
Word for the surgical opening of the stomach	Gastrotomy

Surgical creation of an opening (anastomosis) between the common bile duct and jejunum	Choledochojejunostomy
Surgical creation of an opening (anastomosis) between the stomach and jejunum	Gastrojejunostomy (you get the picture)

12 Preoperative 101

When can a patient eat prior to major surgery?

The patient should be NPO after midnight the night before or at least for 8 hrs before surgery.

What risks should be discussed with all patients and documented on the consent form for a surgical procedure?

Bleeding, infection, anesthesia; other risks are specific to the individual procedure

If a patient is on antihypertensive medications, should the patient take them on the day of the procedure?

Yes, the patient should take antihypertensives on the day of the procedure.

If a patient is on an oral hypoglycemic agent (OHA), should the patient take the OHA on the day of surgery?

Not if the patient is to be NPO on the day of surgery

If a patient is taking insulin, should the patient take it on the day of surgery?

No, only half of a long-acting insulin (e.g., lente) and start D5 NS IV; check glucose levels often preoperatively, operatively, and postoperatively

Should a patient who smokes cigarettes stop before an operation?

Yes, improvement is seen in just 2 to 4 weeks after smoking cessation.

What laboratory test must all women of childbearing age have before entering the OR?

Beta-HCG and CBC because of the possibility of pregnancy and anemia from menses

What preoperative procedure should be performed before colon surgery?

Bowel prep with colon cathartic (e.g., GoLYTELY), oral antibiotics (neomycin and erythromycin base), and IV antibiotic before incision

13

Surgical Operations You Should Know

Define the following procedures:

Billroth I

Antrectomy with gastroduodenostomy

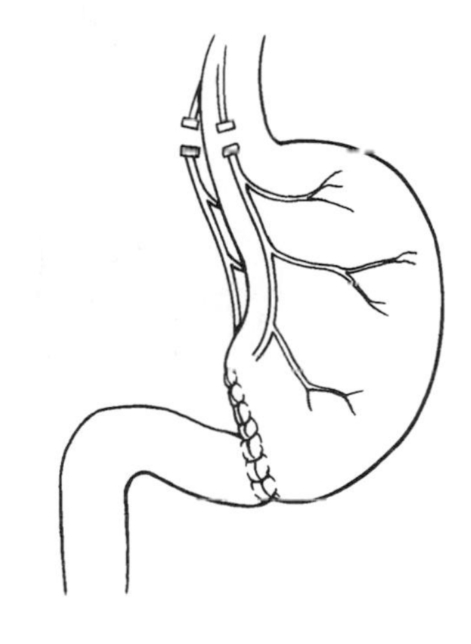

Billroth II

Antrectomy with gastrojejunostomy

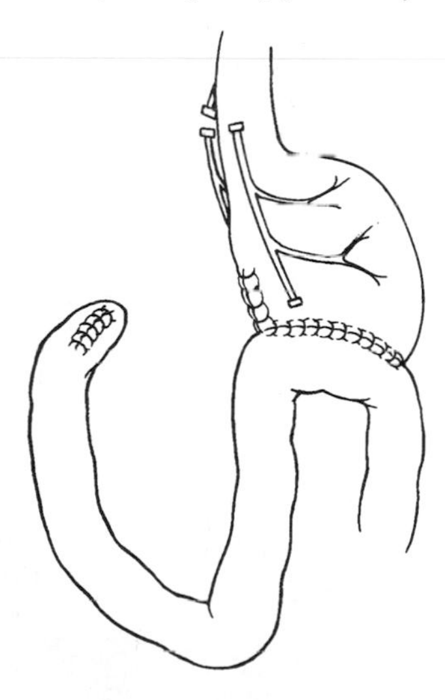

How to remember the difference between a Billroth I and a Billroth II?

Billroth 1 has one limb; Billroth 2 has two limbs.

Roux-en-Y limb

Jejunojejunostomy forming a Y-shaped figure of small bowel; the free end can then be anastomosed to a second hollow structure (e.g., gastrojejunostomy)

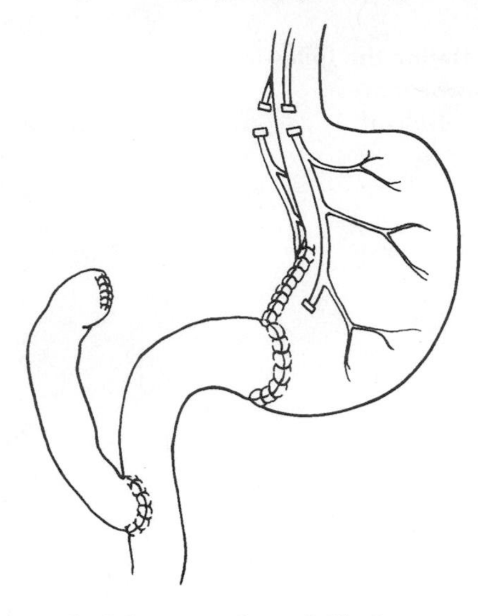

Brooke ileostomy

Standard ileostomy that is **folded on itself** to protrude from the abdomen approximately 2 cm to allow easy appliance placement and collection of succus

CEA

Carotid **E**nd**a**rterectomy; removal of atherosclerotic plaque from a carotid artery

Bassini herniorrhaphy

Repair of inguinal hernia by approximating transversus abdominis aponeurosis and the conjoint tendon to the reflection of **Poupart's** (inguinal) ligament

McVay herniorrhaphy

Repair of inguinal hernia by approximating the transversus abdominis aponeurosis and the conjoint tendon to **Cooper's** ligament (which is basically the superior pubic bone periosteum)

Lichtenstein herniorrhaphy
"Tension-free" inguinal hernia repair using **synthetic** graft material

Shouldice herniorrhaphy
Repair of inguinal hernia by **imbrication** of the transversalis fascia, transversus abdominis aponeurosis, and the conjoint tendon and approximation of the transversus abdominis aponeurosis and the conjoint tendon to the inguinal ligament

Plug and patch hernia RX
Prosthetic plug pushes hernia sac in and then is covered with a prosthetic patch to repair inguinal hernias

APR
Abdomino**P**erineal **R**esection; removal of the rectum and sigmoid colon through abdominal and perineal incisions (patient is left with a colostomy); used for low rectal cancers less than 8 cm from the anal verge

LAR
Low **A**nterior **R**esection; **resection** of **low** rectal tumors through an **anterior** abdominal incision

Hartmann's procedure
1. Proximal colostomy
2. Distal stapled-off colon or rectum that is left in peritoneal cavity

Mucus fistula
Distal end of the colon is brought to the abdominal skin as a stoma (proximal end is brought up to skin as an end colostomy)

Kocher maneuver
Dissection of the duodenum from the right-sided peritoneal attachment to allow mobilization and visualization of the back of the duodenum/pancreas

Seldinger technique
Placement of a central line by first placing a wire in the vein, followed by placing the catheter over the wire

Puestow procedure — Side-to-side anastomosis of the pancreas and jejunum (pancreatic duct is filleted open)

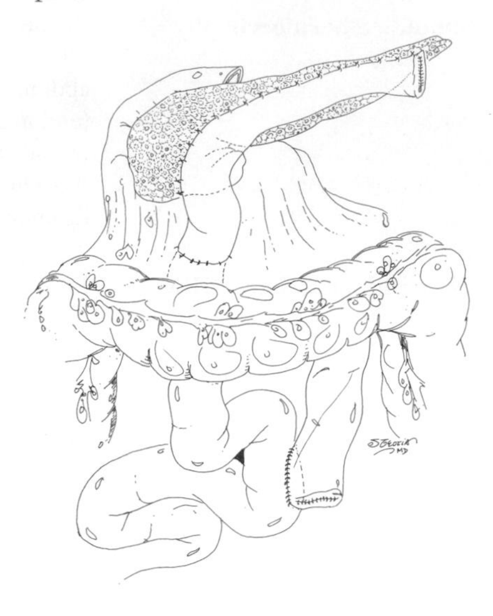

Stamm gastrostomy — Gastrostomy placed by open surgical incision and tacked to the abdominal wall

Highly selective vagotomy — Transection of vagal fibers to the body of the stomach without interruption of fibers to the pylorus (does not need pyloroplasty or other drainage procedure because the pylorus should still function)

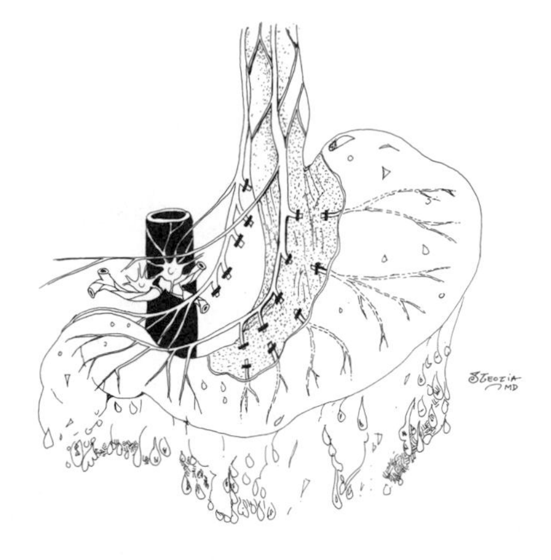

Enterolysis	Lysis of peritoneal adhesions
LOA	**L**ysis **o**f **A**dhesions (enterolysis)
Appendectomy	Removal of the appendix
Lap appy	Laparoscopic removal of the appendix
Cholecystectomy	Removal of the gallbladder
Lap chole	Laparoscopic removal of the gallbladder
Nissen	Nissen fundoplication; 360° wrap of the stomach by the fundus of the stomach around the distal esophagus to prevent reflux

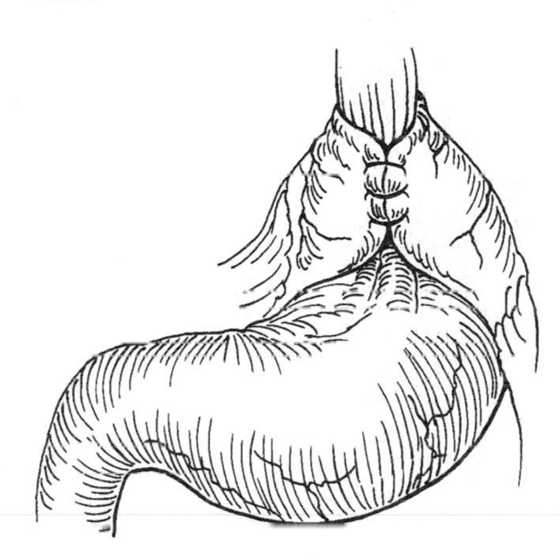

LAP Nissen	Nissen fundoplication with laparoscopy
Simple mastectomy	Removal of breast and nipple without removal of nodes
Choledochojejunostomy	Anastomosis of the common bile duct to the jejunum (end to side)
Graham patch	Placement of omentum with stitches over a gastric or duodenal perforation (i.e., omentum is used to plug the hole)

Heineke-Mikulicz pyloroplasty

Longitudinal incision through all layers of the pylorus, sewing closed in a transverse direction to make the pylorus non-functional (used after truncal vagotomy)

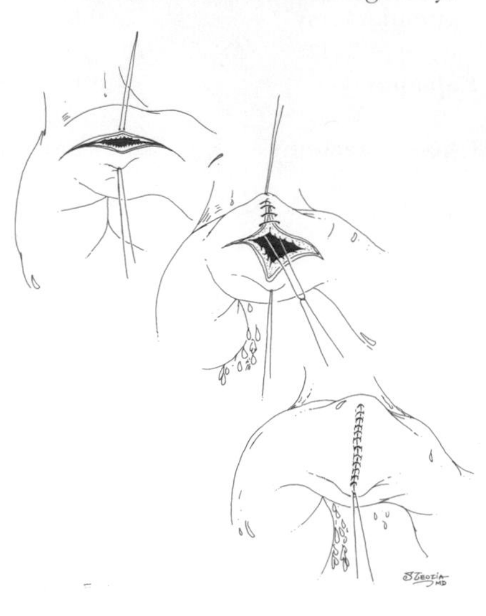

Pringle maneuver

Temporary occlusion of the porta hepatis (for temporary control of liver blood flow when liver parenchyma is actively bleeding)

Modified radical mastectomy

Removal of the breast, nipple, **and axillary lymph nodes** (no muscle is removed)

Lumpectomy and radiation

Removal of breast mass and axillary lymph nodes; normal surrounding breast tissue is spared; patient then undergoes postoperative radiation treatments

I and D

Incision and **d**rainage of pus; the wound is then packed open

PEG

Percutaneous **E**ndoscopic **G**astrostomy; the endoscope is placed in the stomach, which is then inflated with air. A needle is passed into the stomach percutaneously, string is passed through the needle traversing the abdominal wall, and gastrostomy is then placed by using the Seldinger technique over the wire.

Exploratory laparotomy

Laparotomy to explore the peritoneal cavity looking for the cause of pain, peritoneal signs, obstruction, hemorrhage, etc.

TURP

Trans**U**rethral **R**esection of the **P**rostate; removal of obstructing prostatic tissue via scope in the urethral lumen

Fem pop bypass

Femoral artery to **pop**liteal artery bypass using synthetic graft or saphenous vein; used to bypass blockage in the femoral artery

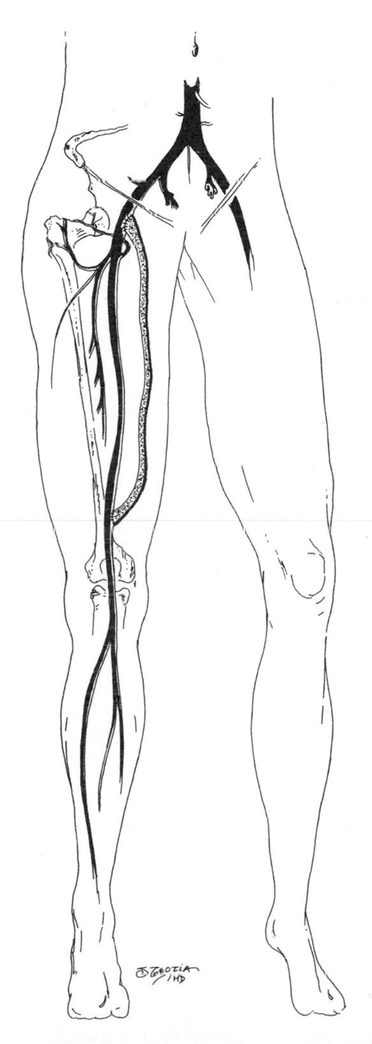

AX FEM

Long prosthetic graft tunneled under the skin placed from the **ax**illary artery to the **fem**oral artery

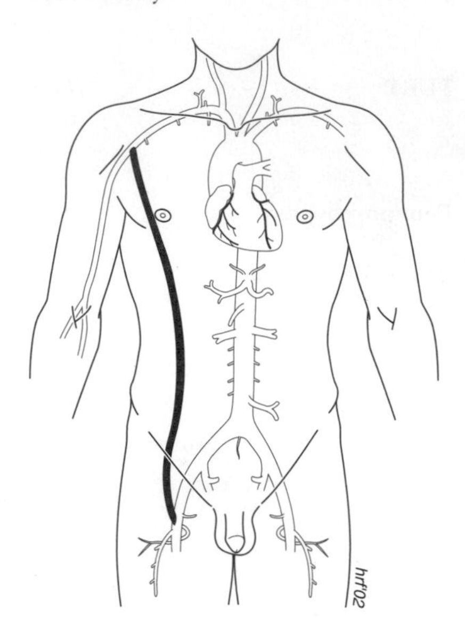

Triple A repair

Repair of an AAA (**A**bdominal **A**ortic **A**neurysm). Open aneurysm and place prosthetic graft. Then close old aneurysm sac around graft.

CABG

Coronary **A**rtery **B**ypass **G**rafting; via saphenous vein graft or internal mammary artery bypass grafts to coronary arteries from aorta (cardiac revascularization)

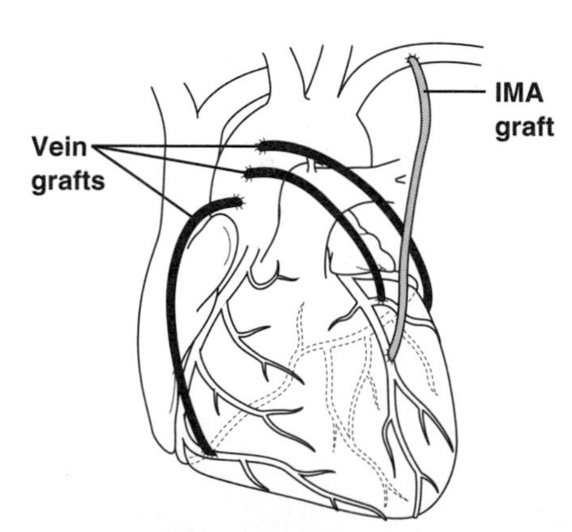

Hartmann's pouch

Oversewing of a rectal stump (or distal colonic stump) after resection of a colonic segment; patient is left with a proximal colostomy

Ileoanal pull-through

Anastomosis of the ileum to the anus after total proctocolectomy

Hemicolectomy

Removal of a colonic segment (i.e., partial colectomy)

Truncal vagotomy

Transection of the vagus nerve trunks; must provide drainage procedure to stomach (e.g., gastrojejunostomy or pyloroplasty) because after truncal vagotomy, the **pylorus does not relax**

Antrectomy

Removal of stomach antrum

Whipple procedure

Pancreaticoduodenectomy:
- Cholecystectomy
- Truncal vagotomy
- Antrectomy
- Pancreaticoduodenectomy—removal of the head of the pancreas and duodenum
- Choledochojejunostomy
- Pancreaticojejunostomy (anastomosis of distal pancreas remnant to the jejunum)
- Gastrojejunostomy (anastomosis of stomach to jejunum)

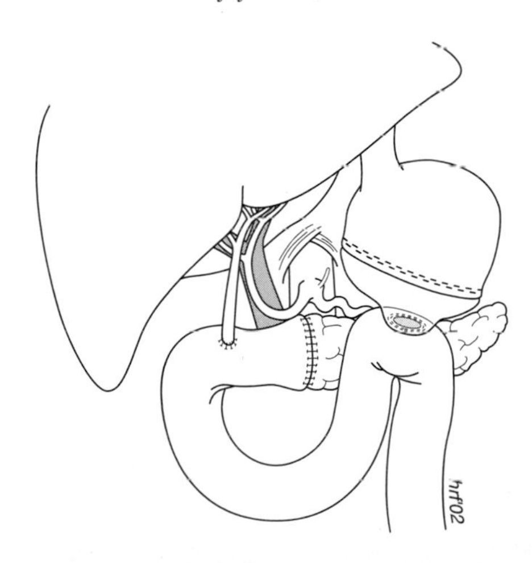

Excisional biopsy	Biopsy with complete excision of all suspect tissue (mass)
Incisional biopsy	Biopsy with incomplete removal of suspect tissue (incises tissue from mass)
Tracheostomy	Placement of airway tube into trachea surgically or percutaneously

14 Wounds, Drains, and Tubes

Define the following terms:

Primary wound closure

Suture wound closes immediately (A.K.A. first intention).

Secondary wound closure

Wound is left open and heals over time **without sutures;** it heals by granulation, contraction, and epithelialization over weeks (leaves a larger scar).

Delayed primary closure (DPC)

Suture wound closes 3 to 5 days AFTER incision (classically 5 days).

How long until a sutured wound epithelializes?

~ 48 hours

After a primary closure, when should the dressing be removed?

Postoperative day 2

When can a patient take a shower after a primary closure?

Anytime after postoperative day 2 (after wound epithelializes)

What is a wet-to-dry dressing?

A damp (not wet) gauze dressing placed over a granulating wound and then allowed to dry to the wound; removal allows for debridement of the wound

What inhibits wound healing?

Infection, ischemia, diabetes mellitus, malnutrition, anemia, steroids, cancer, radiation

What reverses the deleterious effects of steroids on wound healing?

Vitamin A

What is an abdominal wound dehiscence?

Opening of the fascial closure (not skin); treat by returning to the OR for immediate fascial reclosure

What is Dakin solution?

Dilute sodium hypochlorite (**bleach**) used in contaminated wounds

What is the purpose of drains?

1. Withdrawal of fluids
2. Apposition of tissues to remove a potential space by suction

What is a Jackson-Pratt (JP) drain?

A closed drainage system attached to a suction bulb ("grenade")

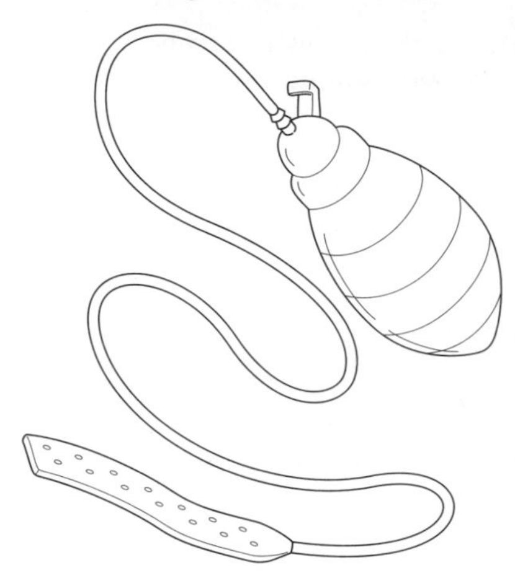

What are the "three S's" of Jackson-Pratt drain removal?

1. **S**titch removal
2. **S**uction discontinuation
3. **S**low, steady pull

What is a Penrose drain?

An open drainage system composed of a thin rubber hose; associated with increased infection rate in clean wounds

Define the following terms:

G-tube

Gastrostomy tube; used for drainage or feeding

J-tube

Jejunostomy tube; used for feeding; may be a small-needle catheter (remember to flush after use or it will clog) or a large, red rubber catheter

Cholecystostomy tube

Tube placed surgically or percutaneously with ultrasound guidance to drain the gallbladder

T-tube

A tube placed in the common bile duct with an ascending and descending limb that forms a "T"

Drains percutaneously
Usually placed after common bile duct exploration

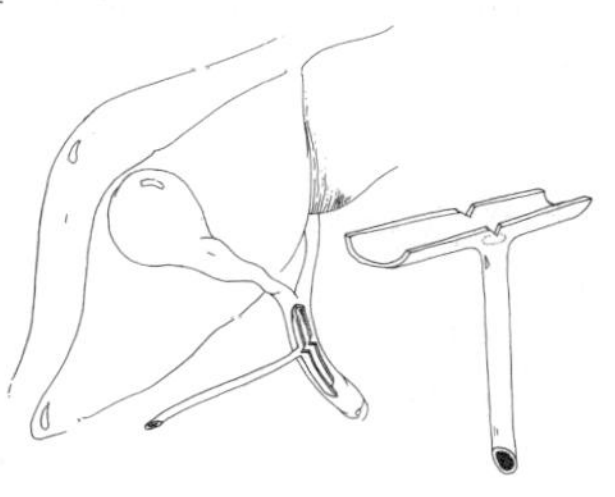

Define the following terms:
Thoracostomy tube — **Chest tube**

What is the purpose of a chest tube?
To appose the parietal and visceral pleura by draining blood, pus, fluid, chyle, or air

CHEST TUBES

How is a chest tube inserted?

1. Administer local anesthetic.
2. Incise skin in the fourth or fifth intercostal space between the mid- and anterior-axillary lines.
3. Perform blunt Kelly-clamp dissection **over** the rib into the pleural space.
4. Perform finger exploration to confirm intrapleural placement.
5. Place tube posteriorly and superiorly.

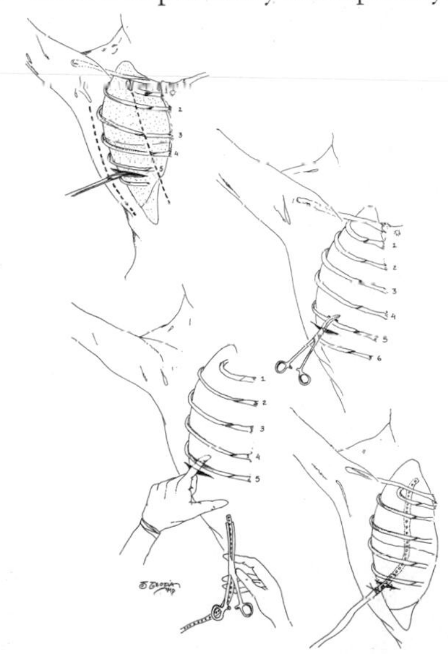

What are the goals of chest tube insertion?

Drain the pleural cavity
Appose parietal and visceral pleura to seal any visceral pleural holes

In most cases, where should the chest tube be positioned?

Posteriorly into the apex

How can you tell on CXR if the last hole on the chest tube is in the pleural cavity?

The last hole is cut through the radiopaque line in the chest tube and is seen on CXR as a break in the line, which should be within the pleural cavity.

What is the chest tube connected to?

A Pleuravac® (three-chambered box)

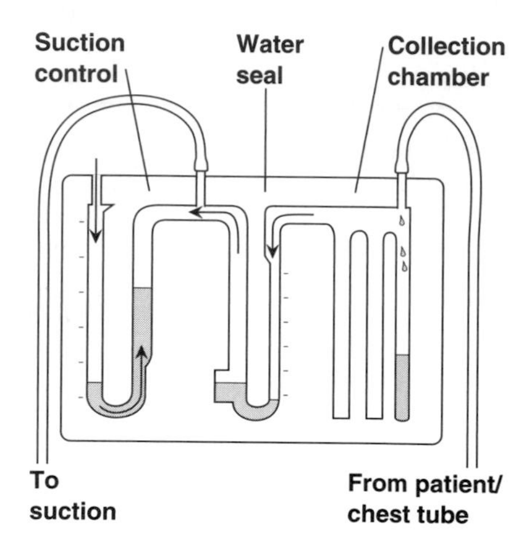

What are the three chambers of the Pleuravac®?

1. Collection chamber
2. Water seal
3. Suction control

Describe how each chamber of the Pleuravac® box works as the old three-bottle system:

Collection chamber

Collects fluid, pus, blood, or chyle and measures the amount
Connects to the water seal bottle and to the chest tube

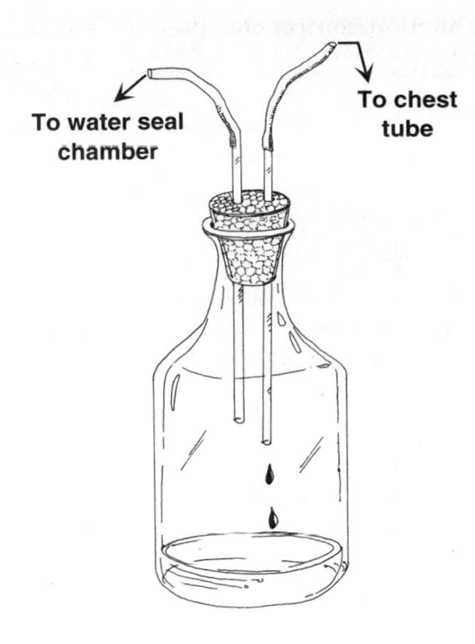

Water-seal chamber

One-way valve—allows air to be removed from the pleural space; does not allow air to enter pleural cavity; connects to the suction control bottle and to the collection chamber

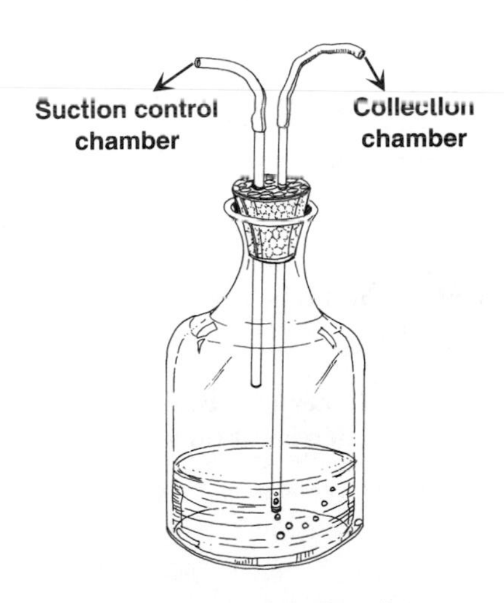

Suction-control chamber

Controls the amount of suction by the height of the water column
Sucking in room air releases excessive suction
Connects to wall suction and to the water seal bottle

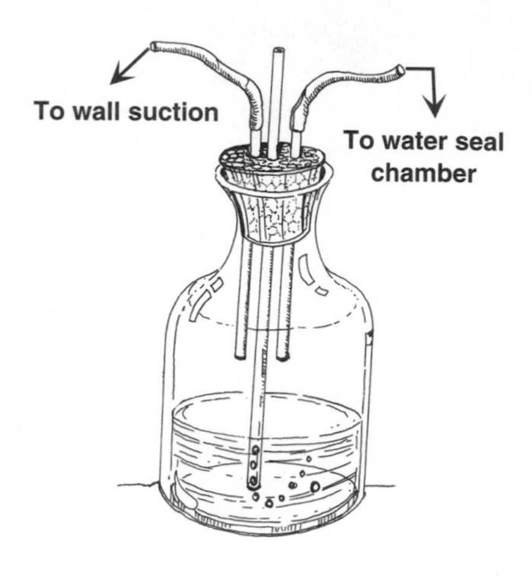

Give a good example of a water seal

Place a straw in a cup of water—you can blow air out but if you suck in, the straw fills with water and thus forms a one-way valve for air just like the chest tube water seal.

How is a chest tube placed on water seal?

By removing the suction; a tension pneumothorax (PTX) cannot form because the one-way valve (water seal) allows release of air buildup

Should a chest tube ever be clamped off?

No, except to "run the system" **momentarily**

What does it mean "to run the system" of a chest tube?

To see if the air leak is from a leak in the pleural cavity (i.e., visceral hole) or from a leak in the tubing
Momentarily occlude the chest tube and if the air leak is still present, it is from the tubing or tubing connection, not from the chest.

How can you tell if the chest tube is "tidling"?

Take the Pleuravac® off of suction and look at the water seal chamber—the fluid should move with respiration/ ventilation—this is called "tidling." This decreases and ceases if the pleura seals off the chest tube.

How can you check for an air leak?

Look at the water seal chamber on suction; if bubbles pass through the water seal fluid, a large air leak (i.e., air leaking into chest tube) is present. If no air leak is evident on suction, remove suction and ask the patient to cough. If air bubbles through the water seal, a small air leak is present.

What is the usual course for removing a chest tube placed for a PTX?

1. Suction until the PTX resolves and the air leak is gone.
2. Water seal for 24 hours.
3. Remove the chest tube if no PTX or air leak is present after 24 hours of water seal.

How fast is a small, stable PTX absorbed?

Approximately 1% daily; therefore, a 10% PTX by volume will absorb in 10 days

How should a chest tube be removed?

1. Cut the stitch.
2. Ask the patient to exhale or inhale maximally
3. Rapidly remove the tube (split second) and at same time, place petroleum jelly gauze covered by 4 × 4's and then tape.
4. Obtain a CXR.

NASOGASTRIC TUBES (NGT)

How should an NGT be placed?

1. Use lubrication and have suction up on the bed.
2. Use anesthetic to numb nose.
3. Place head in flexion.
4. Ask patient to drink a small amount of water when the tube is in the back of the throat and to swallow the tube; if the patient can talk without difficulty and succus returns, the tube should be in the stomach (get an x-ray if there is any question).

How should an NGT be removed?

Give patient a tissue, discontinue suction, untape nose, remove quickly, and tell patient to blow nose.

What test should be performed before feeding via any tube?

High abdominal x-ray to confirm placement into the GI tract (past the pylorus in most cases)

How does an NGT work?

Sump pump, dual lumen tube—the large clear tube is hooked to suction and the small blue tube allows for air sump (i.e., circuit sump pump with air in the blue tube and air and succus sucked out through the large clear lumen)

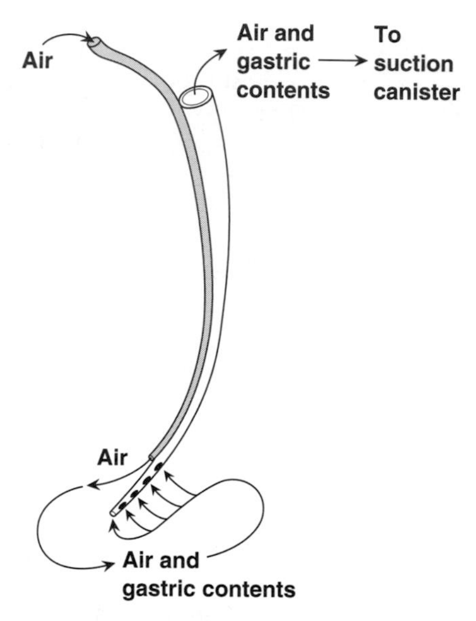

How can you check to see if the NGT is working?

The blue port will make a sucking noise. Always keep the blue port opening above the stomach.

Should an NGT be placed on continuous or intermittent suction?

Continuous low suction—side holes disengage if they are against mucosa because of the sump mechanism and multiple holes

What happens if the NGT is clogged?

The tube will not decompress the stomach and will keep the low esophageal sphincter (LES) open (i.e., a setup for aspiration).

How should an NGT be unclogged?

Saline-flush the clear port, reconnect to suction, and flush air down the blue sump port.

What is a common cause of excessive NGT drainage?

The tip of the NGT is inadvertently placed in the duodenum and drains the pancreatic fluid and bile; an x-ray should be taken and the tube repositioned into the stomach.

What is the difference between a feeding tube (Dobbhoff tube) and an NGT?

A feeding tube is a thin tube weighted at the end that is not a sump pump but a simple catheter. It must be placed past the pylorus, which is facilitated by the weighted end and peristalsis.

FOLEY CATHETER

What is a Foley catheter?

Catheter into the bladder, allowing accurate urine output determination

What is a coudé catheter?

A Foley catheter with a small, curved tip to help maneuver around a large prostate

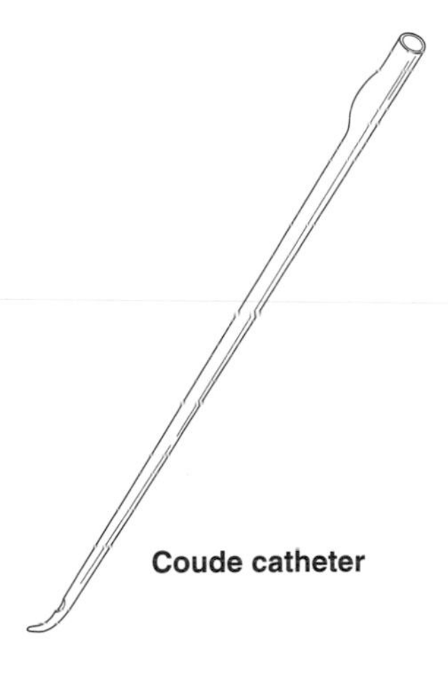

If a Foley catheter cannot be inserted, what are the next steps?

1. Anesthetize the urethra with a sterile local anesthetic (e.g., lidocaine jelly).
2. Try a **larger** Foley catheter.

CENTRAL LINES

What are they?

Catheters placed into the major veins (central veins) via subclavian-, internal-jugular-, or femoral-vein approaches

What major complications result from placement?

PTX (always obtain postplacement CXR), bleeding, malposition (e.g., into the neck from subclavian approach), dysrhythmias

In long-term central lines, what does the "cuff" do?

Allows ingrowth of fibrous tissue, which:
- Holds the line in place
- Forms a barrier to the advance of bacteria

What is a Hickman® or Hickman-type catheter?

External central line tunneled under the skin with a "cuff"

What is a Port-A-Cath®?

Central line that has a port buried under the skin that must be accessed through the skin (percutaneously)

MISCELLANEOUS

How can diameter in mm be determined from a French measurement?

Divide the French size by pi or 3.14 (e.g., a 15 French tube has a diameter of 5 mm).

How can needle-gauge size be determined?

A 14-gauge needle is 1/14 of an inch (and thus a 14-gauge needle is larger than a 21-gauge needle).

What is a Tenckhoff catheter?

Catheter placed into the peritoneal cavity for peritoneal dialysis

15 Surgical Anatomy Pearls

What is the drainage of the left testicular vein?
Left renal vein

What is the drainage of the right testicular vein?
IVC

What is Gerota's fascia?
Fascia surrounding the kidney

What are the prominent collateral circulations seen in portal hypertension?
Esophageal varices, hemorrhoids (inferior hemorrhoidal vein to internal iliac vein), patent umbilical vein (caput medusa), and retroperitoneal vein via lumbar tributaries

What parts of the GI tract are retroperitoneal?
Most of the duodenum, the ascending colon, the descending colon, and the pancreas

What is the gubernaculum?
Embryologic structure that adheres the testes to the scrotal sac; used to help manipulate the testes during indirect hernia repair

Which artery bleeds in bleeding duodenal ulcers?
Gastroduodenal artery

What is the name of the lymph nodes between the pectoralis minor and major muscles?
Rotter's lymph nodes

Is the left vagus nerve anterior or posterior?
Anterior; remember the esophagus rotates during development

What is Morrison's pouch?
The hepatorenal recess; the most posterior cavity within the peritoneal cavity

Give the locations of the following structures:

Foregut — Mouth to ampulla of Vater

Midgut — Ampulla of Vater to distal third of transverse colon

Hindgut — Distal third of transverse colon to the anus

Where are the blood vessels on a rib?

The vein, artery, and nerve (VAN) are underneath the rib (thus, place chest tubes and thoracentesis needles above the rib!).

What is the order of the femoral vessels?

The femoral vein is medial to the femoral artery (think: **NAVEL** for the order of the right femoral vessels—**n**erve, **a**rtery, **v**ein, **e**xtralymphatic tissue, **l**ymphatics).

What is Hesselbach's triangle?

The area bordered by:
1. Inguinal ligament
2. Epigastric vessels
3. Lateral border of the rectus sheath

What nerve is located on top of the spermatic cord?

Ilioinguinal nerve

What is Calot's triangle?

The area bordered by:
1. Cystic duct
2. Common hepatic duct
3. Cystic artery

What is Calot's node?

Lymph node found in Calot's triangle

What separates the right and left lobes of the liver?

Cantle's line—a line drawn from the IVC to just left of the gallbladder fossa

What is the gastrinoma triangle?

A triangle where more than 90% of gastrinomas are located, bordered by:
1. Junction of the second and third portions of the duodenum
2. Cystic duct
3. Pancreatic neck

Which artery is responsible for anterior spinal syndrome?

Artery of Adamkiewicz

Where is McBurney's point?	One-third the distance from the anterior superior iliac spine to the umbilicus (estimate of the position of the appendix)
How can you find the appendix after you find the cecum?	Trace the taenia back as they converge on the origin of the appendix.
Where is the space of Retzius?	The preperitoneal space anterior to the bladder
What are the white lines of Toldt?	The lateral peritoneal reflections of the ascending and descending colon
What is the strongest layer of the small bowel?	Submucosa (not the serosa, think: SUbmucosa = SUperior)
Which parts of the GI tract do not have a serosa?	Esophagus Middle and distal rectum
What is the vein that overlies the pylorus?	Vein of Mayo
What is the pouch of Douglas?	Pouch between the rectum and bladder or uterus
What does the thoracic duct empty into?	Left subclavian vein; left internal jugular vein junction
What is the coronary vein?	Left gastric vein
What is the hypogastric artery?	Internal iliac artery
What is longer, the left or right renal vein?	The left
What are the layers of the abdominal wall?	1. Skin, then fat 2. Scarpa's fascia, then more fat 3. External oblique 4. Internal oblique 5. Transversus abdominis 6. Transversalis fascia 7. Preperitoneal fat 8. Peritoneum
What are the plicae circulares?	Plicae = folds, circulares = circular; thus, the circular folds of mucosa of the small bowel

What is another name for the plicae circulares?

Valvulae conniventes

What are the major structural differences between the jejunum and ileum?

Jejunum—long vasa rectae; large plicae circulares; thicker wall
Ileum—shorter vasa rectae; smaller plicae circulares; thinner wall (think: **I**leum = **I**nferior vasa rectae, **I**nferior plicae circulares, and **I**nferior wall)

What are the major anatomic differences between the colon and the small bowel?

The colon has taenia coli, haustra, and appendices epiploicae (fat appendages), whereas the small intestine is smooth.

How far up does the diaphragm extend?

To the nipples in men (fourth intercostal space; thus, the abdomen extends to the level of the nipples)

What dermatome is at the umbilicus?

T10

16

Fluids and Electrolytes

What are the two major body fluid compartments?	1. Intracellular 2. Extracellular
What are the two subcompartments of extracellular fluid?	1. Interstitial fluid (in between cells) 2. Intravascular fluid (plasma)
What percentage of body weight is in fluid?	60%
What percentage of body fluid is intracellular?	66%
What percentage of body fluid is extracellular?	33%
What is the composition of body fluid?	Fluids = 60% total body weight Intracellular = 40% total body weight Extracellular = 20% total body weight (think: 60, 40, 20)
On average, what percentage of body weight does blood account for in adults?	~ 7%
How many liters of blood are in a 70-kg man?	0.07 × 70 = 5 liters
What are the fluid requirements every 24 hours for each of the following substances:	
Water	~ 30 to 35 ml/kg
Sodium and potassium	~ 1 mEq/kg
Chloride	~ 1.5 mEq/kg

What are the levels and sources of normal daily water loss?

Urine—1200 to 1500 ml (25–30 ml/kg)
Sweat—200 to 400 ml
Respiratory losses—500 to 700 ml
Feces—100 to 200 ml

What are the levels and sources of normal daily electrolyte loss?

Sodium and potassium = 100 mEq
Chloride = 150 mEq (40 mEq/l sodium and chloride lost as sweat)

What is the physiologic response to hypovolemia?

Sodium/H_2O retention via renin → aldosterone, water retention via ADH, vasoconstriction via angiotensin II and sympathetics, low urine output and tachycardia (early), hypotension (late)

THIRD SPACING

What is it?

Fluid accumulation in the interstitium of tissues, as in edema, e.g., loss of fluid into the interstitium and lumen of a paralytic bowel following surgery (think of the intravascular and intracellular spaces as the first two spaces)

When does "third-spacing" occur postoperatively?

Third-spaced fluid tends to mobilize back into the intravascular space around the third postoperative day; beware of fluid overload once the fluid begins to return to the intravascular space. Switch to hypotonic fluid and decrease IV rate.

What are the classic signs of third spacing?

Tachycardia
Decreased urine output

What is the treatment?

IV hydration with isotonic fluids

What are the surgical causes of the following conditions:

Metabolic acidosis

Loss of bicarbonate: diarrhea, ileus, fistula, high-output ileostomy, carbonic anhydrase inhibitors
Increase in acids: lactic acidosis (ischemia), ketoacidosis, renal failure, necrotic tissue

Hypochloremic alkalosis

NGT suction, loss of gastric HCl through vomiting/NGT

Metabolic alkalosis	Vomiting, NG suction, diuretics, alkali ingestion, mineralocorticoid excess
Respiratory acidosis	Hypoventilation (e.g., CNS depression), drugs (e.g., morphine), PTX, pleural effusion, parenchymal lung disease, acute airway obstruction
Respiratory alkalosis	Hyperventilation (e.g., anxiety, pain, fever, wrong ventilator settings)
What is the "classic" acid-base finding with significant vomiting or NGT suctioning?	Hypokalemic hypochloremic metabolic alkalosis
Why hypokalemia with NGT suctioning?	Loss in gastric fluid—loss of HCl causes alkalosis, driving K^+ into cells; K^+ loss into urine exchange for Na^+
What is the treatment for hypokalemic hypochloremic metabolic alkalosis?	IVF, Cl^-/K^+ replacement
What is paradoxic alkalotic aciduria?	Seen in severe hypokalemic hypochloremic metabolic alkalosis with paradoxic metabolic alkalosis of serum and acidic urine
How does paradoxic alkalotic aciduria occur?	H^+ is lost in the urine in exchange for Na^+ in an attempt to restore volume.
With paradoxic alkalotic aciduria, why is H^+ preferentially lost?	H^+ is exchanged preferentially into the urine instead of K+ because of the low concentration of K^+.
What can be followed to assess fluid status?	Urine output, vital signs, **weight changes,** skin turgor, jugular venous distention (JVD), mucosal membranes, rales (crackles), central venous pressure, PCWP, chest x-ray findings
With hypovolemia, what changes occur in vital signs?	Tachycardia, tachypnea, initial rise in diastolic blood pressure because of clamping down (peripheral vasoconstriction) with subsequent decrease in both systolic and diastolic blood pressures

What are the insensible fluid losses?

Loss of fluid not measured:
Feces—100 to 200 ml/24 hours
Breathing—500 to 700 ml/24 hours (**Note:** increases with fever and tachypnea)
Skin—approximately 300 ml/24 hours, increased with fever; thus, insensible fluid loss is not directly measured

What are the quantities of daily secretions?

Bile—approximately 1000 ml/24 hours
Gastric—approximately 2000 ml/24 hours
Pancreatic—approximately 600 ml/24 hours
Small intestine—approximately 3000 ml/day
Saliva—approximately 1500 ml/24 hours
Note: almost all secretions are reabsorbed

How can the estimated levels of daily secretions from bile, gastric, and small-bowel sources be remembered?

Alphabetically and numerically: B, G, S and 1, 2, 3; or B1, G2, S3 as bile, gastric, and small bowel produce roughly 1 L, 2 L, and 3 L, respectively!

What are the principles of fluid and electrolyte replacement?

1. Replace deficits.
2. Fulfill daily maintenance requirements.
3. Replace ongoing losses.

COMMON IV REPLACEMENT FLUIDS (ALL VALUES ARE PER LITER)

What comprises normal saline (NS)?

154 mEq of Cl^-
154 mEq of Na^+

What comprises ½ NS?

77 mEq of Cl^-
77 mEq of Na^+

What comprises ¼ NS?

39 mEq of Cl^-
39 mEq of Na^+

What comprises lactated Ringer's (LR)?

130 mEq Na^+
110 mEq Cl^-
28 mEq lactate
4 mEq K^+
3 mEq Ca+

What comprises D5W?	5% dextrose (50 g) in H_2O
What accounts for tonicity?	Mainly electrolytes; thus, NS and LR are both isotonic, whereas ½ NS is hypotonic to serum
What happens to the lactate in LR in the body?	Converted into bicarbonate; thus, LR cannot be used as a maintenance fluid because patients would become alkalotic

CALCULATION OF MAINTENANCE FLUIDS

What is the 100/50/20 rule?	Maintenance IV fluids for a 24-hour period 100 ml/kg for the first 10 kg 50 ml/kg for the next 10 kg 20 ml/kg for every kg over 20 (divide by 24 for hourly rate)
What is the 4/2/1 rule?	Maintenance IV fluids—hourly rate 4 ml/kg for the first 10 kg 2 ml/kg for the next 10 kg 1 ml/kg for every kg over 20
What is the maintenance for a 70-kg man?	Using 100/50/20: 100 × 10 kg = 1000 50 × 10 kg = 500 20 × 50 kg = 1000 Total = 2500 Divided by 24 hours: 104 ml/hr maintenance rate Using 4/2/1: 4 × 10 kg = 40 2 × 10 kg = 20 1 × 50 kg = 50 Total = 110 ml/hr maintenance rate
What is the common adult maintenance fluid?	D5 1/2 NS with 20 mEq KCl/L
What is the common pediatric maintenance fluid?	D5 1/4 NS with 20 mEq KCl/L (use 1/4 NS because of the decreased ability of children to concentrate urine)
Why should sugar (dextrose) be added to maintenance fluid?	To inhibit muscle breakdown

What is the best way to assess fluid status?	Urine output (unless the patient has cardiac or renal dysfunction, in which case central venous pressure or wedge pressure is often used)
What is the minimal urine output for an adult on maintenance IV?	30 ml/hr (0.5 cc/kg/hr)
What is the minimal urine output for an adult trauma patient?	50 ml/hr
How many ml are in 12 oz (beer can)?	356 ml
How many ml are in 1 oz?	30 ml
How many ml are in 1 tsp?	5 ml
What are common isotonic fluids?	NS, LR
What is a bolus?	A volume of fluid given IV in a rapid manner (e.g., 1 L over 1 hour); used for increasing intravascular volume, and isotonic fluids should be used (i.e., NS or LR)
Why not combine bolus fluids with dextrose?	Hyperglycemia may result.
What is the possible consequence of hyperglycemia in the patient with hypovolemia?	Osmotic diuresis
Why not combine bolus fluids with a significant amount of potassium?	Hyperkalemia may result (the potassium in LR is very low: 4 mEq/L).
Why should isotonic fluids be given for resuscitation (i.e., to restore intravascular volume)?	If hypotonic fluid is given, the tonicity of the intravascular space will be decreased and H_2O will freely diffuse into the interstitial and intracellular spaces. Thus, use isotonic fluids to expand the intravascular space.

What portion of 1 L NS will stay in the intravascular space after a laparotomy?	In 5 hours, only approximately 200 cc (or 20%) will remain in the intravascular space!
What is the most common trauma resuscitation fluid?	LR
What is the most common postoperative IV fluid after a laparotomy?	D5LR for 24 to 36 hours, followed by maintenance fluid
After a laparotomy, when should a patient's fluid be "mobilized"?	Classically, postoperative day 3; the patient begins to "mobilize" the third-space fluid back into the intravascular space

ELECTROLYTE IMBALANCES

What is a common cause of electrolyte abnormalities?	Lab error!

HYPERKALEMIA

What is the normal range for potassium level?	3.5–5.0 mEq/L
What are the surgical causes of hyperkalemia?	Iatrogenic overdose, blood transfusion, renal failure, diuretics, acidosis, tissue destruction (injury/hemolysis)
What are the signs/ symptoms?	Decreased deep tendon reflex (DTR) or areflexia, weakness, paraesthesia, paralysis, respiratory failure
What are the EKG findings?	**Peaked T waves,** depressed ST segment, prolonged PR, wide QRS, bradycardia, ventricular fibrillation
What are the critical values?	$K^+ > 6.5$
What is the urgent treatment?	IV calcium (cardioprotective), EKG monitoring Sodium bicarbonate IV (alkalosis drives K^+ intracellularly) Glucose and insulin Albuterol Sodium polystyrene sulfonate (Kayexalate) and **furosemide** (Lasix) Dialysis

What is the nonacute treatment?	Furosemide (Lasix), sodium polystyrene sulfonate (Kayexalate)
What is the acronym for the treatment of acute symptomatic hyperkalemia?	**C BILD:** **C=C**alcium **B=B**icarbonate **I=I**nsulin/dextrose **L=L**asix **D=D**ialysis
What is "pseudohyperkalemia"?	Spurious hyperkalemia as a result of falsely elevated K^+ in sample from sample hemolysis
What acid-base change lowers the serum potassium?	Alkalosis (thus, give bicarbonate for hyperkalemia)

HYPOKALEMIA

What are the surgical causes?	Diuretics, certain antibiotics, steroids, alkalosis, diarrhea, intestinal fistulae, NG aspiration, vomiting, insulin, insufficient supplementation, amphotericin
What are the signs/ symptoms?	Weakness, tetany, nausea, vomiting, **ileus,** paraesthesia
What are the EKG findings?	**Flattening of T waves, U waves,** ST segment depression, PAC, PVC, atrial fibrillation
What is the rapid treatment?	KCl IV
What is the maximum amount that can be given through a peripheral IV?	10 mEq/hour
What is the maximum amount that can be given through a central line?	20 mEq/hour
What is the chronic treatment?	KCl PO

What is the most common electrolyte-mediated ileus in the surgical patient?	Hypokalemia
What electrolyte condition exacerbates digitalis toxicity?	Hypokalemia

HYPERNATREMIA

What is the normal range for sodium level?	135–145 mEq/L
What are the surgical causes?	Inadequate hydration, diabetes insipidus, diuresis, vomiting, diarrhea, diaphoresis, tachypnea, iatrogenic (e.g., TPN)
What are the signs/ symptoms?	Seizures, confusion, stupor, pulmonary or peripheral edema, tremors, respiratory paralysis
What is the treatment supplementation slowly over days?	D5W or 1/2 NS

HYPONATREMIA

What are the surgical causes of the following types:	
Hypovolemic?	Diuretic excess, hypoaldosteronism, vomiting, NG suction, burns, pancreatitis, diaphoresis
Euvolemic?	SIADH, CNS abnormalities, drugs
Hypervolemic?	Renal failure, CHF, liver failure (cirrhosis), iatrogenic fluid overload (dilutional)
What are the signs/ symptoms?	Seizures, coma, nausea, vomiting, ileus, lethargy, confusion, weakness
What is the treatment of the following types:	
Hypovolemic?	NS IV, correct underlying cause
Euvolemic?	SIADH: furosemide and NS acutely, fluid restriction

Hypervolemic?	Dilutional: fluid restriction and diuretics
What may occur if you correct hyponatremia too quickly?	Central pontine myelinosis!
What is the most common cause of mild postoperative hyponatremia?	Fluid overload

"PSEUDOHYPONATREMIA"

What is it?	Spurious lab value of hyponatremia as a result of hyperglycemia, hyperlipidemia, or hyperproteinemia

HYPERCALCEMIA

What are the causes?	"CHIMPANZEES": **C**alcium supplementation IV **H**yperparathyroidism (1°/3°) hyperthyroidism **I**mmobility/iatrogenic (thiazide diuretics) **M**ets/Milk alkali syndrome **P**aget's disease (bone) **A**ddison's disease/acromegaly **N**eoplasm (colon, lung, breast, prostate, multiple myeloma) **Z**ollinger-Ellison syndrome (as part of MEN I) **E**xcessive vitamin D **E**xcessive vitamin A **S**arcoid
What are the signs/ symptoms?	Hypercalcemia—"Stones, bones, abdominal groans, and psychiatric overtones" Polydipsia, polyuria, constipation
What are the EKG findings?	Short QT interval, prolonged PR interval
What is the acute treatment of hypercalcemic crisis?	Volume expansion with NS, diuresis with furosemide (not thiazides)
What are other options for lowering Ca^+ level?	Steroids, calcitonin, bisphosphonates (pamidronate, etc.), mithramycin, dialysis (last resort)

HYPOCALCEMIA

How can the calcium level be determined with hypoalbuminemia?	(4-measured albumin level) × 0.8, then add this value to the measured calcium level
What are the surgical causes?	Short bowel syndrome, intestinal bypass, vitamin D deficiency, sepsis, acute pancreatitis, osteoblastic metastasis, aminoglycosides, diuretics, renal failure, hypomagnesemia, rhabdomyolysis
What is Chvostek's sign?	Facial muscle spasm with tapping of facial nerve
What is Trousseau's sign?	Carpal spasm after occluding blood flow in forearm with blood pressure cuff
What are the signs/ symptoms?	Chvostek's and Trousseau's signs, paraesthesia (early), increased deep tendon reflexes (late), confusion, abdominal cramps, laryngospasm, stridor, seizures, tetany, psychiatric abnormalities (e.g., paranoia, depression, hallucinations)
What are the EKG findings?	Prolonged QT and ST interval (peaked T-waves are also possible, as in hyperkalemia)
What is the acute treatment?	Calcium gluconate IV
What is the chronic treatment?	Calcium PO, vitamin D
What is the possible complication of infused calcium if the IV infiltrates?	**Tissue necrosis;** never administer peripherally unless absolutely necessary (calcium gluconate is less toxic than calcium chloride during an infiltration)

HYPERMAGNESEMIA

What is the normal range for magnesium level?	1.5–2.5 mEq/L
What is the surgical cause?	TPN, renal failure, IV over supplementation

What are the signs/ symptoms?	Respiratory failure, CNS depression, decreased deep tendon reflexes (Remember on obstetrics-gynecology)
What is the treatment?	Calcium gluconate IV, insulin plus glucose, dialysis (similar to treatment of hyperkalemia), furosemide (Lasix)

HYPOMAGNESEMIA

What are the surgical causes?	TPN, hypocalcemia, gastric suctioning, aminoglycosides, renal failure, diarrhea, vomiting
What are the signs/ symptoms?	Increased deep tendon reflexes, tetany, asterixis, tremor, Chvostek's sign, ventricular ectopy, vertigo, tachycardia, dysrhythmias
What is the acute treatment?	$MgSO_4$ IV
What is the chronic treatment?	Magnesium oxide PO (side effect: diarrhea)
Hypomagnesemia may make it impossible to correct what other electrolyte abnormality?	Hypokalemia (always fix hypomagnesemia with hypokalemia)

HYPERGLYCEMIA

What are the surgical causes?	Diabetes (poor control), infection, stress, TPN, drugs, lab error (drawing over IV site)
What are the signs/ symptoms?	Polyuria, hypovolemia, confusion/coma, polydipsia, ileus, DKA (Kussmaul breathing), abdominal pain, hyporeflexia
What is the treatment?	IVF, insulin, monitoring of glucose and electrolytes
What is the Weiss protocol?	Sliding scale insulin

HYPOGLYCEMIA

What are the surgical causes?	Excess insulin, decreased caloric intake, insulinoma, drugs, liver failure, adrenal insufficiency, gastrojejunostomy

What are the signs/ symptoms?

Sympathetic response (diaphoresis, tachycardia, palpitations), confusion, coma, headache, diplopia, neurologic deficits, seizures

What is the treatment?

Glucose (IV or PO)

HYPOPHOSPHATEMIA

What is the normal range for phosphorus level?

2.5–4.5 mg/dl

What are the signs/ symptoms of hypophosphatemia?

Weakness, cardiomyopathy, neurologic dysfunction (e.g., ataxia), rhabdomyolysis, hemolysis, poor pressor response

What are the causes?

GI losses, inadequate supplementation, medications, sepsis, alcohol abuse, renal loss

What is the critical value?

< 1.0 mg/dl

What is the treatment?

Supplement with sodium phosphate or potassium phosphate IV (depending on potassium level).

HYPERPHOSPHATEMIA

What are the signs/ symptoms?

Calcification (ectopic), heart block

What are the causes?

Renal failure, sepsis, chemotherapy, hyperthyroidism

What is the treatment?

Aluminum hydroxide (binds phosphate)

MISCELLANEOUS

This EKG pattern is consistent with which electrolyte abnormality?

Hyperkalemia: Peaked T-waves

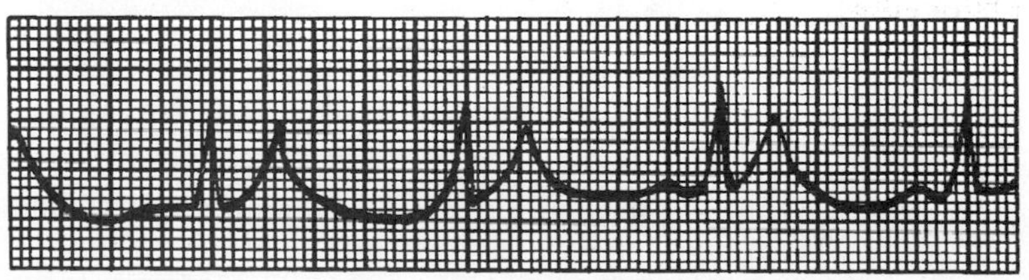

If hyperkalemia is left untreated, what can occur?

Ventricular tachycardia/fibrillation → death

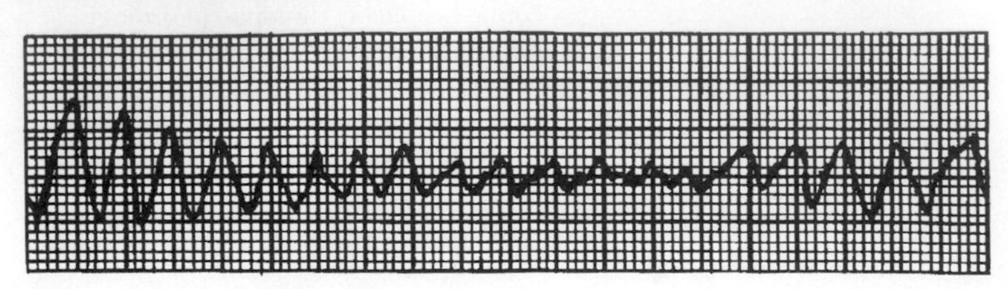

Which electrolyte is an inotrope?

Calcium

What are the major cardiac electrolytes?

Potassium (dysrhythmias), magnesium (dysrhythmias), calcium (dysrhythmias/inotrope)

Which electrolyte must be monitored closely in patients on digitalis?

Potassium

What is the most common cause of electrolyte-mediated ileus?

Hypokalemia (low potassium level)

What is a colloid fluid?

Protein-containing fluid (albumin)

What is the rationale for using an albumin-furosemide "sandwich"?

The albumin will pull interstitial fluid into the intravascular space and the furosemide will then help excrete the fluid as urine.

An elderly patient goes into CHF (congestive heart failure) on postoperative day 3 after a laparotomy. What is going on?

Mobilization of the "third-space" fluid into the intravascular space, resulting in fluid overload and resultant CHF (but, also must rule out MI)

What fluid is used to replace NGT (gastric) aspirate?

D5 ½ NS with 20 KCL

17

Blood and Blood Products

Define the following terms:

PT	**P**rothrombin **T**ime: tests extrinsic coagulation pathway
PTT	**P**artial **T**hromboplastin **T**ime: tests intrinsic coagulation pathway
INR	**I**nternational **N**ormalized **R**atio (reports PT results)
Whole blood	One unit = 450 ml (± 50 ml); deficient in platelets and clotting factors V, VIII, and XI; **rarely used**
Packed red blood cells (PRBCs)	One unit ~ 300 ml (± 50 ml); no platelets or clotting factors; can be mixed with NS to infuse faster
Platelets	Replace platelets with units of platelets (6–10 units from single donor or random donors)
Fresh frozen plasma (FFP)	Replaces **clotting factors;** no RBCs/WBCs/platelets
Cryoprecipitate (cryo)	Replaces fibrinogen, Von Willebrand factor, and some clotting factors

Which electrolyte is most likely to fall with the infusion of stored blood? Why?

Ionized calcium; the citrate preservative used for the storage of blood binds serum calcium

What changes occur in the storage of whole blood?

↓ Ca^+, ↑ K^+, ↓ 2,3-DPG, ↑ H^+ (↓ pH), ↓ clotting factors (V, VII, & XI), ↓ PMNs

What are general guidelines for blood transfusion?
Acute blood loss, Hgb < 10, and history of CAD/COPD **or** healthy symptomatic patient with Hgb < 8

What is the rough formula for converting Hgb to Hct?
Hgb × 3 = Hct

One unit of PRBC increases Hct by how much?
~ 3% to 4%

Which blood type is the universal donor?
O negative

What is a type and screen?
Patient's blood type is determined and the blood is screened for antibodies; a type and cross from that sample can then be ordered if needed later.

What is a type and cross?
Patient's blood is sent to the blood bank and cross-matched for **specific donor units for possible blood transfusion.**

Define thrombocytopenia.
Low platelet count (<100,000)

What are the common causes of thrombocytopenia in the surgical patient?
Sepsis, H_2 blockers, heparin, massive transfusion, DIC, antibiotics, spurious lab value, Swann-Ganz catheter

What can be given to help correct platelet dysfunction from uremia, aspirin, or bypass?
DDAVP (desmopressin)

What common medication causes platelets to irreversibly malfunction?
Aspirin (inhibits cyclo-oxygenase)

What platelet count is associated with spontaneous bleeding?
Less than 20,000

What should the platelet count be before surgery?
Greater than 50,000

When should "prophylactic" platelet transfusions be given?
With platelets below 10,000 (old recommendation was 20,000)

What is microcytic anemia "until proven otherwise" in a man or postmenopausal woman?	Colon cancer
Why not infuse PRBCs with lactated Ringer's?	The calcium in LR may result in coagulation within the IV line.
For how long can packed RBCs be stored?	About 6 weeks (42 days)
What is the most common cause of transfusion hemolysis?	ABO incompatibility as a result of **clerical error**
What is the risk of receiving a unit of blood infected with HIV?	Approximately 1 in 1,000,000
What are the symptoms of a transfusion reaction?	**Fever,** chills, nausea, hypotension, lumbar pain, chest pain, abnormal bleeding
What is the treatment for transfusion hemolysis?	**Stop** transfusion; provide fluids; perform diuresis (Lasix) to protect kidneys; alkalinize urine (bicarbonate); give pressors as needed
What component of the blood transfusion can cause a fever?	WBC
What is widely stated to be the "optimal" Hct?	Approximately 30%
What is the optimal Hct in a patient with a history of heart disease or stroke?	Approximately 30%
When should aspirin administration be discontinued preoperatively?	At 1 week because platelets live 7 to 10 days (must use judgment if patient is at risk for stroke, MI, or both; it may be better to continue and use excellent surgical hemostasis in these patients)
What can move the oxyhemoglobin dissociation curve to the right?	Acidosis, 2,3-DPG, fever, elevated P_{CO_2} (to the right means greater ability to release the O_2)

What is the normal life of RBCs?	120 days
What is the normal life of platelets?	7 to 10 days
What factor is deficient in hemophilia A?	Factor VIII
How do you remember the clotting factor for hemophilia A?	Think: "**eight**" sounds like "**A**"
What is the preoperative treatment of hemophilia A?	Factor VIII infusion to ≥ 100% normal preoperative levels
What coagulation study is elevated with hemophilia A?	PTT
How do you remember which coagulation study is affected by the hemophilias?	There are two major hemophilias and two t's in PTT.
What factor is deficient in hemophilia B?	Factor IX
How do you remember which factors are deficient with hemophilia A and hemophilia B?	Alphabetically and chronologically: A before B and VIII before IX; thus, hemophilia A is factor VIII and hemophilia B is factor IX
How are hemophilias A and B inherited?	Sex-linked recessive
What is Von Willebrand's disease?	Deficiency of Von Willebrand factor (vWF) and factor VIII:C
How is Von Willebrand's disease inherited?	Autosomal dominant
What to use to correct Von Willebrand's disease?	DDAVP or cryo
What coagulation is abnormal with the following disorders:	
Hemophilia A?	PTT (elevated)

Hemophilia B?	PTT (elevated)
Von Willebrand's disease?	Bleeding time
What is the effect on the coagulation system if the patient has a deficiency in protein C, protein S, or antithrombin III?	A hypercoagulable state
What is a "left shift" on a CBC?	Juvenile polymorphonuclear leukocytes (bands); legend has it that the old counters for all the blood cells had the lever for bands on the LEFT of the counter
What is the usual "therapeutic" PT?	With coumadin, usually shoot for an INR of 2.0–3.0.
What is the acronym basis for the word WARFARIN?	Wisconsin Alumni Research Foundation-arin

18 Surgical Hemostasis

What motto is associated with surgical hemostasis?

"All bleeding stops."

What is the most immediate method to obtain hemostasis?

Pressure (finger)

What is the "Bovie"?

Electrocautery (designed by Bovie with Cushing for neurosurgery in the 1920s)

What is the CUT mode on the Bovie?

Continuous electrical current (20,000 Hz); cuts well with a decreased ability to coagulate

What is the COAG mode on the Bovie?

Intermittent electrical current (20,000 Hz); results in excellent vessel coagulation with decreased ability to cut

Where should a Bovie be applied to a clamp or pick-up to coagulate a vessel?

Anywhere on the clamp/pick-up

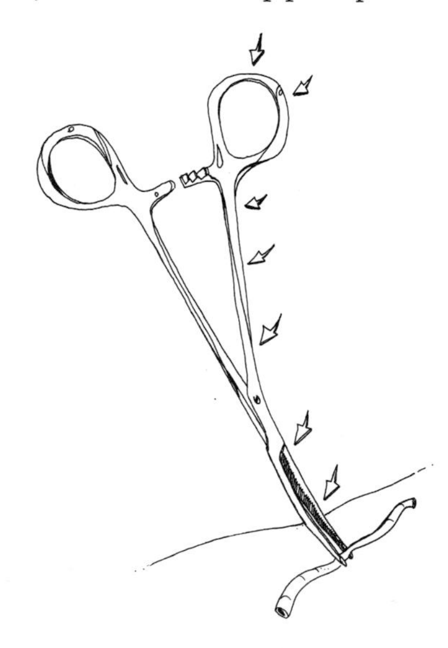

Define the following terms:

Figure-of-eight suture

Suture ligature placed **twice** in the tissue prior to being tied

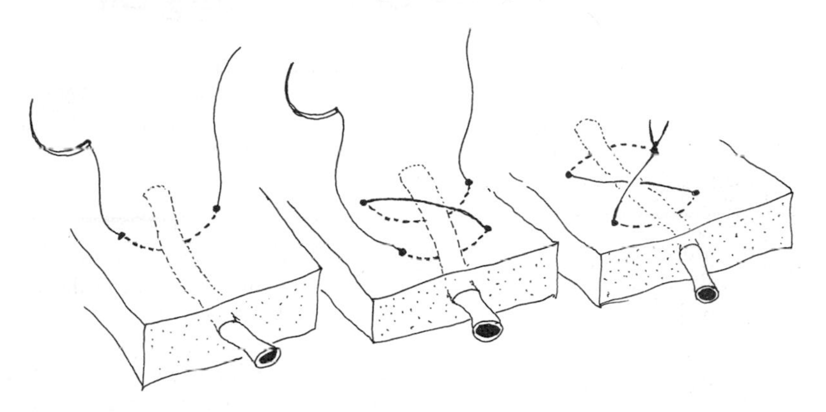

Vessel "tied in continuity"

Tie, tie, cut in between

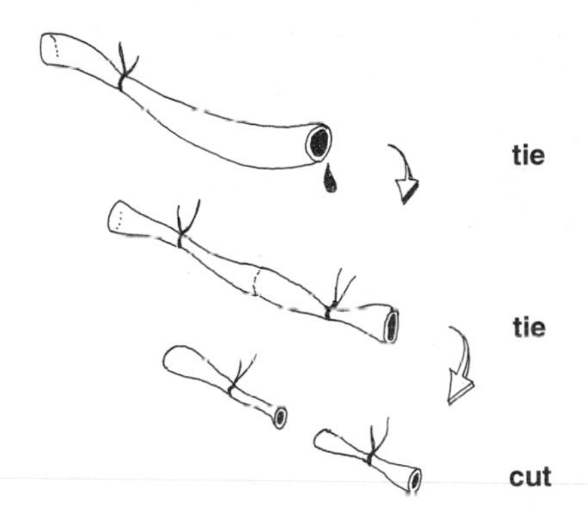

Surgicel®

Cellulose sheets—act as a framework for clotting factors/platelets to adhere to (**Think:** Surg**icel** = **cel**lulose)

Fibrin glue

Fibrinogen and thrombin sprayed simultaneously and mixed to produce a fibrin "glue"

Harmonic scalpel

Ultrasonic scalpel that vibrates more than 50,000 times per second; seals vessels and cuts tissue

Clips

Metallic clips for clipping vessels

19 Common Surgical Medications

ANTIBIOTICS

Which antibiotics are commonly used for anaerobic infections?

Metronidazole, clindamycin, cefoxitin, cefotetan, imipenem, ticarcillin-clavulanic acid, Unasyn®, Augmentin®

Which antibiotics are commonly used for gram-negative infections?

Gentamicin and other aminoglycosides, ciprofloxacin, aztreonam, third-generation cephalosporins, sulfamethoxazole-trimethoprim

Which antibiotic, if taken with alcohol, will produce a disulfiram-like reaction?

Metronidazole (Flagyl) (disulfiram is Antabuse)

What is the drug of choice for treating amoebic infections?

Metronidazole (Flagyl)

Which antibiotic is associated with cholestasis?

Ceftriaxone (Rocephin)

Which antibiotic cannot be given to children or pregnant women?

Ciprofloxacin (interferes with the growth plate)

With which antibiotics must serum levels be determined?

Aminoglycosides—some experts also believe in determining serum levels with vancomycin

Is rash (only) in response to penicillins a contraindication to cephalosporins?

No, but breathing problems, urticaria, and edema in response to penicillins are contraindications to the cephalosporins.

Describe the following medications:	
Augmentin®	Amoxicillin and clavulanic acid
Unasyn®	Ampicillin and sulbactam
Cefazolin (Ancef®)	First-generation cephalosporin; surgical prophylaxis for **skin flora**
Cefoxitin (Mefoxin®)	Second-generation cephalosporin; used for mixed aerobic/anaerobic infections; effective against *Bacteroides fragilis* and anaerobic bacteria
Ceftazidime (Ceftaz®)	Third-generation cephalosporin; strong activity against *Pseudomonas*
Clindamycin	Strong activity against gram-negative **anaerobes,** such as *B. fragilis;* adequate gram-positive activity
Gentamicin	Aminoglycoside used to treat **gram-negative** bacteria; nephrotoxic, ototoxic; blood peak/trough levels should be monitored
Imipenem and cilastatin (Primaxin®)	Often used as a last resort against serious, multiresistant organisms Usually combined with cilastin, which inhibits renal excretion of imipenem Has a very wide spectrum
Metronidazole (Flagyl®)	Used for serious **anaerobic** infections (e.g., diverticulitis); also used to treat amebiasis; patient must abstain from alcohol use during therapy
Nafcillin (Nafcil®)	Antistaphylococcal penicillin commonly used for cellulites
Vancomycin	Used to treat methicillin-resistant *Staphylococcus aureus* (MRSA); used orally to treat *C. difficile* pseudomembranous colitis (poorly absorbed from the gut); with IV administration, peak/trough levels should be monitored

Percocet®	PO narcotic pain reliever with acetaminophen and oxycodone
Ciprofloxacin (Cipro®)	Quinoline antibiotic with broad-spectrum activity, especially against gram-negative bacteria, including *Pseudomonas*
Aztreonam (Azactam®)	Monobactam with gram-negative spectrum
Amphotericin	IV antifungal antibiotic associated with renal toxicity
Dantrolene (Dantrium®)	Medication used to treat malignant hyperthermia
Fluconazole (Diflucan®)	Antifungal agent (IV or PO) **not** associated with renal toxicity
Nystatin	PO and topical antifungal

STEROIDS

What are the side effects?	Adrenal suppression, immunosuppression, weight gain with central obesity, cushingoid facies, acne, hirsutism, purple striae, hyperglycemia, sodium retention/ hypokalemia, hypertension, osteopenia, myopathy, ischemic bone necrosis (avascular necrosis of the hip), GI perforations
What are its uses?	Immunosuppression (transplant), autoimmune diseases, hormone replacement (Addison's disease), spinal cord trauma
Can steroids be stopped abruptly?	**No, steroids should never be stopped abruptly; always taper.**
Which patients need stress-dose steroids before surgery?	Those who are on steroids, have suspected hypoadrenalism, or are about to undergo adrenalectomy
What is the "stress dose" for steroids?	**100** mg of hydrocortisone IV every 8 hours and then taper (adults)

Which vitamin helps counteract the deleterious effects of steroids on wound healing?	Vitamin A

HEPARIN

Describe the action.	Heparin binds with and activates antithrombin III.
What are its uses?	Prophylaxis/treatment—DVT, pulmonary embolism, stroke, atrial fibrillation, acute arterial occlusion, cardiopulmonary bypass
What are the side effects?	Bleeding complications; can cause thrombocytopenia
What reverses the effects?	**Protamine** IV (**1:100, 1** mg of protamine to every **100** units of heparin)
What laboratory test should be used to follow effect?	aPTT—activated partial thromboplastin time
What is the standard lab target for therapeutic heparinization?	1.5–2.5 times control
Who is at risk for a protamine anaphylactic reaction?	Patients with type 1 diabetes mellitus, s/p prostate surgery
What is the half-life of heparin?	Approximately 90 minutes (1–2 hours)
How long before surgery should it be discontinued?	From 4 to 6 hours preoperatively
Does heparin dissolve clots?	No; it stops the progression of clot formation and allows the body's own fibrinolytic systems to dissolve the clot.
What is LMWH?	**L**ow **m**olecular **w**eight **h**eparin
What laboratory test do you need to follow LMWH?	None, except in children, patients with obesity, and those with renal failure, which is the major advantage of LMWH

WARFARIN (COUMADIN)

ACRONYM basis for name?	**W**isconsin **A**lumni **R**esearch **F**oundation
Describe its action.	**Inhibits vitamin K-dependent clotting factors II, VII, IX, X,** (i.e., 2, 7, 9, **10** [think 2+7=9 and 10]), produced in the liver
What are its uses?	Long-term anticoagulation (PO)
What are its associated risks?	Bleeding complications, teratogenic in pregnancy, skin necrosis, dermatitis
What laboratory test should be used to follow its effect?	PT (prothrombin time) as reported as INR
What is INR?	International normalized ratio
What is the classic therapeutic INR?	INR of 2–3
What is the half-life of effect?	40 hours; thus, it takes about 2 days to observe a change in the PT
What reverses the action?	**Cessation,** vitamin K, fresh-frozen plasma (in emergencies)
How long before surgery should it be discontinued?	From 3 to 5 days preoperatively and IV heparin should be begun; heparin should be discontinued from 4 to 6 hours preoperatively and can be restarted postoperatively; coumadin can be restarted in a few days

MISCELLANEOUS AGENTS

Describe the following drugs:

Sucralfate (Carafate®)	Treats peptic ulcers by forming an acid-resistant barrier; binds to ulcer craters; needs acid to activate and thus should not be used with H_2 blockers
Cimetidine (Tagamet®)	H_2 blocker (ulcers/gastritis)
Ranitidine (Zantac®)	H_2 blocker (ulcers/gastritis)

Omeprazole (Prilosec®)	Gastric acid–secretion inhibitor; works by inhibiting the **K^+/H^+-ATPase**
Promethazine (Phenergan®)	Acute antinausea agent; used postoperatively
Metoclopramide (Reglan®)	Increases gastric emptying with increase in LES pressure; **dopamine antagonist;** used in diabetic gastroparesis and to help move feeding tubes past the pylorus
Albumin	5% albumin—expands plasma volume 25% albumin—draws extravascular fluid into intravascular space by oncotic pressure
Famotidine (Pepcid®)	H_2 blocker
Aspirin	Irreversibly inhibits platelets by irreversibly inhibiting cyclo-oxygenase
Furosemide (Lasix®)	Loop diuretic (watch for hypokalemia)

If the patient does not respond to a dose of furosemide, should the dose be repeated, increased, or decreased?

The dose should be doubled if there is no response to the initial dose.

What medication is used to treat promethazine-induced dystonia?

Diphenhydramine hydrochloride IV (Benadryl)

Which medication is classically associated with mesenteric ischemia?

Digitalis

What type of antihypertensive medication is contraindicated in patients with renal artery stenosis?

Ace inhibitors

Does acetaminophen (Tylenol®) inhibit platelets?

No

What medications are used to stop seizures?
Benzodiazepines (e.g., lorazepam [Ativan]); phenytoin (Dilantin)

List the preop antibiotics for:

Vascular prosthetic graft
Ancef® (gm+ coverage)

Appendectomy
Cefoxitin, cefotetan, Unasyn® (anaerobic coverage)

Colon surgery
Cefoxitin, cefotetan, Unasyn® (anaerobic coverage)

NARCOTICS

What are common postoperative IV narcotics?
Morphine (most common), meperidine (Demerol®), fentanyl

What is Demerol's claim to fame?
It is used commonly with acute pancreatitis/biliary pathology because morphine may cause sphincter of Oddi spasm/constriction.

What are side effects of narcotics?
Respiratory depression, hypotension, itching, bradycardia, nausea

What is the danger of prolonged use of Demerol?
Accumulation of metabolite normeperidine (especially with renal/hepatic dysfunction), which may result in oversedation, hallucinations, and seizures!

What medication reverses the effects of narcotic overdose?
Naloxone (Narcan®), 0.4 mg IV

MISCELLANEOUS

What reverses the effects of benzodiazepines?
Flumazenil (Romazicon®) 0.2 mg IV

What is Toradol®?
Ketorolac IV NSAID

What are the risks of Toradol®?
GI bleed, renal injury, platelet dysfunction

Why give a patient IV Cipro when he is eating a regular diet?
No reason—500 mg of Cipro PO gives the same serum level as 400 mg Cipro IV! And PO is much cheaper!

20 Complications

ATELECTASIS

What is it?
Collapse of the alveoli

What is the etiology?
Inadequate alveolar expansion (i.e., poor ventilation of lungs during surgery, inability to fully inspire secondary to pain), high levels of inspired oxygen

What are the signs?
Fever, decreased breath sounds with rales, tachypnea, tachycardia, and increased density on CXR

What are the risk factors?
Chronic obstructive pulmonary disease (COPD), smoking, abdominal or thoracic surgery, oversedation, poor pain control (**patient cannot breathe deeply secondary to pain on inspiration**)

What is its claim to fame?
Most common cause of fever during postoperative days 1 to 2

What prophylactic measures can be taken?
Preoperative smoking cessation, incentive spirometry, good pain control

What is the treatment?
Postoperative **incentive spirometry,** deep breathing, coughing, early ambulation, postural drainage, suctioning, and chest PT

POSTOPERATIVE RESPIRATORY FAILURE

What is it?
Respiratory impairment with increased respiratory rate, shortness of breath, dyspnea

What is the differential diagnosis?
Hypovolemia, pulmonary embolism, administration of supplemental O_2 to a patient with COPD, atelectasis, pneumonia, aspiration, pulmonary edema, abdominal compartment syndrome, pneumothorax, chylothorax, hemothorax, narcotic overdose, mucus plug

What is the treatment?
Supplemental O_2, chest PT; suctioning, intubation, and ventilation if necessary

What is the initial workup?
ABG, CXR, EKG, Sat monitor, PE

What are the indications for intubation and ventilation?
Cannot protect airway (unconscious), excessive work of breathing, progressive **hypoxemia** ($paO_2 < 55$ despite supplemental O_2), progressive **acidosis** (pH < 7.3 and $PCO_2 > 50$), RR > 35

What are the possible causes of postoperative pleural effusion?
Diaphragmatic inflammation with possible subphrenic abscess formation, fluid overload, pneumonia

What is the treatment of postoperative wheezing?
Albuterol nebulizer

Why may it be dangerous to give a patient with chronic COPD supplemental oxygen?
This patient uses relative hypoxia for respiratory drive, and supplemental O_2 may remove this drive!

PULMONARY EMBOLISM

What is a pulmonary embolism (PE)?
DVT that embolizes to the pulmonary arterial system

What is DVT?
Deep **V**enous **T**hrombosis—a clot forming in the pelvic or lower extremity veins

Is DVT more common in the right or left iliac vein?
Left is more common (4 to 1) because the aortic bifurcation crosses and possibly compresses the left iliac vein.

What are the signs/ symptoms of DVT?
Lower extremity pain, swelling, tenderness, Homan's sign, pulmonary embolus (PE)
Up to 50% can be asymptomatic!

What is Homan's sign? Calf pain with dorsiflexion of the foot seen classically with DVT, but actually found in fewer than one-third of patients with DVT

What test is used to evaluate for DVT? Duplex ultrasonography

What is Virchow's triad? Stasis, endothelial injury, hypercoagulable state (risk factors for thrombosis)

What are the risk factors for DVT and PE? Postoperative status, multiple trauma, paralysis, immobility, CHF, obesity, BCP/tamoxifen, cancer, advanced age, polycythemia, MI, HIT syndrome, hypercoagulable state (protein C/protein S deficiency)

What are the signs/ symptoms? Shortness of breath, tachypnea, hypotension, CP, occasionally fever, tender LE, loud pulmonic component of S2, hemoptysis with pulmonary infarct

What are the associated lab findings? ABG—decreased PO_2 and PCO_2 (from hyperventilation)

Which diagnostic tests are indicated? V-Q scan (ventilation-perfusion scan), pulmonary A-gram is the gold standard

What are the associated CXR findings?

1. Westermark's sign (wedge-shaped area of decreased pulmonary vasculature resulting in hyperlucency)
2. Opacity with base at pleural edge from pulmonary infarction

What are the associated EKG findings? More than 50% are abnormal; classic finding is cor pulmonale (S1Q3T3 RBBB and right-axis deviation); EKG most commonly shows flipped T waves or ST depression.

What is a "saddle" embolus? PE that "straddles" the pulmonary artery and is in the lumen of both the right and left pulmonary arteries

What is the treatment if the patient is stable? Anticoagulation (heparin followed by long-term [3–6 months] coumadin) or Greenfield filter

What is a Greenfield filter?

Metallic filter placed into IVC via jugular vein to catch emboli prior to lodging in the pulmonary artery

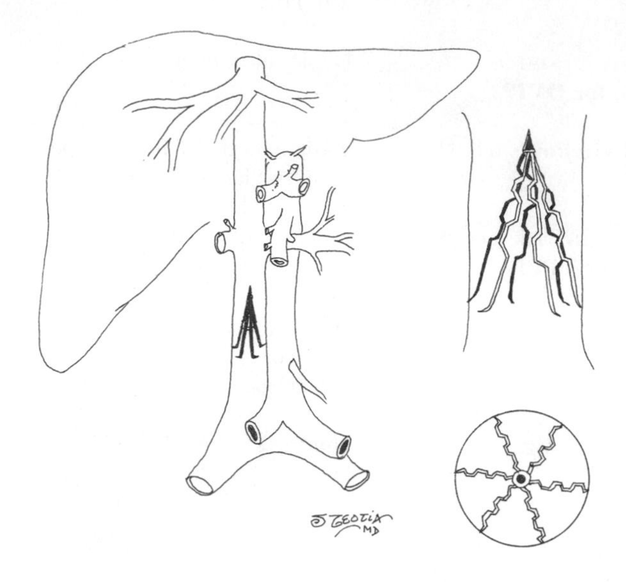

When is a Greenfield filter indicated?

If anticoagulation is contraindicated or patient has further PE on adequate anticoagulation

What is the treatment if the patient's condition is unstable?

Consider thrombolytic therapy; consult thoracic surgeon for possible Trendelenburg operation; consider catheter suction embolectomy.

What is the Trendelenburg operation?

Pulmonary artery embolectomy

What prophylactic measures can be taken for DVT/PE?

Sub-Q heparin (5,000 units sub-Q every 8–12 hrs; must be started preoperatively), sequential compression device BOOTS beginning in OR (often used with sub-Q heparin), compression hose, early ambulation

ASPIRATION PNEUMONIA

What is it?

Pneumonia following aspiration of vomitus

What are the risk factors?

Intubation/extubation, impaired consciousness (i.e., drug or ETOH overdose), dysphagia (esophageal disease), nonfunctioning NGT, Trendelenburg position, OR emergent intubation with full stomach

What are the signs/ symptoms?

Respiratory failure, CP, increased sputum production, fever, cough, mental status changes, tachycardia, cyanosis, infiltrate on CXR

What are the associated CXR findings?

Early—fluffy infiltrate or normal CXR
Late—pneumonia, ARDS

Which lobes are commonly involved?

Supine—RUL
Sitting/semirecumbent—RLL

Which organisms are commonly involved?

Community acquired—gram-positive/mixed
Hospital/ICU—gram-negative rods

Which diagnostic tests are indicated?

CXR, sputum, Gram stain, sputum culture, bronchoalveolar lavage

What is the treatment?

Bronchoscopy, antibiotics if pneumonia develops, intubation if respiratory failure occurs, ventilation with PEEP if ARDS develops

What is Mendelson's syndrome?

Chemical pneumonitis secondary to aspiration of stomach contents (i.e., gastric acid)

GASTROINTESTINAL COMPLICATIONS

What are possible NGT complications?

Aspiration-pneumonia/atelectasis (especially if NGT is clogged)
Sinusitis
Minor UGI bleeding
- Epistaxis
- Pharyngeal irritation

GASTRIC DILATATION

What are the risk factors?

Abdominal surgery, gastric outlet obstruction, splenectomy

What are the signs/ symptoms?	Abdominal distension, hiccups, electrolyte abnormalities, nausea
What is the treatment?	NGT decompression
What do you do if you have a patient with high NGT output?	Check high abdominal x-ray and, if the NGT is in duodenum, pull back the NGT into the stomach.

POSTOPERATIVE PANCREATITIS

What is it?	Pancreatitis resulting from manipulation of the pancreas during surgery or low blood flow during the procedure (i.e., cardiopulmonary bypass), gallstones, hypercalcemia, medications, idiopathic
What lab tests are performed?	Amylase and lipase
What is the initial treatment?	Same as that for the other causes of pancreatitis (e.g., NPO, aggressive fluid resuscitation, ± NGT)

CONSTIPATION

What are the postoperative causes?	Narcotics, immobility
What is the treatment?	OBR
What is OBR?	**O**rtho **B**owel **R**outine: docusate sodium (daily), dicacodyl suppository if no bowel movement occurs, Fleet® enema if suppository is ineffective

SHORT BOWEL SYNDROME

What is it?	Malabsorption and diarrhea resulting from extensive bowel resection (approximately >/= 120 cm of small bowel remaining)
What is the initial treatment?	TPN early, followed by many small meals chronically

POSTOPERATIVE SMALL BOWEL OBSTRUCTION (SBO)/ILEUS

What causes are related to SBO?

Adhesions (most of which resolve spontaneously), incarcerated hernia (internal or fascial/dehiscence)

What causes are related to ileus?

Adynamic ileus (normal after laparotomy), ileus from hypokalemia or narcotics, intraperitoneal infection

What are the signs of resolving ileus/SBO?

Flatus PR, stool PR

What is the order of recovery of bowel function after abdominal surgery?

First—small intestine
Second—stomach
Third—colon

When can a postoperative patient be fed through a J tube?

From 12 to 24 postoperative hours because the small intestine recovers function first in that period

JAUNDICE

What are the causes of the following types of postoperative jaundice:

Prehepatic?

Hemolysis (prosthetic valve), resolving hematoma, transfusion reaction, postcardiopulmonary bypass, blood transfusions (decreased RBC compliance leading to cell rupture)

Hepatic?

Drugs, hypotension, hypoxia, sepsis, hepatitis, "sympathetic" hepatic inflammation from adjacent right lower lobe infarction of the lung or pneumonia, preexisting cirrhosis, right-sided heart failure, hepatic abscess, pylephlebitis (thrombosis of portal vein), Gilbert syndrome, Crigler-Najjar syndrome, Dubin-Johnson syndrome, fatty infiltrate from TPN

Posthepatic?

Obstruction (stone), cholangitis, cholecystitis, biliary-duct injury, pancreatitis, sclerosing cholangitis, tumors (e.g., cholangiocarcinoma, pancreatic cancer, gallbladder cancer, metastases), biliary stasis (e.g., ceftriaxone [Rocephin])

What blood tests would support the assumption that hemolysis was causing jaundice in a patient?	**Decreased**—Haptoglobin, Hct **Increased**—LDH, reticulocytes Also, fragmented RBCs on a peripheral smear

BLIND LOOP SYNDROME

What is it?	Bacterial overgrowth in the small intestine
What are the causes?	Anything that disrupts the normal flow of intestinal contents (i.e., causes stasis)
What are the surgical causes of B_{12} deficiency?	Gastrectomy (decreased secretion of intrinsic factor) and excision of the terminal ileum (site of B_{12} absorption)

POSTVAGOTOMY DIARRHEA

What is it?	Diarrhea after a truncal vagotomy
What is the cause?	It is thought that after truncal vagotomy, a rapid transport of bile salts to the colon results in osmotic inhibition of water absorption in the colon, leading to diarrhea.

DUMPING SYNDROME

What is it?	Delivery of **hyperosmotic** chyme to the small intestine causing massive fluid shifts into the bowel (normally the stomach will decrease the osmolality of the chyme prior to its emptying)
With what conditions is it associated?	Any procedure that bypasses the pylorus or compromises its function (i.e., gastroenterostomies or pyloroplasty); thus, "dumping" of chyme into small intestine
What are the signs/ symptoms?	Postprandial diaphoresis, tachycardia, abdominal pain/distention, emesis, increased flatus, dizziness, weakness
How is the diagnosis made?	History; hyperosmolar glucose load will elicit similar symptoms

What is the medical treatment?	Small, multiple, low-fat/carbohydrate meals that are high in protein content; also, **avoidance of liquids** with meals to slow gastric emptying; surgery is a last resort
What is the surgical treatment?	Conversion to Roux-en-Y (± reversed jejunal interposition loop)
What is a reversed jejunal interposition loop?	A segment of jejunum is cut and then reversed to allow for a short segment of reversed peristalsis to slow intestinal transit.

ENDOCRINE COMPLICATIONS

DIABETIC KETOACIDOSIS (DKA)

What is it?	Deficiency of body insulin, resulting in hyperglycemia, formation of ketoacids, osmotic diuresis, and metabolic acidosis
What are the signs of DKA?	Polyuria, tachypnea, dehydration, confusion
What are the associated lab values?	Elevated glucose, increased anion gap, hypokalemia, urine ketones, acidosis
What is the treatment?	Insulin drip, IVF rehydration, K^+ supplementation ± bicarbonate IV
What electrolyte must be monitored closely in DKA?	Potassium and HYPOkalemia (Remember correction of acidosis and GLC/Insulin drive K^+ into cells and are treatment for HYPERkalemia!)

ADDISONIAN CRISIS

What is it?	Acute adrenal insufficiency in the face of a stressor (i.e., surgery, trauma, infection)
What is the cause?	Postoperatively, inadequate cortisol release usually results from steroid administration in the past year.
What are the signs/ symptoms?	Tachycardia, nausea, vomiting, diarrhea, **abdominal pain,** ± fever, progressive lethargy, **hypotension, eventual hypovolemic shock**

What is its clinical claim to infamy?	Tachycardia and hypotension refractory to IVF and pressors!
Which lab values are classic?	Decreased sodium, increased K^+ (secondary to decreased aldosterone)
What is the treatment?	IVFs (D5 NS), hydrocortisone IV, fludrocortisone PO
What is fludrocortisone?	Mineralocorticoid replacement (aldosterone)

SIADH

What is it?	**S**yndrome of **I**nappropriate **A**nti**D**iuretic **H**ormone (ADH) secretion (think of **in-appropriate increase** in ADH secretion)
What does ADH do?	ADH increases NaCl and H_2O resorption in the kidney, increasing intravascular volume (released from posterior pituitary).
What are the causes?	**Mainly lung**/CNS: CNS trauma, oat-cell lung cancer, pancreatic cancer, duodenal cancer, pneumonia/lung abscess, increased PEEP, stroke, general anesthesia, idiopathic, postoperative, morphine
What are the associated lab findings?	Low sodium, chloride, and serum osmolality; increased urine osmolality
What is the treatment?	Treat the primary cause and restrict fluid intake.

DIABETES INSIPIDUS (DI)

What is it?	Decreased release of ADH, resulting in massive I's and O's (think: **D**iabetes = **D**ecreased ADH)
What are the risk factors?	Central DI—head trauma, intracranial disorder Nephrogenic DI—renal disease, electrolyte disorders, medications
What is the treatment?	Vasopressin (IV, SQ, or intranasal) to replace the deficiency and massive quantities of IV fluids

CARDIOVASCULAR COMPLICATIONS

What are the arterial line complications?

Infection; thrombosis, which can lead to finger/hand necrosis; death/hemorrhage from catheter disconnection (remember to perform and document the **Allen test** before inserting an arterial line or obtaining a blood gas sample)

What is an Allen test?

Measures for adequate collateral blood flow to the hand via the ulnar artery: patient clenches fist, then both radial and ulnar arteries are occluded; patient opens the blanched hand. The ulnar artery is released. If the palm has an immediate strong blush, the ulnar artery should be adequate collateral flow if the radial artery thromboses.

What are the common causes of dyspnea following central line placement?

Pneumothorax, pericardial tamponade, carotid puncture (which can cause a hematoma that compresses the trachea), air embolism

What is the differential diagnosis of postoperative chest pain?

MI, atelectasis, pneumonia, pleurisy, esophageal reflux, PE, musculoskeletal pain, subphrenic abscess, aortic dissection, pneumo/chyle/hemothorax, gastritis

What is the differential diagnosis of postoperative atrial fibrillation?

Fluid overload, PE, MI, pain (excess catecholamines), atelectasis, pneumonia, digoxin toxicity, hypoxemia, thyrotoxicosis, hypercapnia, idiopathic, acidosis, electrolyte abnormalities

MYOCARDIAL INFARCTION (MI)

What is the most dangerous period for a postoperative MI following a previous MI?

Six months after an MI

What are the risk factors for postoperative MI?

History of MI, angina, Q's on EKG, S3, JVD, CHF, aortic stenosis, advanced age, extensive surgical procedure, MI within 6 months, EKG changes

How do postoperative MIs present?

Often without chest pain
New onset **CHF,** new onset **cardiac dysrhythmia,** hypotension, chest pain, tachypnea, tachycardia, nausea/vomiting, bradycardia, neck pain, arm pain

What EKG findings are associated with cardiac ischemia/MI?

Flipped T waves, ST elevation, ST depression, Q waves (usually late), dysrhythmias (e.g., new onset a fib, PVC, V tach)

Which lab tests are indicated?

Cardiac isoenzymes (elevated CK mb fraction), troponin I

What is the treatment of postoperative MI?

Nitrates (paste or drip), as tolerated
Aspirin
Oxygen
Pain control with IV morphine
β-blocker, as tolerated
Heparin (possibly; thrombolytics are contraindicated in the postoperative patient)
ICU monitoring
(Memory aid for treating cardiac ischemia/MI: **BEMOAN**—**Be** = **B**eta blocker [as tolerated], **M** = **M**orphine, **O** = Oxygen, **A** = **A**spirin, **N** = **N**itrates [IV or paste])

When do postoperative MIs occur?

Two-thirds occur on postoperative days 2 to 5 (often silent and present with **dyspnea** or **dysrhythmia**).

What is the first thing to do if a patient is found unresponsive after a cardiac event?

Establish an AIRWAY! Always remember A, B, C first!

POSTOPERATIVE CVA

What is a CVA?

Cerebrovascular accident (stroke)

What are the signs/symptoms?

Aphasia, motor/sensory deficits usually lateralizing

What is the workup?

Head CT; must rule out hemorrhage if anticoagulation is going to be used; carotid Doppler ultrasound study to evaluate for carotid occlusive disease

What is the treatment?

ASA, ± heparin if thrombotic as feasible postoperatively
Thrombolytic therapy is not usually postoperative option.

What is the perioperative prevention?

Avoid hypotension; continue aspirin therapy preoperatively in high-risk patients if feasible.

MISCELLANEOUS

POSTOPERATIVE RENAL FAILURE

What is it?

Urine output less than 25 ml/hr (30 ml/hr is minimum adult output), increased creatinine and BUN

What is the differential diagnosis?

Prerenal?

Inadequate blood perfusing kidney: inadequate fluids, hypotension, cardiac pump failure (CHF)

Renal?

Kidney parenchymal dysfunction: acute tubular necrosis, nephrotoxic dyes or drugs

Postrenal?

Obstruction to outflow of urine from kidney: Foley catheter obstruction/stone, ureteral/urethral injury, BPH, bladder dysfunction (e.g., medications, spinal anesthesia)

What is the work up?

Lab tests: electrolytes, BUN, Cr, urine lytes/Cr, FENa, urinalysis, renal ultrasound

What is FENa?

Fractional excretion of Na^+ (sodium)

What is the formula for FENa?

"YOU NEED PEE"

$$\frac{\mathbf{Una} + \times \mathbf{Pcr}}{Ucr \times Pna} \times 100$$

(U = urine, CR^+ creatinine, Na^+ = sodium, P = plasma)

Define the lab results with prerenal vs renal failure:

BUN/Cr ratio

Prerenal: $> 20:1$
Renal: $< 20:1$

Specific gravity

Prerenal: > 1.020 (as the body tries to hold on to fluid)
Renal < 1.020 (kidney has decreased ability to concentrate urine)

FeNa

Prerenal FENa < 1
Renal > 1

Urine Na+ (sodium)

Prerenal < 20
Renal > 40

Urine osmolality

Prerenal > 500
Renal < 350 mOsm/Kg

What are the indications for dialysis?

Fluid overload, refractory hyperkalemia, BUN > 130, acidosis, uremic encephalopathy

DIC

What is it?

Activation of the coagulation cascade leading to **thrombosis** and **consumption** of clotting factors and platelets and activation of fibrinolytic system (fibrinolysis), resulting in **bleeding**

What are the causes?

Tissue necrosis, septic shock, massive large-vessel coagulation, shock, allergic reactions, massive blood transfusion reaction, cardiopulmonary bypass, cancer, obstetric complications, snakebites, trauma, burn injury, prosthetic material, liver dysfunction

What are the signs/ symptoms?

Acrocyanosis or other signs of thrombosis, then diffuse bleeding from incision sites, venipuncture sites, catheter sites, or mucous membranes

What are the associated lab findings?

Increased fibrin-degradation products, elevated PT/PTT, decreased platelets, decreased fibrinogen (level correlates well with bleeding), presence of schistocytes (fragmented RBCs), increased D-dimer

What is the treatment?

Removal of the cause; otherwise supportive: IVFs, O_2, platelets, FFP, cryoprecipitate (fibrin), Epsilon-aminocaproic acid, as needed in predominantly thrombotic cases

Use of heparin is indicated in cases that are predominantly thrombotic with anti-thrombin III supplementation as needed.

How should one treat abdominal wound dehiscence?

Emergently to OR for fascial reclosure

ABDOMINAL COMPARTMENT SYNDROME

What is it?

Increased intra-abdominal pressure usually seen after laparotomy

What are the signs/ symptoms?

Tight distended abdomen, decreased urine output, increased airway pressure, **increased intra-abdominal pressure**

How to measure intra-abdominal pressure?

Read intrabladder pressure (Foley catheter hooked up to manometry after instillation of 50–100 cc of water).

What is normal intra-abdominal pressure?

< 15 mm Hg

What intra-abdominal pressure indicates need for treatment?

25 mm Hg especially if signs of compromise

What is the treatment?

Release the pressure by opening the abdomen and place a sheet of synthetic material to the skin to allow for more intra-abdominal volume.

What is a "Bogata Bag"?

A sheet of plastic (empty urology irrigation bag or IV bag) used to temporarily close the abdomen to allow for more intra-abdominal volume

URINARY RETENTION

What is it?

Enlarged urinary bladder resulting from medications or spinal anesthesia

How is it diagnosed? Physical exam (palpable bladder), bladder residual volume upon placement of a Foley catheter

What is the treatment? Foley catheter

WOUND INFECTION**

What are the signs/ symptoms? Erythema, swelling, pain, heat, (rubor, tumor, calor, dolor)

What is the treatment? Open wound, leave open with wet to dry dressing changes, antibiotics if cellulitis present

WOUND HEMATOMA***

What is it? Collection of blood (blood clot) in operative wound

What is the treatment? Acute: remove with hemostasis
Subacute: observe (heat helps resorption)

WOUND SEROMA

What is it? Postoperative collection of lymph and serum in the operative wound

What is the treatment? Needle aspiration, repeat if necessary (prevent with closed drain)

PSEUDOMEMBRANEOUS COLITIS

What is it also called? Antibiotic-associated diarrhea

What are the signs/ symptoms? **Diarrhea,** fever, hypotension/tachycardia

How is it diagnosed? *C. difficile* toxin in stool, fecal WBC, flex sig (see a mucus pseudomembrane in lumen of colon = hence the name)

What is the treatment?

1. Flagyl (PO or IV)
2. Vancomycin if refractory to Flagyl

21 Common Causes of Ward Emergencies

What can cause hypotension?

Hypovolemia (iatrogenic, hemorrhage), MI, cardiac dysrhythmia, hypoxia, false reading (e.g., wrong cuff/arterial line twist or clot), pneumothorax, PE, cardiac tamponade, medications (e.g., morphine)

How do you act?

A, B, C's, examine, recheck BP, IV access, labs (e.g. HCT), EKG, pulse ox/vital signs monitoring, CXR, supplemental oxygen, check medications/history

What are the common causes of postoperative hypertension?

Pain (from catecholamine release), anxiety, hypercapnia, hypoxia (which may also cause hypotension), preexisting condition, bladder distention

What can cause hypoxia/ shortness of breath?

Atelectasis, pneumonia, mucous plug, pneumothorax, PE, MI/dysrhythmia, venous blood in ABG syringe, SAT% machine malfunction/probe malposition, iatrogenic (wrong ventilator settings), severe anemia/hypovolemia, low cardiac output, CHF, ARDS, fluid overload

How do you act?

A, B, C's, physical exam, vital signs/pulse oximetry monitoring, supplemental oxygen, IV access, ABG, EKG, CXR

What can cause mental status change?

Hypoxia until ruled out, hypotension (e.g., cardiogenic shock), hypovolemia, iatrogenic (narcotics/benzodiazepines), drug reaction, alcohol withdrawal, drug withdrawal, seizure, ICU psychosis, stroke, sepsis, metabolic derangements, intracranial bleeding, **urinary retention in the elderly**

What are the signs of alcohol withdrawal?
Confusion, tachycardia/autonomic instability, seizure, hallucinations

What are the causes of tachycardia?
Hypovolemia/third-spacing, pain, alcohol withdrawal, anxiety/agitation, urinary retention, cardiac dysrhythmia (e.g., sinoventricular tachycardia, atrial fibrillation with rapid rate), MI, PE, β-blocker withdrawal

What are the causes of decreased urine output?
Hypovolemia, urinary retention, Foley catheter malfunction, cardiac failure, MI, acute tubular necrosis (ATN), ureteral/urethral injury

How do you act initially?
A, B, C's, examine, vital signs, check or place Foley catheter, irrigate Foley catheter, fluid bolus

22 Surgical Nutrition

What is the motto of surgical nutrition?
If the gut works, use it.

What are the normal daily dietary requirements for adults of the following:

Protein?
1 g/kg/day

Calories?
35 kcal/kg/day

By how much is basal energy expenditure (BEE) increased or decreased in the following cases:

Severe head injury?
Increased ≈1.7 ×

Severe burns?
Increased ≈2–3 ×

What are the calorie contents and metabolic by-products of the following substances:

Fat?
9 kcal/g; [CO_2 + H_2O]

Protein?
4 kcal/g; [ammonia]

Carbohydrate?
4 kcal/g; [CO_2 + H_2O]

What is the formula for converting nitrogen requirement/loss to protein requirement/loss?
Nitrogen × 6.25 = protein

What is RQ?
Respiratory quotient: the ratio of CO_2 produced to O_2 consumed

What is the normal RQ?
0.8

What can be done to decrease the RQ?
More fat, less carbohydrates

What dietary change can be made to decrease CO_2 production in a patient in whom CO_2 retention is a concern?
Decrease carbohydrate calories and increase calories from fat

What lab tests are used to monitor nutritional status?
Blood levels of:
↓ **Prealbumin** (T 1/2 ≈2–3 days)—acute change determination
↓ Transferrin (T 1/2 ≈8–9 days)
↓ Albumin (T 1/2 ≈14–20 days)—more chronic determination
Total lymphocyte count < 1800
Anergy
↓ Retinol-binding protein (T 1/2 ≈12 hours)

Where is iron absorbed?
Duodenum (some in proximal jejunum)

Where is vitamin B_{12} absorbed?
Terminal ileum

What are the surgical causes of vitamin B_{12} deficiency?
Gastrectomy, excision of terminal ileum, blind loop syndrome

Where are bile salts absorbed?
Terminal ileum

Where are fat-soluble vitamins absorbed?
Terminal ileum

Which vitamins are fat soluble?
K, A, D, E ("KADE")

What are the signs of the following disorders:

Vitamin A deficiency?
Poor wound healing

Vitamin B_{12}/folate deficiency?
Megaloblastic anemia

Vitamin C deficiency?
Poor wound healing, bleeding gums

Vitamin K deficiency? ↓ in the vitamin K–dependent clotting factors (II, VII, IX, and X); bleeding; elevated PT

Chromium deficiency? Diabetic state

Zinc deficiency? Poor wound healing, alopecia, dermatitis, taste disorder

Fatty acid deficiency? Dry, flaky skin; alopecia

What vitamin increases the PO absorption of iron? PO vitamin C (ascorbic acid)

What vitamin lessens the deleterious effects of steroids on wound healing? Vitamin A

What are the common indications for total parenteral nutrition (TPN)?

NPO more than 7 days
Enterocutaneous fistulas
Short bowel syndrome
ATN
Burns
Prolonged ileus
Severe weight loss
Before surgery
Pancreatitis

What is TPN? Total parenteral nutrition = IV nutrition

What is in TPN?

Protein
Carbohydrates
Lipids
(H_2O, electrolytes, minerals/vitamins, ± insulin, ± H_2 blocker)

How much of each in TPN:

Lipids? 20% to 30% of calories (lipid from soybeans, etc.)

Protein? 1.7g/kg/day (10–20% of calories) as amino acids

Carbohydrates? 50% to 60% of calories as dextrose

What are the possible complications of TPN?	Line infection, fatty infiltration of the liver, electrolyte/glucose problems, pneumothorax during placement of central line, loss of gut barrier, acalculus cholecystitis, refeeding syndrome, hyperosmolality
What are the advantages of enteral feeding?	Keeps gut barrier healthy, thought to lessen translocation of bacteria, not associated with complications of line placement, associated with fewer electrolyte/glucose problems
What is the major nutrient of the gut (small bowel)?	Glutamine
What is "refeeding syndrome"?	Decreased serum **potassium, magnesium,** and **phosphate** after refeeding (via TPN or enterally) a starving patient
What are the vitamin K–dependent clotting factors?	2,7,9,10 (think: 2 + 7 = 9, and then 10)
What is an elemental tube feed?	Very low residue tube feed in which almost all the tube feed is absorbed
Where is calcium absorbed?	Duodenum (actively) Jejunum (passively)
What is the major nutrient of the colon?	**Butyrate** (and other short-chain fatty acids)
What must bind B_{12} for absorption?	Intrinsic factor from the gastric parietal cells
What sedative medication has caloric value?	Propofol delivers 1 kcal/cc in the form of lipid!
Why may all the insulin placed in a TPN bag not get to the patient?	Insulin will bind to the IV tubing.
What is the best way to determine the caloric requirements of a patient on the ventilator?	Metabolic cart

How can serum bicarbonate be increased in patients on TPN?

Increase acetate (which is metabolized into bicarbonate)

What are "trophic" tube feeds?

Very low rate of tube feeds (i.e., approximately 10 cc/hr), which are thought to keep mucosa alive and healthy

When should PO feedings be started after a laparotomy?

After flatus or stool PR (usually postoperative days 3–5)

23 Shock

What is the definition of shock?

Inadequate tissue perfusion

What are the different types (5)?

Hypovolemic
Septic
Cardiogenic
Neurogenic
Anaphylactic

What are the signs of shock?

Pale, diaphoretic, cool skin
Hypotension, tachycardia, tachypnea
↓ mental status and pulse pressure
Poor capillary refill
Poor urine output

What are the best indicators of tissue perfusion?

Urine output, mental status

What lab tests help assess tissue perfusion?

pH from ABG (acidosis associated with inadequate tissue perfusion), lactic acid (elevated with inadequate tissue perfusion), base deficit

HYPOVOLEMIC SHOCK

What is the definition?

Decreased intravascular volume

What are the common causes?

Hemorrhage
Burns
Bowel obstruction
Crush injury
Pancreatitis

What are the signs?

Early—Orthostatic hypotension, mild tachycardia, anxiety, diaphoresis, vasoconstriction (decreased pulse pressure with increased diastolic pressure)

Late—Changed mental status, decreased BP, marked tachycardia

What are the signs/ symptoms with:

Class I hemorrhage (750 cc or 15% or less blood loss)?

Mild anxiety, normal vital signs

Class II hemorrhage (15–30% or 750–1500 cc blood loss)?

Normal systolic BP with decreased pulse pressure, tachycardia, tachypnea, anxiety

Class III hemorrhage (30–40% or 1500–2000 cc blood loss)?

Tachycardia (heart rate > 120), tachypnea (respiratory rate > 30), **decreased systolic BP,** decreased pulse pressure, confusion

Class IV hemorrhage (> 40% or > 2000 cc blood loss)?

Decreased systolic BP, tachycardia (heart rate > 140), tachypnea (respiratory rate > 35), decreased pulse pressure, confused and lethargic, no urine output

What is the treatment?

1. **Stop the bleeding**
2. **Volume:** IVF (isotonic LR) then blood as needed

What is irreversible shock?

Loss of blood that is lethal even if the patient is fully resuscitated

How is the effectiveness of treatment evaluated:

Bedside indicator?

Urine output, BP, heart rate, mental status, extremity warmth, capillary refill

Labs?

pH, base deficit, and lactate level

What usually causes failure of resuscitation?

Persistent massive hemorrhage, requiring emergent surgical procedure

Why does decreased pulse pressure occur with early hypovolemic shock?

Pulse pressure (systolic–diastolic BP) decreases because of vasoconstriction, resulting in an elevated diastolic BP.

What is the most common vital sign change associated with early hypovolemic shock?

Tachycardia

What type of patient does not mount a normal tachycardiac response to hypovolemic shock?
Patients on β-blockers, spinal shock (loss of sympathetic tone), endurance athletes

Should vasopressors be used to treat hypovolemic shock?
No

SEPTIC SHOCK

What is the definition?
Documented infection, organ dysfunction, and hypotension refractory to fluid resuscitation

What is the specific etiology?
Most common—gram-negative septicemia
Less common—gram-positive septicemia

What factors increase the susceptibility to septic shock?
Any mechanism that increases susceptibility to infection (e.g., trauma, immunosuppression, corticosteroids, hematologic disease, diabetes)

What complications are major risks in septic shock?
Multiple organ failure, DIC, **death**

What are the signs/ symptoms?
Initial—vasodilation, resulting in warm skin and full pulses; normal urine output
Delayed—vasoconstriction and poor urine output; mental status changes; hypotension

What percentage of blood cultures are positive in patients with bacterial septic shock?
Only about 50%!

What are the associated findings?
Fever, hyperventilation, tachycardia

Which are the associated lab findings?
Early—hyperglycemia/glycosuria, respiratory alkalosis, hemoconcentration, leukopenia
Late—leukocytosis, acidosis, elevated lactic acid
Note: Identifying organism is important to direct treatment.

What is the treatment?

1. Volume (IVF)
2. Antibiotics
3. Drainage of infection
4. Pressors PRN

CARDIOGENIC SHOCK

What is the definition?

Cardiac insufficiency; left ventricular failure (usually), resulting in inadequate tissue perfusion

What are the causes?

MI, papillary muscle dysfunction, massive cardiac contusion, cardiac tamponade, tension pneumothorax, cardiac valve failure

What are the signs/ symptoms on exam?

Dyspnea
Rales
Pulsus alternans (increased pulse with greater filling following a weak pulse)
Loud pulmonic component of S_2
Gallop rhythm

What are the associated vital signs/parameters?

Hypotension, decreased cardiac output, elevated CVP/wedge pressure, decreased urine output (low renal blood flow), tachycardia (possibly)

What are the signs on CXR?

Pulmonary edema

What is the treatment?

Based on diagnosis/mechanism:
1. CHF: diuretics and vasodilators, with or without pressors
2. Left ventricular failure (MI): pressors, afterload reduction

What are the last resort support mechanisms?

Intraaortic balloon pump (IABP), ventricular assist device (VAD)

NEUROGENIC SHOCK

What is the definition?

Inadequate tissue perfusion from loss of sympathetic vasoconstrictive tone

What are the common causes?

Spinal trauma
- Complete transection of spinal cord
- Partial cord injury with spinal shock
- Spinal anesthesia

What are the signs/ symptoms?
Hypotension and **bradycardia,** neurologic deficit

Why are heart rate and BP decreased?
Loss of sympathetic tone (but hypovolemia [e.g., hemoperitoneum] must be ruled out)

What are the associated findings?
Neurologic deficits suggesting cord injury

What is the treatment?
IV fluids (vasopressors reserved for hypotension refractory to fluid resuscitation)

What percentage of patients with hypotension and spinal neurologic deficits have hypotension of purely neurogenic origin?
About two thirds (67%) of patients

What is spinal shock?
Complete flaccid paralysis immediately following spinal cord injury; may or may not be associated with circulatory shock

What is the lowest reflex available to the examiner?
Bulbocavernous reflex: checking for contraction of the anal sphincter upon compression of the glans penis or clitoris

What is the lowest level voluntary muscle?
External anal sphincter

What are the classic findings associated with spinal cord shock?
Hypotension
Bradycardia or lack of compensatory tachycardia

24 Surgical Infection

What are the classic signs/ symptoms of inflammation/ infection?	Tumor (mass = swelling/edema) Calor (heat) Dolor (pain) Rubor (redness = erythema)
Define:	
Bacteremia	Bacteria in the blood
SIRS	**S**ystemic **I**nflammatory **R**esponse **S**yndrome (fever, tachycardia, tachypnea, leukocytosis)
Sepsis	Documented infection and SIRS
Septic shock	Sepsis and hypotension refractory to fluid resuscitation
Cellulitis	**Blanching erythema** from superficial dermal/epidermal infection (usually strep > staph)
Abscess	Collection of pus within a cavity
Superinfection	A new infection arising while a patient is receiving antibiotics for the original infection at a different site (e.g., *C. difficile* colitis)
Nosocomial infection	Infection originating in the hospital
What is the most common nosocomial infection?	Urinary tract infection (UTI)
What is the most common nosocomial infection causing death?	Respiratory tract infection

URINARY TRACT INFECTIONS (UTIS)

What diagnostic tests are used?

Urinalysis, culture, urine microscopy for WBC

What constitutes a POSITIVE urine analysis?

Positive nitrite (from bacteria)
Positive leukocyte esterase (from WBC)
More than 10 WBC/HPF
Presence of bacteria (supportive)

What number of colony-forming units (CFU) confirms the diagnosis of UTI?

On urine culture, classically 100,000 or 10^5 CFU

What are the common organisms?

Escherichia coli, Klebsiella, Proteus (*Enterococcus, Staphylococcus aureus*)

What is the treatment?

Antibiotics with gram-negative spectrum (e.g., sulfamethoxazole/trimethoprim [Bactrim], gentamicin, ciprofloxacin, aztreonam); check culture and sensitivity

What is the treatment of bladder candidiasis?

1. Remove or change Foley catheter.
2. Administer systemic fluconazole or amphotericin bladder washings.

CENTRAL LINE INFECTIONS

What are the signs of a central line infection?

Unexplained hyperglycemia, fever, mental status change, hypotension, tachycardia → **shock,** pus, and erythema at central line site

What is the treatment?

Remove line; administer antibiotics.

When should a central line be changed over a wire?

Fever without obvious external signs (pus, erythema at central line site) of infection; send tip of catheter to the lab for culture

When should a central line changed over a wire be left in place?

If culture of previous line returns less than 15 CFU

When should a central line changed over a wire be pulled and a central line placed at a different site?

If the previous line culture returns more than 15 CFU

WOUND INFECTION

What is it?
Infection in an operative wound

When do these infections arise?
Classically, postoperative days 5 to 7

What are the signs/ symptoms?
Pain at incision site, erythema, drainage, induration, warm skin, fever

What is the treatment?
Remove skin sutures/staples, perform digital examination to rule out fascial dehiscence, pack wound open, send wound culture, administer antibiotics.

What are the most common bacteria found in postoperative wound infections?
Staphylococcus aureus (20%)
Escherichia coli (10%)
Enterococcus (10%)
Other causes: *Staphylococcus epidermidis*, *Pseudomonas*, anaerobes, other gram-negative organisms, *Streptococcus*

Which bacteria will cause fever and wound infection in the first 24 hours after surgery?
1. *Streptococcus*
2. *Clostridium* (bronze-brown weeping tender wound)

CLASSIFICATION OF OPERATIVE WOUNDS

What is a "clean" wound?
Elective, nontraumatic wound without acute inflammation; usually closed primarily without the use of drains

What is the infection rate of a clean wound?
Less than 1.5%

What is a clean-contaminated wound?
Operation on the GI or respiratory tract without unusual contamination or entry into the biliary or urinary tract

Without infection present, what is the infection rate of a clean-contaminated wound?
Less than 3%

What is a contaminated wound?	Acute inflammation, traumatic wound, GI tract spillage, or a major break in sterile technique
What is the infection rate of a contaminated wound?	Approximately 5%
What is a dirty wound?	Pus present, perforated viscus, or dirty traumatic wound
What is the infection rate of a dirty wound?	Approximately 33%
What are the possible complications of wound infections?	Fistula, sinus tracts, sepsis, abscess, suppressed wound healing, superinfection (i.e., a new infection that develops during antibiotic treatment for the original infection)
What factors influence the development of infections?	A foreign body (e.g., suture, drains, grafts) Decreased blood flow (poor delivery of PMNs and antibiotics) Strangulation of tissues with excessively tight sutures Necrotic tissue or excessive local tissue destruction (e.g., too much Bovie) Long operations (> 2 hrs) Hypothermia Hematomas or seromas Dead space that prevents the delivery of phagocytic cells to bacterial foci Poor approximation of tissues
What patient factors influence the development of infections?	Uremia Hypovolemic shock Vascular occlusive states Advanced age Immunosuppressed states: immunosuppressant treatment, chemotherapy, systemic malignancy, trauma or burn injury, diabetes mellitus, obesity, malnutrition, AIDS, uremia, distant area of infection
Which lab tests are indicated?	Leukocytosis or leukopenia (as an abscess may act as a WBC sink), blood cultures, imaging studies (i.e., CT to locate an abscess)

What is the treatment?

Incision and drainage—an abscess must be drained (**Note:** fluctuation is a sign of a subcutaneous abscess. Most abdominal abscesses are drained percutaneously.)
Antibiotics

PERITONEAL ABSCESS

What is a peritoneal abscess?

Abscess within the peritoneal cavity

What are the causes?

Postoperative status after a laparotomy, ruptured appendix, peritonitis, any inflammatory intraperitoneal process, anastomotic leak

What are the sites of occurrence?

Pelvis, Morison's pouch, subphrenic, paracolic gutters, periappendiceal, lesser sac

What are the signs/ symptoms?

Fever (classically spiking), abdominal pain, mass

How is the diagnosis made?

Abdominal CT (or ultrasound)

When should an abdominal CT be obtained looking for a postoperative abscess?

After postoperative day 7 (otherwise, abscess will not be "organized" and will look like a normal postoperative fluid collection)

What CT findings are associated with abscess?

Fluid collection with fibrous rind, **gas** in fluid collection

What is the treatment?

Percutaneous CT drainage

What is an option for drainage of pelvic abscess?

Transrectal drainage (or transvaginal)

All abscesses must be drained except which type?

Amebiasis!

What is a "stitch" abscess?

Subcutaneous abscess centered around a subcutaneous stitch, which is a "foreign body"; treat with drainage and stitch removal

NECROTIZING FASCITIS

What is it?	Bacterial infection of underlying fascia (spreads rapidly along fascial planes)
What are the causative agents?	Classically, *Streptococcus*, but most often polymicrobial with anaerobes/gram-negative organisms
What are the signs/ symptoms?	Fever, pain, crepitus, cellulitis, skin discoloration, blood blisters (hemorrhagic bullae), weeping skin, increased WBCs, subcutaneous air on x-ray, septic shock
What is the treatment?	IV antibiotics and aggressive early extensive surgical debridement, cultures, tetanus prophylaxis

CLOSTRIDIAL MYOSITIS

What is it?	Clostridial muscle infection
What is another name for this condition?	Gas gangrene
What is the most common causative organism?	*Clostridium perfringens*
What are the signs/ symptoms?	Pain, fever, shock, crepitus, foul-smelling brown fluid, subcutaneous air on x-ray
What is the treatment?	IV antibiotics, aggressive surgical debridement of involved muscle, tetanus prophylaxis

SUPPURATIVE HIDRADENITIS

What is it?	Infection/abscess formation in **apocrine** sweat glands
In what (3) locations does it occur?	Perineum/buttocks, inguinal area, axilla (site of apocrine glands)
What is the most common causative organism?	*Staphylococcus aureus*
What is the treatment?	Antibiotics Incision and drainage (excision of skin for chronic infections)

PSEUDOMEMBRANOUS COLITIS

What is it?

Antibiotic-induced colonic overgrowth of *C. difficile*, secondary to loss of competitive nonpathogenic bacteria that comprise the normal colonic flora

Note: it can be caused by any antibiotic, but especially penicillins, cephalosporins, and clindamycin.

What are the signs/symptoms?

Diarrhea, ± fever, ± increased WBCs, ± abdominal cramps, ± abdominal distention

What causes the diarrhea?

Exotoxin released by *C. difficile*

How is the diagnosis made?

Assay stool for exotoxin titer; fecal leukocytes may or may not be present; on colonoscopy, there is an exudate that looks like a membrane (hence, "pseudomembranous").

What is the treatment?

PO vancomycin (97% sensitive) or PO metronidazole (Flagyl; 93% sensitive); discontinuation of causative agent

Never give antiperistaltics.

PROPHYLACTIC ANTIBIOTICS

What are the indications for prophylaxis (IV antibiotics)?

Accidental wounds with heavy contamination and tissue damage

Accidental wounds requiring surgical therapy that has had to be delayed

Injuries in which adequate debridement cannot be performed

Known gross bacterial contamination in any wound

Prosthetic heart valve

Penetrating injuries of hollow intra-abdominal organs

Large bowel resections and anastomosis (cathartics, PO neomycin plus erythromycin on the day prior to surgery, and cefoxitin preoperatively)

Some clean-contaminated procedures (e.g., common bile duct exploration)

Patient with pre-existing valvular heart disease

Cardiovascular surgery with the use of a prosthesis/vascular procedures
Patients with open fractures (start in ER)
Traumatic wounds occurring more than 8 hours prior to medical attention

What must a prophylactic antibiotic cover for procedures on the large bowel/abdominal trauma/ appendicitis?

Anaerobes

What commonly used antibiotics offer anaerobic coverage?

Cefoxitin (Mefoxin), clindamycin, metronidazole (Flagyl), cefotetan, ampicillin-sulbactam (Unasyn)

What antibiotic is used prophylactically for vascular surgery?

Ancef (if patient is significantly allergic to PCN—hives/swelling/shortness of breath—then erythromycin or clindamycin)

When is the appropriate time to administer prophylactic antibiotics?

Must be in adequate levels in the blood stream **prior to surgical incision!**

PAROTITIS

What is it?

Infection of the parotid gland

What is the most common causative organism?

Staphylococcus

What are the associated risk factors?

Age older than 65 years, malnutrition, poor oral hygiene, presence of NG tube, NPO, dehydration

What is the most common time of occurrence?

Usually 2 weeks postoperative

What are the signs?

Hot, red, tender parotid gland and increased WBCs

What is the treatment?

Antibiotics, operative drainage as necessary

MISCELLANEOUS

Which bacteria can be found in the stool (colon)?

Anaerobic—*Bacteroides fragilis*
Aerobic—*Escherichia coli*

Which bacteria are found in infections from human bites?
Streptococcus viridans, S. aureus, Peptococcus, Eikenella

What is the most common ICU pneumonia bacteria?
Gram-negative organisms

What is Fournier's gangrene?
Perineal infection starting classically in the scrotum in patients with diabetes; treat with triple antibiotics and wide debridement (± colostomy to divert stool from area)

Does adding antibiotics to peritoneal lavage solution lower the risk of abscess formation?
No ("Dilution is the solution to pollution.")

What is the classic finding associated with a *Pseudomonas* infection?
Green exudate and "fruity" smell

What are the classic antibiotics for "triple" antibiotics?
Ampicillin, gentamycin, and metronidazole (Flagyl)

Which antibiotic is used to treat ameba infection?
Metronidazole (Flagyl)

Which bacteria commonly infect prosthetic material and central lines?
Staphylococcus epidermis

What is the antibiotic of choice for *Actinomyces*?
Penicillin G (exquisitely sensitive)

What is a furuncle?
A staphylococcal abscess that forms in a hair follicle (think: **f**ollicle = **f**uruncle)

What is a carbuncle?
A subcutaneous staphylococcal abscess (usually an extension of a furuncle), most commonly seen in patients with diabetes (i.e., rule out diabetes)

What is a felon?
Infection of the finger pad (think, **f**elon = **f**inger printing)

What microscopic finding is associated with *Actinomyces*?
Sulfur granules

What organism causes tetanus?
Clostridium tetani

What are the signs of tetanus?
Lockjaw, muscle spasm, laryngospasm, convulsions, respiratory failure

What are the appropriate prophylactic steps in tetanus-prone (dirty) injury in the following patients:

Three previous immunizations?
None (tetanus toxoid only if > 5 years since last toxoid)

Two previous immunizations?
Tetanus toxoid

One previous immunization?
Tetanus immunoglobulin IM and tetanus toxoid IM (at different sites!)

No previous immunizations?
Tetanus immunoglobulin IM and tetanus toxoid IM (at different sites!)

What is Fitz-Hugh-Curtis syndrome?
Right upper quadrant pain from gonococcal perihepatitis in women

What is bacterial translocation?
Bacteria gain access to lymphatics and blood stream from the colon via compromised mucosal barrier.

25 Fever

Define postoperative fever.	Temperature > 38.5° C or 101.5° F
What are the classic W's of postoperative fever? (5)	**W**ind—atelectasis **W**ater—urinary tract infection (UTI) **W**ound—wound infection **W**alking—DVT/thrombophlebitis **W**onder drugs—drug fever
Give the classic postoperative timing for the following causes of postoperative fever:	
Atelectasis (Wind)	First 24 to 48 hours
UTI (Water)	Anytime after postoperative day 3
Wound infection (Wound)	Anytime after postoperative day 5
DVT/PE/thrombophlebitis (Walking)	Postoperative days 7 to 10
Drug fever (Wonder drugs)	Anytime
What is the most common cause of fever on postoperative days 1 to 2?	Atelectasis
What is a "complete" fever work up?	Physical exam (look at wound, etc.), CXR, urinalysis, blood cultures, CBC
What causes fever before 24 postoperative hours?	Atelectasis, β-hemolytic streptococcal or clostridial wound infections, anastomotic leak
What causes fever from postoperative days 3 to 5?	UTI, pneumonia, IV site infection, wound infection

What is an anesthetic cause of fever INTRAoperatively?	Malignant hyperthermia—treat with **dantrolene**
What causes fever from postoperative days 5 to 10?	Wound infection, pneumonia, abscess, infected hematoma, *C. difficile* colitis, anastomotic leak **DVT, peritoneal abscess, drug fever** Pulmonary embolism, abscess, parotitis
What causes wound infection on postoperative days 1 to 2?	*Streptococcus* Clostridia (painful bronze-brown weeping wound)

26 Surgical Prophylaxis

What medications provide protection from postoperative GI bleeding?

H_2 blockers (e.g., ranitidine or cimetidine), sucralfate (binds ulcer craters), antacids

What measures provide protection from postoperative atelectasis/ pneumonia?

Incentive spirometry, coughing, **smoking cessation**, ambulation

What treatments provide protection from postoperative DVT?

Subcutaneous low-dose heparin, sequential compression device (SCD) for lower extremities, or both; early ambulation

What measures provide protection from wound infection?

Shower the night before surgery with chlorhexidine scrub.
Never use a razor for hair removal (electric shavers only).
Ensure adequate skin prep in OR.
Do not close the skin in a contaminated case.
Ensure preoperative antibiotics in the bloodstream **before incision.**
Ensure no excess Bovie (necrotic tissue).

Why not use a razor to remove hair?

The micro cuts are a nidus for bacteria and subsequent wound infection.

How long should you give "prophylactic antibiotics"?

<24 hrs

What treatment provides protection from oral/ esophageal fungal infection during IV antibiotic treatment?

PO nystatin

What measure provides protection from infection after colon surgery?

1. Bowel prep: lower bacterial count in colon by catharsis (GoLYTELY or Fleets)
2. PO antibiotics (neomycin, erythromycin) preoperatively
3. Preoperative IV antibiotic with spectrum versus anaerobes (e.g., Cefoxitin)

What treatment provides protection from OPSS after splenectomy?

Immunization versus *H. influenza*, *Streptococcus*, *Meningococcus*, and penicillin when illness/fever occurs

What treatment provides protection from endocarditis with faulty heart valve or prosthetic heart valve?

Antibiotics prior to dental procedure or any surgery

What treatment provides protection from tetanus infection?

Tetanus toxoid (and tetanus immune globulin, if one or no previous toxoid with dirty wound)

What treatment provides protection from ETOH withdrawal?

Chlordiazepoxide (Librium®), also give Rally pack)

What treatment provides protection from Wernicke's encephalopathy?

Rally pack (A.K.A. banana bag since the IV is yellow with the vitamins in it); pack includes thiamine, folate, and magnesium

What is Wernicke's encephalopathy?

Condition resulting from thiamine deficiency in patients with alcoholism, causing a **triad** of symptoms:

1. Confusion
2. Ataxia
3. Ophthalmoplegia

What treatment decreases the risk of perioperative adrenal crisis in a patient on chronic steroids?

"Stress-dose" steroids: 100 mg hydrocortisone administered preoperatively, continued postoperatively, and then tapered off

27 Surgical Radiology

CHEST

What defines a technically adequate CXR?

The film must be **RIPE:**

- **R**otation: Clavicular heads are equidistant from the thoracic spinous processes.
- **I**nspiration: Diaphragm is at or below ribs 8–10 posteriorly and ribs 5–6 anteriorly.
- **P**enetration: Disk spaces are visible but there is no bony detail of the spine; bronchovascular structures are seen through the heart.
- **E**xposure: Make sure all of the lung fields are visible.

How should a CXR be read?

Check the following:

- **Tubes and lines:** Check placement
- **Patient data:** Name, date, history number
- **Orientation:** Up/down, left-right
- **Technique:** AP or PA, supine or erect, decubitus
- **Trachea:** Midline or deviated, caliber
- **Lungs:** CHF, mass
- **Pulmonary vessels:** Artery or vein enlargement
- **Mediastinum:** Aortic knob, nodes
- **Hila:** Masses, lymphadenopathy
- **Heart:** Transverse diameter should be ≤ half the transthoracic diameter
- **Pleura:** Effusion, thickening, pneumothorax
- **Bones:** Fractures, lesions
- **Soft tissues:** Periphery and below the diaphragm

What CXR is better: P-A or A-P?	P-A, less magnification of the heart (heart is closer to the x-ray plate)
Classically, how much pleural fluid can the diaphragm hide on upright CXR?	It is said that the diaphragm can overshadow up to 500 cc (but probably closer to 200 cc in reality).
How can CXR confirm that the last hole on a chest tube is in the pleural cavity?	The last hole is through the radiopaque line on the chest tube; thus, look for the break in the radiopaque line to be in the rib cage.
How can a loculated pleural effusion be distinguished from a free-flowing pleural effusion?	Ipsilateral decubitus CXR; if fluid is not loculated (or contained) it will layer out
How do you recognize a pneumothorax on CXR?	Air without lung markings is seen outside the white pleural line—best seen in the apices on an upright CXR.
What x-ray should be obtained before feeding via a nasogastric or nasoduodenal tube?	Low CXR to ensure the tube is in the GI tract and not in the lung
What C-spine views are used to rule out bony injury?	A-P, lateral, **open mouth odontoid** views
What plain x-rays are used to look for ligamentous C-spine injury?	Lateral flex and extension C-spine films
What CXR findings may provide evidence of traumatic aortic injury?	Widened mediastinum > 8 cm (most common) Apical pleural capping Loss of aortic knob Inferior displacement of left main bronchus; NG tube displaced to the right, tracheal deviation, hemothorax

ABDOMEN

How should an abdominal X-ray (AXR) be read?	Check the following: Patient data: Name, date, history number

Orientation: up/down, left-right
Technique: AP or PA, supine or erect, decubitus
Air: free air under diaphragm, air-fluid levels,
Gas dilatation (3,6,9 rule)
Borders: psoas shadow, preperitoneal fat stripe
Mass: look for organomegaly, kidney shadow
Stones/calcification: urinary, biliary, fecalith
Stool
Tubes
Bones
Foreign bodies

How can you tell the difference between a small bowel obstruction (SBO) and an ileus?

In SBO there is a transition point (cut-off sign) between the distended proximal bowel and the distal bowel of normal caliber. The distal bowel may be gasless. The bowel in ileus is *diffusely* distended.

What is the significance of an air-fluid level?

Seen in obstruction or ileus on an upright x-ray; intraluminal bowel diameter increases, allowing for separation of fluid and gas

What are the normal calibers of the small bowel, transverse colon, and cecum?

Use the **"3, 6, 9 rule."**
Small bowel < 3 cm
Transverse colon < 6 cm
Cecum < 9 cm

What is the "rule of 3s" for the small bowel?

The bowel wall should be less than 3 mm thick.
The bowel folds should be less than 3 mm thick.
The bowel diameter should be less than 3 cm wide.

How can the small and large bowel be distinguished on AXR?

By the intraluminal folds; the small bowel plicae circulares are complete, whereas the plicae semilunares of the large bowel are only partially around the inner circumference of the lumen

Where does peritoneal fluid accumulate in the supine position?	Morrison's pouch (hepatorenal recess), the space between the anterior surface of the right kidney and the posterior surface of the right lobe of the liver
What percentage of kidney stones are radiopaque?	Approximately 90%
What percentage of gallstones are radiopaque?	Approximately 10%
What percentage of patients with acute appendicitis have a radiopaque fecalith?	Approximately 5%
What are the radiographic signs of appendicitis?	Fecalith; sentinel loops; scoliosis away from the right because of pain; mass effect (abscess); loss of psoas shadow; loss of preperitoneal fat stripe; and, very rarely, a small amount of free air, if perforated
What does KUB stand for?	**K**idneys, **U**reters, and **B**ladder—commonly used term for a plain film AXR (abdominal flat plate)
What is the "parrot's beak" or "bird's beak" sign?	Evidence of sigmoid volvulus on barium enema; evidence of achalasia on barium swallow
What is a "cut-off sign"?	Seen in obstruction, bowel distention, and distended bowel that is "cut-off" from normal bowel
What are "sentinel loops"?	Distention or air-fluid levels (or both) near a site of abdominal inflammation (e.g., seen in RLQ with appendicitis)
What is loss of the psoas shadow?	Loss of the clearly defined borders of the psoas muscle on AXR; loss signifies inflammation or ascites
What is loss of the peritoneal fat stripe (A.K.A. preperitoneal fat stripe)?	Loss of the lateral peritoneal/ preperitoneal fat interface; implies inflammation

What is "thumbprinting"?

Nonspecific colonic mucosal edema resembling thumb indentations on AXR

What is pneumatosis intestinalis?

Gas within the intestinal wall (usually means dead gut) that can be seen in patients with congenital variant or chronic steroids

What is free air?

Air free within the peritoneal cavity (air or gas should be seen only within the bowel or stomach); usually results from bowel or stomach perforation

What is the best position for the detection of FREE AIR (free intraperitoneal air)?

Upright CXR—air below the right diaphragm

If you cannot get an upright CXR, what is the second best plain x-ray for free air?

Left lateral decubitus, because it prevents confusion with gastric air bubble; with free air **both** sides of the bowel wall can be seen; can detect as little as 1 cc of air

How long after a laparotomy can there be free air on AXR?

Usually 7 days or less

What is Chilaiditi's syndrome?

Transverse colon over the liver simulating free air

When should a postoperative abdominal/pelvic CT looking for a peritoneal abscess be performed?

Postoperative day 7 or later, to give time for the abscess to form

What is the best test to evaluate the biliary system and gallbladder?

Ultrasound (U/S)

What is the normal diameter of the common bile duct with gallbladder present?

$<$ 4 mm until age 40, then add 1 mm per decade (e.g., 7 mm at age 70)

What is the normal common bile duct diameter after removal of the gallbladder?

8 to 10 mm

What U/S findings are associated with acute cholecystitis?

Gallstones, thickened gallbladder wall (> 3 mm), distended gallbladder (> 4 cm A-P), impacted stone in gallbladder neck, pericholecystic fluid

What type of kidney stone is not seen on AXR?

Uric acid (think: **u**ric acid = **u**nseen)

What medication should be given prophylactically to a patient with a true history of contrast allergy?

Methylprednisolone or dexamethasone; the patient should also receive nonionic contrast (associated with one-fifth as many reactions as ionic contrast, the less expensive standard)

What is a C-C mammogram?

A cranio-caudal mammogram, in which the breast is compressed top to bottom

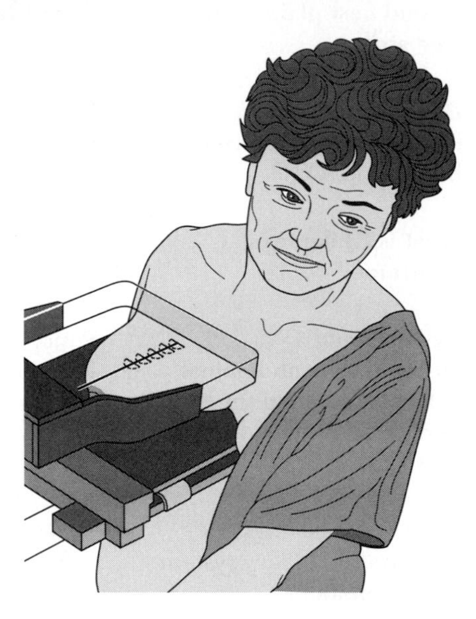

What is an MLO mammogram?

Medio-lateral oblique mammogram, in which the breast is compressed in a 45° angle from the axilla to the lower sternum

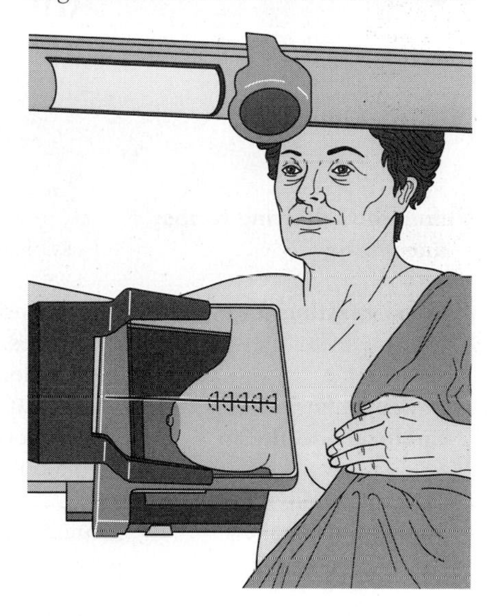

What are the best studies to evaluate for a pulmonary embolus?

V-Q ventilation-perfusion scan, spiral thoracic CT scan, pulmonary angiogram (gold standard)

28 Anesthesia

Define the following terms:

Anesthesia — Loss of sensation/pain

Local anesthesia — Anesthesia of a small confined area of the body (i.e., lidocaine for an elbow laceration)

Epidural anesthesia — Anesthetic drugs/narcotics infused into epidural space

Spinal anesthesia — Anesthetic agents injected into the thecal sac

Regional anesthesia — Blocking of the sensory afferent nerve fibers from a **region** of the body (i.e., radial nerve block)

General anesthesia — Unconsciousness/amnesia (inhalational anesthetics)

GET or GETA — General endotracheal anesthesia

Give examples of the following terms:

Local anesthetic — Lidocaine, bupivacaine (Marcaine)

Regional anesthetic — Lidocaine, bupivacaine (Marcaine)

General anesthesia — Isoflurane, enflurane, sevoflurane, desflurane, nitrous oxide, halothane

Dissociative agent — Ketamine (children/burn patients)

What is cricoid pressure? — Manual pressure on cricoid cartilage occluding the esophagus and thus decreasing the chance of aspiration of gastric contents during intubation

What is "rapid-sequence" anesthesia induction?

1. Oxygenation and short-acting induction agent
2. Muscle relaxant
3. Cricoid pressure
4. Intubation
5. Inhalation anesthetic (rapid: boom, boom, boom → to lower the risk of aspiration during intubation)

Give examples of induction agents.

Propofol, midazolam, sodium thiopental

What are contraindications of the depolarizing agent succinylcholine?

Patients with burns, neuromuscular diseases/paraplegia, eye trauma, or increased ICP

Why is succinylcholine contraindicated in these patients?

Depolarization can result in life-threatening **hyperkalemia; succinylcholine also increases intraocular pressure.**

Why doesn't lidocaine work in an abscess?

Lidocaine does not work in an acidic environment.

Why does lidocaine burn on injection and what can be done to decrease the burning sensation?

Lidocaine is acidic, which causes the burning; add sodium bicarbonate to decrease the burning sensation.

Why does some lidocaine come with epinephrine?

Epinephrine is meant to vasoconstrict the small vessels and thus decrease bleeding and washing out of the lidocaine from the area, prolonging its effect.

In what locations is lidocaine with epinephrine contraindicated?

Fingers, toes, penis, etc., because of the possibility of ischemic injury/necrosis resulting from vasoconstriction

What are the contraindications to nitrous oxide?

Nitrous oxide is poorly soluble in serum and thus expands into any air-filled body pockets; avoid in patients with middle ear occlusions, **pneumothorax, small bowel obstruction,** etc.

What is the feared side effect of bupivacaine (Marcaine)?

Cardiac dysrhythmia after intravascular injection leading to fatal refractory dysrhythmia

What are the side effects of morphine?	Constipation, respiratory failure, hypotension (from histamine release), spasm of sphincter of Oddi (use demerol in pancreatitis and biliary surgery), decreased cough reflex
What are the side effects of meperidine?	Similar to those of morphine but causes less sphincteric spasm and can cause tachycardia and seizures
Limit to the duration of Demerol postoperatively?	Build up of the metabolites (normeperidine)
What medication is a contraindication to demerol?	Monoamine oxidase inhibitor
What metabolite of demerol breakdown causes side effects (e.g., seizures)?	Normeperidine
What is the treatment of life-threatening respiratory depression with morphine or demerol?	**Narcan** IV (Naloxone)
What are the side effects of epidural analgesia?	**Orthostatic hypotension,** decreased motor function, urinary retention
What is the advantage of epidural analgesia?	Analgesia without decreased cough reflex
What must be taken out only after removal of the epidural catheter?	The Foley catheter should be removed after the epidural is removed; otherwise, patient is likely to suffer from urinary retention.
What are the side effects of spinal anesthesia?	**Urinary retention** Hypotension (neurogenic shock)
What is the side effect of inhalational (volatile) anesthesia?	Halothane—**hypotension** (cardiac depression, decreased baroreceptor response to hypotension, and peripheral vasodilation), malignant hyperthermia

MALIGNANT HYPERTHERMIA

What is it?

Inherited predisposition to an anesthetic Rxn, causing uncoupling of the excitation-contraction system in skeletal muscle, which in turn causes **malignant hyperthermia;** hypermetabolism is fatal if untreated

What is the incidence?

Very rare

What are the causative agents?

General anesthesia, succinylcholine

What are the signs/ symptoms?

Increased body temperature; hypoxia; acidosis; tachycardia, leading to death if untreated

What is the treatment?

IV dantrolene, body cooling, discontinuation of anesthesia

MISCELLANEOUS

What are some of the nondepolarizing muscle blockers?

Vecuronium
Pancuronium

What is the antidote to the nondepolarizing neuromuscular blocking agents?

Edrophonium
Neostigmine
Pyridostigmine

How do these agents work?

They inhibit anticholinesterase.

Which muscle blocker is depolarizing?

Succinylcholine

What is the duration of action of succinylcholine?

Less than 6 minutes

What is the antidote to reverse succinylcholine?

Time; endogenous blood pseudocholinesterase (patients deficient in this enzyme may be paralyzed for hours!)

What is the maximum dose of lidocaine?

5 mg/kg

What is the duration of lidocaine local anesthesia?

30 to 60 minutes (up to 4 hours with epinephrine)

What are the early signs of lidocaine toxicity?

Tinnitus, perioral/tongue numbness, metallic taste, blurred vision, muscle twitches, drowsiness

What are the signs of lidocaine toxicity with large overdose (> 10 mcg/ml)?

Seizures, coma, respiratory arrest
Loss of consciousness
Apnea

When should the Foley catheter be removed in a patient with an epidural catheter?

Several hours **after** the epidural catheter is removed

What is a PCA pump?

Patient-**C**ontrolled **A**nalgesia; a pump delivers a set amount of pain reliever when the patient pushes a button (e.g., 1 mg of morphine every 6 minutes)

What are the advantages of PCA pump?

Better pain control
Patients actually use less pain medication with a PCA!
If given a moderate dose without a basal rate, patients should not be able to overdose (they will fall asleep and not be able to push the button!)

What is a "basal rate" on the PCA?

A steady continuous infusion rate of the narcotic (e.g., 1–2 mg of morphine) continuously infused per hour; patient can supplement with additional doses as needed

What is used to reverse narcotics?

Naloxone (Narcan)

What is used to reverse benzodiazepines?

Flumazenil

What is fentanyl?

Very potent narcotic (number one drug of abuse by anesthesiologists)

Name an IV NSAID.

Ketorolac (has classic side effects of NSAIDs: PUD, renal insufficiency)

What is an option to endotracheal intubation as a general anesthetic when patient has no history of GERD?

LMA—**L**aryngeal **M**ask **A**irway (does not protect against aspiration of gastric contents)

What is a feared but very rare complication of halothane anesthetic?

Halothane hepatitis

29 Surgical Ulcers

Define the following terms:

Peptic ulcer	General term for gastric/duodenal ulcer disease
Duodenal ulcer	Ulcer in the duodenum
Gastric ulcer	Ulcer in the stomach
Curling's ulcer	Gastric ulcer after burn injury (think: Curling's—curling iron burn—burn)
Cushing's ulcer	Peptic ulcer after neurologic insult (think: Cushing—famous neurosurgeon)
Dieulafoy's ulcer	Pinpoint gastric mucosal defect bleeding from underlying arterial vessel malformation
Marjolin's ulcer	Squamous cell carcinoma ulceration overlying chronic osteomyelitis or burn scar
Apthous ulcer	GI tract ulcer seen in Crohn's disease
Marginal ulcer	Mucosal ulcer seen at a site of GI-tract anastomosis
Decubitus ulcer	Skin/subcutaneous ulceration from pressure necrosis, classically on the buttocks/sacrum
Venous stasis ulcer	Skin ulceration on **medial malleolus** caused by venous stasis of a lower extremity
LE arterial insufficiency ulcer	Skin ulcers usually located on the toes/feet

30 Surgical Oncology

Define:	
Surgical oncology	Surgical treatment of tumors
XRT	Radiation therapy
In situ	Not invading basement membrane
Benign	Nonmalignant tumor—does not invade or metastasize
Malignant	Tumors with anaplasia that invade and metastasize
Adjuvant RX	Treatment that aids or assists surgical treatment = Chemo or XRT
Neoadjuvant RX	Chemo, XRT, or both BEFORE surgical resection
Brachytherapy	XRT applied directly or very close to the target tissue (e.g., implant)
Metachronous tumors	Tumors occurring at different times
Synchronous tumors	Tumors occurring at the same time
What does the T, M, and N stand for in TMN staging?	**T: T**umor size **M: M**ets (distant) **N: N**odes

What tumor marker is associated with colon cancer?

CEA

What tumor marker is associated with hepatoma?

Alpha-fetoprotein

What is paraneoplastic syndrome?

Syndromes of dysfunction not directly associated with tumor mass or mets (autoimmune or released substance)

Section II General Surgery

31

GI Hormones and Physiology

GASTRIC PHASES

Name the three phases of acid secretion.	1. Cephalic 2. Gastric 3. Intestinal
What stimulates the cephalic phase?	The thought, sight, or smell of food; mediated by the vagus nerve
What stimulates the gastric phase?	Food entering the stomach (i.e., gastric distention, decreased pH); mediated by gastrin
What stimulates the intestinal phase?	The entry of products of digestion into the duodenum
Define the products of the following stomach cells:	
Gastric parietal cells	HCl Intrinsic factor
Chief cells	Pepsinogen (think: "a peppy chief")
G cells	Gastrin, G cells are found in the antrum (think: G – Gastrin)
Mucous neck cells	Bicarbonate mucus
What is pepsin?	A proteolytic enzyme that hydrolyzes peptide bonds
What is intrinsic factor?	A protein secreted by the parietal cells that combines with vitamin B_{12} and enables absorption in the terminal ileum

Name three receptors on the parietal cell that stimulate HCl release.

1. Histamine
2. Acetylcholine
3. Gastrin

What is the enterohepatic circulation?

Circulation of bile acids from the liver to the gut and back to the liver via the portal vein

Where are most of the bile acids absorbed?

The terminal ileum

How many times is the entire bile acid pool circulated during a typical meal?

Two times

What are the stimulators of gallbladder emptying?

Cholecystokinin Vagal input

What are the inhibitors of gallbladder emptying?

Somatostatin Sympathetics (it is impossible to flee and digest food at the same time) VIP

CHOLECYSTOKININ

What is its source?

Duodenal mucosal cells

What stimulates its release?

Fat, protein, amino acids, HCl

What inhibits its release?

Trypsin and chymotrypsin

What are its actions?

Empties gallbladder
Opens ampulla of Vater
Slows gastric emptying
Stimulates pancreatic acinar cell growth and release of exocrine products

SECRETIN

What is its source?

Duodenal cells (specifically the argyrophil S cells)

What stimulates its release?

pH less than 4.5 (acid) Fat in the duodenum

What inhibits its release?

High pH in the duodenum

What are its actions?	Releases pancreatic bicarbonate/enzymes/H_2O Releases bile/bicarbonate Decreases LES Decreases release of gastric acid

GASTRIN

What is its source?	Gastric antrum G cells
What stimulates its release?	Stomach peptides/amino acids Vagal input Calcium
What inhibits its release?	pH less than 3.0 Somatostatin
What are its actions?	Release of HCl from parietal cells Trophic effect on mucosa of the stomach and small intestine

SOMATOSTATIN

What is its source?	Pancreatic D cells
What stimulates its release?	Food
What are its actions?	Globally inhibits GI function

MISCELLANEOUS

What is the purpose of the colon?	Reabsorption of H_2O and storage of stool
What is the main small bowel nutritional source?	Glutamine
What is the main nutritional source of the colon?	Butyrate (short-chain fatty acid)
Where is calcium absorbed?	Duodenum actively, jejunum passively
Where is iron absorbed?	Duodenum

Where is vitamin B_{12} absorbed?	Terminal ileum
Which hormone primarily controls gallbladder contraction?	CCK
What supplement does a patient need after removal of the terminal ileum or stomach?	B_{12}
Name the main constituents of bile.	Water, phospholipids (lecithins), bile acids, cholesterol, and bilirubin
What are most gallstones made of?	Cholesterol
How do opiates affect the bowel?	Opiates stimulate sodium absorption and inhibit secretion in the ileum, as well as decreasing GI motility by incoordinated peristalsis. Therefore, place patients on stool softeners when dispensing pain medication.
Which type of muscle fibers, smooth or striated, does the esophagus contain?	Both Upper third—striated muscle control of motor nerves Middle third—mixed Lower third—smooth muscle, primarily under control of vagal motor fibers
Which electrolytes does the colon actively absorb?	Na^+, Cl^-
Which electrolytes does the colon actively secrete?	HCO_3 (plays a role in diarrhea causing the patient to have a normal anion gap acidosis)
Which electrolytes does the colon passively secrete?	K^+
What is the gastrocolic reflex?	Increased secretory and motor functions of the stomach result in increased colonic motility

What is the blood supply to the liver?

Seventy-five percent from the portal vein, rich in products of digestion
Twenty-five percent from the hepatic artery, rich in O_2 (but each provide for 50% of oxygen)

What are Peyer patches?

Nodules of lymphoid tissue with B and T lymphocytes in the small intestine that selectively sample lumenal antigens found in the terminal ileum

32

Acute Abdomen and Referred Pain

What is an "acute abdomen"?

Acute abdominal pain so severe that the patient seeks medical attention (not the same as a "surgical abdomen," because most cases of acute abdominal pain do not require surgical treatment)

What are peritoneal signs?

Signs of peritoneal irritation: extreme tenderness, percussion tenderness, rebound tenderness, voluntary guarding, motion pain, **involuntary** guarding/rigidity (late)

Define the following terms:

Rebound tenderness

Pain upon releasing the palpating hand pushing on the abdomen

Motion pain

Abdominal pain upon moving, pelvic rocking, moving of stretcher, or heel strike

Voluntary guarding

Abdominal muscle contraction with palpation of the abdomen

Involuntary guarding

Rigid abdomen as the muscles "guard" involuntarily

Colic

Intermittent severe pain (usually because of intermittent contraction of a hollow viscus against an obstruction)

What conditions can mask abdominal pain?

Steroids, diabetes, paraplegia, narcotics

What is the most common cause of acute abdominal surgery in the United States?

Acute appendicitis (7% of the population will develop it sometime during their lives)

What important questions should be asked when obtaining the history of a patient with an acute abdomen?

"Have you had this pain before?"
"On a scale from 1 to 10, what would you rank this pain?"
"Fevers/chills?"
"Duration?" (comes and goes vs. constant)
"Quality?" (sharp vs. dull)
"Does anything make the pain better or worse?"
"Migration?"
"Point of maximal pain?"
"Urinary symptoms?"
"Nausea, vomiting, or diarrhea?"
"Anorexia?"
"Constipation?"
"Last bowel movement?"
"Any change in bowel habits?"
"Any relation to eating?"
"Last menses?"
"Last meal?"
"Vaginal discharge?"
"Melena?"
"Hematochezia?"
"Hematemesis?"
"Medications?"
"Allergies?"
"Past medical history?"
"Past surgical history?"
"Family history?"
"Tobacco/ETOH/Drugs?"

What should the acute abdomen physical exam include?

Inspection (e.g., surgical scars, distention)
Auscultation (e.g., bowel sounds, bruits)
Palpation (e.g., tenderness, R/O hernia, CVAT, rectal, pelvic exam, rebound, voluntary guard, motion tenderness)
Percussion (e.g., liver size, spleen size)

What is the classic position of a patient with peritonitis?

Motionless (often with knees flexed)

What is the classic position of a patient with a kidney stone?

Cannot stay still, restless, writhing in pain

What lab tests are used to evaluate the patient with an acute abdomen?

CBC with **differential,** chem-10, amylase, type and screen, urinalysis, LFTs

What is a "left shift" on CBC differential?

Sign of inflammatory response: Immature neutrophils (bands) (today many call more than 80% of WBCs as neutrophils a left shift)

What lab test should every woman of childbearing age with an acute abdomen receive?

Human chorionic gonadotropin (β-hCG) to rule out pregnancy/ectopic pregnancy

Which x-rays are used to evaluate the patient with an acute abdomen?

Upright chest x-ray, upright abdominal film, supine abdominal x-ray (if patient cannot stand, left lateral decubitus abdominal film)

How is free air ruled out if the patient cannot stand?

Left lateral decubitus—free air collects over the liver and does not get confused with the gastric bubble

What diagnosis must be considered in every patient with an acute abdomen?

Appendicitis!

What are the differential diagnoses by quadrant?

RUQ

Cholecystitis, hepatitis, PUD, perforated ulcer, pancreatitis, liver tumors, gastritis, hepatic abscess, choledocholithiasis, cholangitis, pyelonephritis, nephrolithiasis, appendicitis **(especially during pregnancy);** thoracic causes (e.g., pleurisy/pneumonia), PE, pericarditis, MI (especially inferior MI)

LUQ

PUD, perforated ulcer, gastritis, splenic disease or rupture, abscess, reflux, dissecting aortic aneurysm, thoracic causes, pyelonephritis, nephrolithiasis, hiatal hernia (strangulated paraesophageal hernia), Boerhaave's syndrome, Mallory-Weiss tear, splenic artery aneurysm

LLQ

Diverticulitis, sigmoid volvulus, perforated colon, colon cancer, urinary tract infection, small bowel obstruction, inflammatory bowel disease, nephrolithiasis, pyelonephritis, fluid accumulation from aneurysm or perforation, referred hip pain; gynecologic causes (e.g., ectopic pregnancy), PID, mittelschmerz, ovarian cyst, fibroid degeneration, endometriosis, gynecologic tumor, torsion of cyst or fallopian tube

RLQ

Same as LLQ, especially **appendicitis,** also mesenteric lymphadenitis, cecal diverticulitis, Meckel's diverticulum, intussusception

What is the differential diagnosis of gynecologic pain?

Ovarian cyst, ovarian torsion, PID, tubo-ovarian abscess, fibroid, necrotic fibroid, pregnancy, ectopic pregnancy, endometritis, cancer of the cervix/uterus/ovary, endometrioma

What is the differential diagnosis of thoracic causes of abdominal pain?

MI (especially inferior), pneumonia, dissecting aorta, aortic aneurysm, empyema, esophageal rupture/tear, PTX, esophageal foreign body

What is the differential diagnosis of scrotal causes of lower abdominal pain?

Testicular torsion, epididymitis, orchitis, inguinal hernia, referred pain from nephrolithiasis or appendicitis

What are nonsurgical causes of abdominal pain?

Gastroenteritis, DKA, sickle cell crisis, rectus sheath hematoma, acute porphyria, PID, kidney stone, pyelonephritis, hepatitis, pancreatitis, pneumonia, MI, *C. difficile* colitis

What are unique differential diagnoses for the patient with AIDS and abdominal pain?

In addition to all common abdominal conditions:
CMV (most common)
Kaposi's sarcoma
Lymphoma
TB
MAI (*Mycobacterium avium* intracellulare)

What are the possible causes of suprapubic pain?

Cystitis, colonic pain, gynecologic causes (and of course appendicitis)

What causes pain limited to specific dermatomes?

Early zoster before vesicles erupt

What is referred pain?	Pain felt at a site distant from a disease process; caused by the convergence of multiple pain afferents in the posterior horn of the spinal cord
What is gastroenteritis?	Viral or bacterial infection of the GI tract, usually with vomiting and diarrhea, pain (usually **after** vomiting), nonsurgical
What is classically stated to be the "great imitator"?	Constipation can cause nonsurgical abdominal pain.
Name the classic locations of referred pain:	
Cholecystitis	Right subscapular pain (also epigastric)
Appendicitis	Early: periumbilical Rarely: testicular pain
Diaphragmatic irritation (from spleen, perforated ulcer, or abscess)	Shoulder pain (on the left a + Kehr's sign)
Pancreatitis/cancer	Back pain
Rectal disease	Pain in the small of the back
Nephrolithiasis	Testicular pain/flank pain
Rectal pain	Midline small of back pain
Small bowel	Periumbilical
Uterine pain	Midline small of back pain
Give the classic diagnosis for the following cases:	
"Abdominal pain out of proportion to exam"	Rule out mesenteric ischemia
Hypotension and pulsatile abdominal mass	Ruptured AAA; go to the OR
Fever, LLQ pain, and change in bowel habits	Diverticulitis

Give the test of choice for the following conditions:	
Cholelithiasis	Ultrasound (US)
Bile duct obstruction	US
Mesenteric ischemia	Mesenteric A-gram
Ruptured abdominal aortic aneurysm	O.R.
AAA	Abdominal CT or US
Abdominal abscess	Abdominal CT
Severe diverticulitis	Abdominal CT
What is the most common cause of RUQ pain?	Cholelithiasis
What is the most common cause of surgical RLQ pain?	Acute appendicitis
What is the most common cause of GI tract LLQ pain?	Diverticulitis

33 Hernias

What is a hernia?

(L. rupture) The protrusion of a peritoneal sac through a musculoaponeurotic barrier (e.g., abdominal wall); a fascial defect

What is the incidence?

Between 5% and 10% lifetime; 50% are indirect inguinal, 25% are direct inguinal, and approximately 15% are femoral

What are the precipitating factors?

Increased intra-abdominal pressure: straining at defecation or urination (rectal cancer, colon cancer, prostatic enlargement, constipation), obesity, pregnancy, ascites, valsavagenic (coughing) COPD; an abnormal congenital anatomic route (i.e., patent processus vaginalis)

Why should hernias be repaired?

To avoid complications of incarceration/strangulation, bowel necrosis, SBO, pain

What is more dangerous: a small or large hernia defect?

A small defect is more dangerous because a tight defect is more likely to strangulate if incarcerated.

Define the following descriptive terms:

Reducible

The ability to return the displaced organ or tissue/hernia contents to their usual anatomic site

Incarcerated

Swollen or fixed within the hernia sac (incarcerated = imprisoned); may cause intestinal obstruction (i.e., an irreducible hernia)

Strangulated	Incarcerated hernia with resulting ischemia; will result in signs and symptoms of ischemia and intestinal obstruction or bowel necrosis (think: strangulated = choked)
Complete	Hernia sac and its contents protrude all the way through the defect
Incomplete	Defect present without sac or contents protruding completely through it

Define the following types of hernias:

Sliding hernia	Hernia sac partially formed by the wall of a viscus (i.e., bladder/cecum)
Littre's hernia	Hernia involving a Meckel's diverticulum
Spigelian hernia	Hernia through the linea semilunaris (or spigelian fascia); also known as spontaneous lateral ventral hernia
Internal hernia	Hernia into or involving intra-abdominal structure
Obturator hernia	Hernia through obturator canal (females ≥ males)
Lumbar hernia	Petit's hernia or Grynfeltt's hernia
Petit's hernia	(Rare) hernia through Petit's triangle (A.K.A. inferior lumbar triangle) (Think: petit = small = inferior)
Grynfeltt's hernia	Hernia through Grynfeltt-Lesshaft triangle (superior lumbar triangle)
Pantaloon hernia	Hernia sac exists as **both a direct and indirect** hernia straddling the inferior epigastric vessels and protruding through the floor of the canal as well as the internal ring (two sacs separated by the inferior epigastric vessels [the pant crotch] like a pair of pantaloon pants)
Incisional hernia	Hernia through an incisional site; most common cause is a wound infection

Ventral hernia	Incisional hernia in the ventral abdominal wall
Parastomal hernia	Hernia adjacent to an ostomy (e.g., colostomy)
Sciatic hernia	Hernia through the sciatic foramen
Richter's hernia	Incarcerated or strangulated hernia involving only **one sidewall of the bowel,** which can spontaneously reduce, resulting in gangrenous bowel and perforation within the abdomen without signs of obstruction

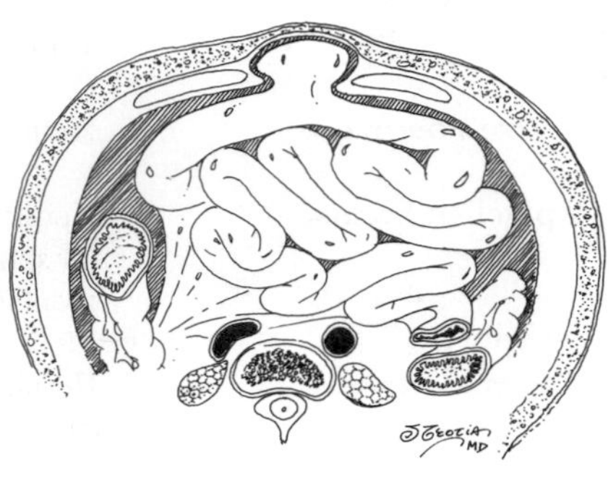

Epigastric hernia	Hernia through the linea alba above the umbilicus
Umbilical hernia	Hernia through the umbilical ring, associated with ascites, pregnancy, and obesity
Intraparietal hernia	Hernia in which abdominal contents migrate between the layers of the abdominal wall
Femoral hernia	Hernia medial to femoral vessels (under inguinal ligament)
Hesselbach's hernia	Hernia under inguinal ligament **lateral** to femoral vessels
Bochdalek's hernia	Hernia through the posterior diaphragm, usually on the left (think: Boch de lek = back to the left on the diaphragm)
Morgagni's hernia	Anterior parasternal diaphragmatic hernia

Properitoneal hernia	Intraparietal hernia between the peritoneum and transversalis fascia
Cooper's hernia	Hernia through the femoral canal and tracking into the scrotum or labia majus
Indirect inguinal	Inguinal hernia lateral to Hesselbach's triangle
Direct inguinal	Inguinal hernia within Hesselbach's triangle
Hiatal hernia	Hernia through esophageal hiatus

What are the boundaries of Hesselbach's triangle?

1. Inferior epigastric vessels
2. Inguinal ligament (Poupart's)
3. Lateral border of the rectus sheath

Floor consists of internal oblique and the transversus abdominis muscle.

What are the layers of the abdominal wall?

Skin
Subcutaneous fat
Scarpa's fascia
External oblique
Internal oblique
Transversus abdominus
Transversalis fascia
Preperitoneal fat
Peritoneum
Note: all three muscle layer aponeuroses form the anterior rectus sheath, with the posterior rectus sheath being deficient below the arcuate line.

GROIN HERNIAS

What are differential diagnoses of a groin mass?

Lymphadenopathy, hematoma, seroma, abscess, hydrocele, femoral artery aneurysm, EIC, undescended testicle, sarcoma, hernias, testicle torsion

DIRECT INGUINAL HERNIA

What is it?

A hernia within the floor of Hesselbach's triangle, i.e., the hernia sac does not traverse the internal ring (think of **directly** through the abdominal wall)

What is the cause?
Acquired defect from mechanical breakdown over the years

What is the incidence?
Approximately 1% of all men; frequency increases with advanced age

What nerve runs with the spermatic cord in the inguinal canal?
Ilioinguinal nerve

INDIRECT INGUINAL HERNIA

What is it?
Hernia through the internal ring of the inguinal canal, traveling down toward the external ring; it may enter the scrotum upon exiting the external ring (i.e., if complete); think of the hernia sac traveling **indirectly** through the abdominal wall from the internal ring to the external ring

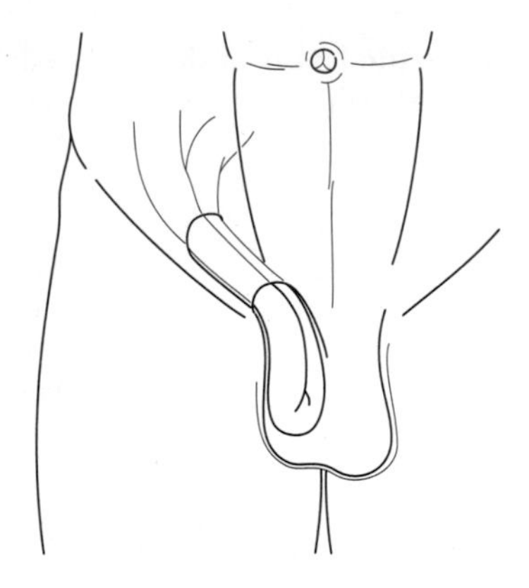

What is the cause?
Patent processus vaginalis (i.e., congenital)

What is the incidence?
Approximately 5% of all men; most common hernia in both men **and** women

How is an inguinal hernia diagnosed?
Relies mainly on history and physical exam with index finger invaginated into the external ring and palpation of hernia; examine the patient standing up if diagnosis is not obvious
Note: if swelling occurs below the inguinal ligament, it is possibly a femoral hernia.

What is the differential diagnosis of an inguinal hernia?

Inguinal lymphadenopathy, femoral lymphadenopathy, psoas abscess, ectopic testis, hydrocele of the cord, saphenous varix, lipoma, varicocele

What is the risk of strangulation?

Higher with indirect than direct inguinal hernia, but highest in femoral hernias

What is the treatment?

Emergent herniorrhaphy is indicated if strangulation is suspected or acute incarceration is present; otherwise, elective herniorrhaphy is indicated to prevent the chance of incarceration/strangulation.

INGUINAL HERNIA REPAIRS

Bassini?

Sutures approximate reflection of inguinal ligament (Poupart's) to the transversus abdominis aponeurosis/ conjoint tendon

McVay?

Cooper's ligament sutured transversus abdominis aponeurosis/conjoint tendon (A.K.A. "tension-free repair")

Lichtenstein?

"Tension-free" repair using mesh

Shouldice?

Imbrication of the floor of the inguinal canal (A.K.A. "Canadian repair")

Plug and patch?

Placing a plug of mesh in hernia defect and then overlaying a patch of mesh over inguinal floor (requires few if any sutures in mesh!)

High ligation?

Ligation and transection of indirect hernia sac without repair of inguinal floor (used only in **children**)

TAPP procedure?

Trans**A**bdominal **P**re**P**eritoneal inguinal hernia repair

TEPA procedure?

Totally **E**xtra**P**eritoneal **A**pproach

What are the indications for laparoscopic inguinal hernia repair?

1. Bilateral inguinal hernias
2. Recurring hernia
3. Need to resume full activity as soon as possible

CLASSIC INTRAOPERATIVE INGUINAL HERNIA QUESTIONS

What is the first subcutaneous named layer?
Scarpa's fascia (thin in adults)

What is the name of the subcutaneous vein that is ligated?
Superficial epigastric vein

What happens if you cut the ilioinguinal nerve?
Numbness of inner thigh or lateral scrotum; usually goes away in 6 months

From what abdominal muscle layer is the cremaster muscle derived?
Internal oblique muscle

From what abdominal muscle layer is the inguinal ligament (A.K.A. Poupart's ligament) derived?
External oblique muscle

To what does the inguinal (Poupart's) ligament attach?
Anterior superior iliac spine to the pubic tubercle

Which nerve travels on the spermatic cord?
Ilioinguinal nerve

What is in the spermatic cord (6)?
1. Cremasteric muscle fibers
2. Vas deferens
3. Testicular artery
4. Testicular pampiniform venous plexus
5. ± hernia sac
6. Genital branch of the genitofemoral nerve

What is the hernia sac made of?
Basically peritoneum or a patent processus vaginalis

What attaches the testicle to the scrotum?
The gubernaculum

What is the most common organ in an inguinal hernia sac in men?
Small intestine

What is the most common organ in an inguinal hernia sac in women?
Ovary/fallopian tube

What lies in the inguinal canal in the female instead of the VAS?

Round ligament

Where in the inguinal canal does the hernia sac lie in relation to the other structures?

Anteromedially

What is a "cord lipoma"?

Preperitoneal fat on the cord structures (pushed in by the hernia sac); not a real lipoma; remove surgically, if feasible

What is a small outpouching of testicular tissue off of the testicle?

Testicular appendage (A.K.A. the appendix testes); remove with electrocautery

What action should be taken if a suture is placed through the femoral artery or vein during an inguinal herniorrhaphy?

Remove the suture as soon as possible and apply pressure (i.e., do not tie the suture down!).

What nerve is found on top of the spermatic cord?

Ilioinguinal nerve

What nerve travels within the spermatic cord?

The genital branch of the genitofemoral nerve

What is Hesselbach's triangle?

1. Epigastric vessels
2. Inguinal ligament
3. Lateral border of the rectus sheath

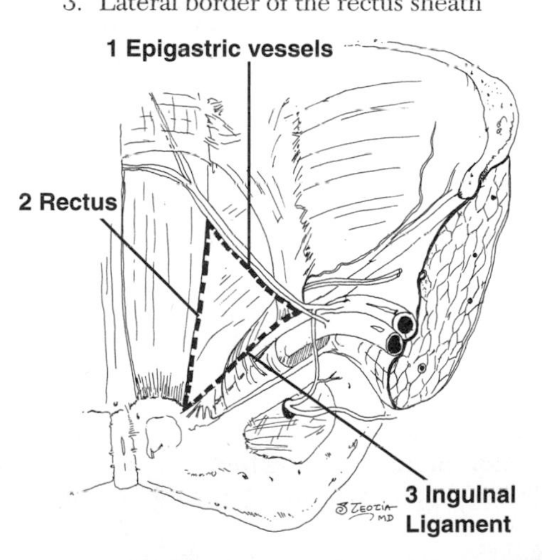

What type of hernia goes through Hesselbach's triangle?

A direct hernia due to a weak abdominal floor

What is a "relaxing incision"?

Incision(s) in the rectus sheath to relax the conjoint tendon so that it can be approximated to the reflection of the inguinal ligament without tension

What is the conjoint tendon?

The aponeurotic attachments of the transversus abdominis to the pubic tubercle (the classic conjoining of the aponeurosis of the internal oblique and transversus aponeurosis attaching to the tubercle is actually very rare [< 4%])

Define inguinal anatomy.

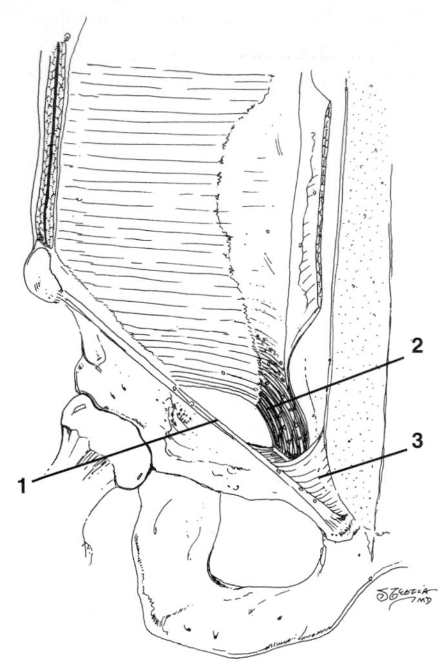

1. Inguinal ligament (Poupart's ligament)
2. Transversus aponeurosis
3. Conjoint tendon

How tight should the new internal inguinal ring be?

Should allow entrance of the tip of a Kelly clamp but not a finger (the new external inguinal ring should not be tight and should allow entrance of a finger)

What percentage of the strength of an inguinal floor repair does the external oblique aponeurosis represent?

ZERO

FEMORAL HERNIA

What is it?

Hernia traveling beneath the inguinal ligament down the femoral canal medial to the femoral vessels

What is the boundary of the femoral canal?

1. Cooper's ligament posteriorly
2. Inguinal ligament anteriorly
3. Femoral vein laterally
4. Lacunar ligament medially

What factors are femoral hernias associated with?

Women, pregnancy, and exertion

What percentage of all hernias are femoral hernias?

5%

What percentage of patients with a femoral hernia are WOMEN?

85%!

What are the complications?

Approximately one-third incarcerate (due to narrow, unforgiving neck).

What is the most common hernia in females?

Indirect inguinal hernia

What is the repair?

McVay (Cooper's ligament repair)

HERNIA REVIEW QUESTIONS

Should elective TURP or elective herniorrhaphy be performed first?

TURP

Which type of esophageal hiatal hernia is associated with GE reflux?

Sliding esophageal hiatal hernia

How can an incarcerated hernia be reduced in the ER?

1. Apply ice to incarcerated hernia.
2. Sedate.
3. Use the Trendelenburg position for inguinal hernias.
4. Apply steady manual pressure.
5. Admit and observe for signs of necrotic bowel after reduction.
6. Perform surgical herniorrhaphy ASAP.

What is the major difference in repairing a pediatric indirect inguinal hernia and an adult inguinal hernia?

In babies and children it is rarely necessary to repair the inguinal floor; repair with "high ligation" of the hernia sac.

What is the Howship-Romberg sign?

Pain along the medial aspect of the proximal thigh from nerve compression caused by obturator hernia

What is the "silk glove" sign?

The inguinal hernia sac in an infant/toddler feels like a finger of a silk glove when rolled under the examining finger.

ESOPHAGEAL HIATAL HERNIAS

What are the types?

1. Paraesophageal
2. Sliding

PARAESOPHAGEAL HIATAL HERNIA

What is it?

Herniation of all or part of the stomach through the esophageal hiatus into the thorax without displacement of the gastroesophageal junction; also known as type II hiatal hernia

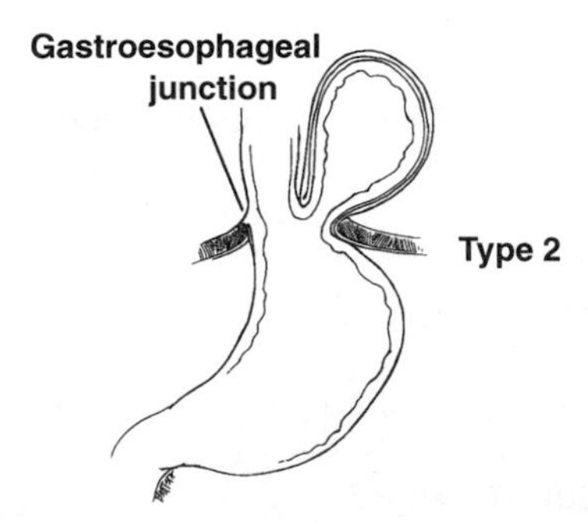

What is the incidence?

Less than 5% of all hiatal hernias (rare)

What are the symptoms?

Derived from mechanical obstruction; emdysphagia, stasis gastric ulcer, and strangulation; many cases are asymptomatic and not associated with reflux because of a relatively normal position of the GE junction

What are the complications?

Hemorrhage, incarceration, obstruction, and strangulation

What is the treatment?

Surgical, because of frequency and severity of potential complications

SLIDING ESOPHAGEAL HIATAL HERNIA

What is it?

Both the stomach and GE junction herniate into the thorax via the esophageal hiatus; also known as type I hiatal hernia.

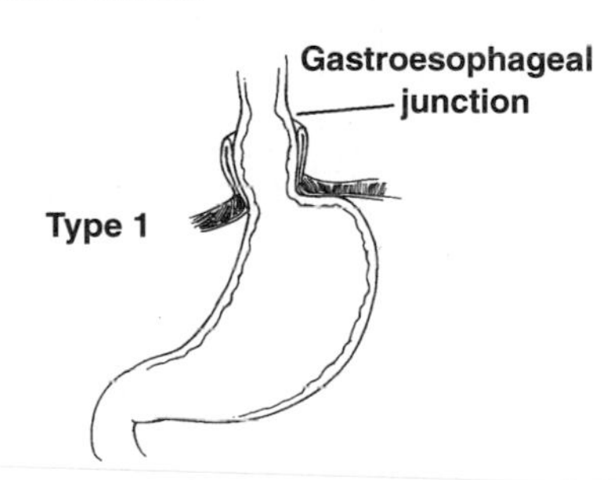

What is the incidence?

More than 90% of all hiatal hernias

What are the symptoms?

Most patients are asymptomatic, but the condition can cause **reflux,** dysphagia (from inflammatory edema), esophagitis, and pulmonary problems secondary to aspiration.

>How is it diagnosed?

UGI series, manometry, EGD with biopsy for esophagitis

What are the complications?

Reflux → esophagitis → Barrett's esophagus → cancer and stricture formation; aspiration pneumonia; it can also result in UGI bleeding from esophageal ulcerations

What is the treatment?

85% of cases treated medically with antacids, H_2 blockers/PPIs, head elevation after meals, small meals, and no food prior to sleeping; 15% of cases require surgery for persistent symptoms despite adequate medical treatment

What is the surgical treatment?

Laparoscopic Nissen fundoplication (LAP NISSEN) involves wrapping the fundus around the LES and suturing it in place

34 Laparoscopy

What is laparoscopy?

Minimally invasive surgical technique using gas to insufflate the peritoneum and instruments manipulated through ports introduced through small incisions with video camera guidance

What gas is used and why?

CO_2 because of better solubility in blood and, thus, less risk of gas embolism, noncombustible

Which operations are performed with the laparoscope?

Frequently—cholecystectomy; appendectomy; inguinal hernia repair; ventral hernia repair, Nissen fundoplication
Infrequently—bowel resection, colostomy, surgery for PUD (PGV, perforation), colectomy, splenectomy

What are the contraindications?

Absolute—hypovolemic shock, severe cardiac decompensation
Relative—extensive intraperitoneal adhesions, diaphragmatic hernia, COPD

What are the associated complications?

Pneumothorax, bleeding, perforating injuries, infection, intestinal injuries, solid organ injury, major vascular injury, **CO_2 embolus,** bladder injury, hernia at larger trocar sites, DVT

What prophylactic measure should every patient get when they are going to have a laparoscopic procedure?

SCD boots—Sequential Compression Device (and most add an OGT to decompress the stomach; Foley catheter is usually used for pelvic procedures)

What are the cardiovascular effects of a pneumoperitoneum?	**Increased afterload** and **decreased preload** (but the CVP and PCWP are deceivingly elevated!)
What is the effect of CO_2 insufflation on end tidal CO_2 levels?	Increased as a result of absorption of CO_2 into the bloodstream; the body compensates with increased ventilation and blows the extra CO_2 off and thus there is no acidosis
What are the advantages over laparotomy?	Shorter hospitalization, less pain and scarring, lower cost, decreased ileus
What is the Veress needle?	Needle with spring-loaded, retractable, blunt inner protective tube that protrudes from the needle end when it enters peritoneal cavity; used for blind entrance and then insufflation of CO_2 through the Veress needle
How can it be verified that the Veress needle is in the peritoneum?	Syringe of saline; saline should flow freely without pressure through the needle "drop test"
If the Veress needle is not in the peritoneal cavity, what happens to the CO_2 flow/pressure?	Flow decreases and pressure is high
What is the Hasson technique?	No Veress needle—cut down and place trocar under **direct visualization**
What is the cause of post-laparoscopic shoulder pain?	Referred pain from CO_2 on diaphragm and diaphragm stretch
What is a laparoscopic-assisted procedure?	Laparoscopic dissection; then, part of the procedure is performed through an open incision
What is FRED®?	**F**og **R**eduction **E**limination **D**evice; sponge with antifog solution used to coat the camera lens
Give some tips for "driving" the camera during laparoscopy.	1. Keep the camera centered on the action. 2. Watch all trocars as they enter the peritoneal cavity (and the tissues beyond, so they can be avoided!).

3. Watch all instruments as they come through the trocars (unless directed otherwise).
4. Ask if you want to come out and clean and re-FRED the lens.
5. Look outside the body at the trocars and instrument angles to reorient yourself.
6. Keep the camera oriented at all times (i.e., up and down); usually the camera cord is on the bottom of the camera—orient yourself to the camera before entering the abdomen.
7. You may clean the camera lens at times by lightly touching the lens to the liver or peritoneum.
8. Never let the camera lens come into contact with the bowel because it may get very hot and you can burn a hole in the bowel or burn the drapes!
9. Put your helmet on (i.e., expect to get yelled at!).
10. Never act agitated when the surgeons are a little abrupt (e.g., "Center—center the camera!").
11. Always watch the trocars as they are removed from the abdominal wall for bleeding from the site and view the layers of the abdominal wall looking for bleeding as you pull the camera trocar out at the end of the case.

At what length must you close trocar sites?

7 mm should be closed.

How do you get the spleen out after a laparoscopic splenectomy?

Crush it in a bag—then pull bag out of a trocar site.

What is an IOC?

Intra**O**perative **C**holangiogram (done during a lap chole to evaluate the thoracic duct anatomy and to look for any retained duct stone)

35 Trauma

What widely accepted protocol does trauma care in the United States follow?

The Advanced Trauma Life Support (ATLS) precepts of the American College of Surgeons

What are the three main elements of the ATLS protocol?

1. Primary survey/resuscitation
2. Secondary survey
3. Definitive care

How and when should the patient history be obtained?

It should be obtained while completing the primary survey; often the rescue squad, witnesses, and family members must be relied upon.

PRIMARY SURVEY

What are the five steps of the primary survey?

A—**A**irway (and C-spine stabilization)
B—**B**reathing
C—**C**irculation
D—**D**isability
E—**E**xposure and **E**nvironment

What principles are followed in completing the primary survey?

Life-threatening problems discovered during the primary survey are **always** addressed **before** proceeding to the next step.

AIRWAY

What are the goals during assessment of the airway?

Securing the airway and protecting the spinal cord

In addition to the airway, what MUST be considered during the airway step?

Spinal immobilization

What comprises spinal immobilization?

Use of a full backboard and rigid cervical collar

In an alert patient, what is the quickest test for an adequate airway?

Ask a question; if the patient can speak, the airway is intact.

What is the first maneuver used to establish an airway?

Chin lift, jaw thrust, or both; if successful, often an oral or nasal airway can be used to temporarily maintain the airway

If these methods are unsuccessful, what is the next maneuver used to establish an airway?

Endotracheal intubation, either nasal or oral (oral if the patient is not breathing with inline C-spine traction)

When is nasotracheal intubation contraindicated?

In patients with maxillofacial fracture or apnea

If all other methods are unsuccessful, what is the definitive airway?

Cricothyroidotomy, A.K.A. "surgical airway": incise the cricothyroid membrane between the cricoid cartilage inferiorly and the thyroid cartilage superiorly and place an endotracheal or tracheostomy tube into the trachea

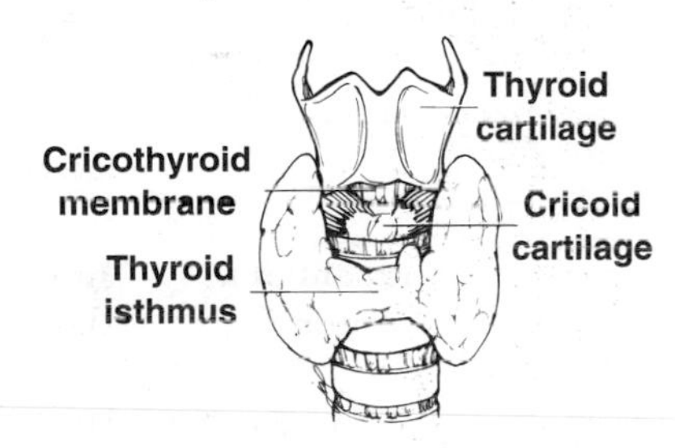

What must always be kept in mind during difficult attempts at establishing an airway?

Spinal immobilization and adequate oxygenation; if at all possible, patients must be adequately ventilated with 100% oxygen using a bag and mask before any attempt at establishing an airway

BREATHING

What are the goals in assessing breathing?

Securing oxygenation and ventilation
Treating life-threatening thoracic injuries

What comprises adequate assessment of breathing?

Inspection—for air movement, respiratory rate, cyanosis, tracheal shift, jugular venous distention, asymmetric chest expansion, use of accessory muscles of respiration, open chest wounds

Auscultation—for breath sounds
Percussion—for hyperresonance or dullness over either lung field
Palpation—for presence of subcutaneous emphysema, flail segments

What are the life-threatening conditions that MUST be diagnosed and treated during the breathing step?

Tension pneumothorax, open pneumothorax, massive hemothorax

Pneumothorax

What is it?

Injury to the lung, resulting in release of air into the pleural space between the normally apposed parietal and visceral pleura

How is it diagnosed?

Tension pneumothorax is a clinical diagnosis: dyspnea, jugular venous distention, tachypnea, anxiety, pleuritic chest pain, unilateral decreased or absent breath sounds, tracheal shift away from the affected side, hyperresonance on the affected side

What is the treatment of a tension pneumothorax?

Immediate decompression by **needle thoracostomy** in the second intercostal space midclavicular line, followed by **tube thoracostomy** placed in the anterior/midaxillary line in the fourth intercostal space (level of the nipple in men)

What is the medical term for a "sucking chest wound"?

Open pneumothorax

How is an open pneumothorax diagnosed and treated?

Diagnosis: usually obvious, with air movement through a chest wall defect and ptx on CXR
Treatment in the ER: +/− intubation with positive-pressure ventilation, tube thoracostomy (chest tube), occlusive dressing over chest wall defect

Flail Chest

What is it?
Two separate fractures in three or more consecutive ribs

How is it diagnosed?
A flail segment of chest wall that moves **paradoxically** (sucks in with inspiration and pushes out with expiration opposite the rest of the chest wall)

What is the major cause of respiratory compromise with flail chest?
Underlying pulmonary contusion!

What is the treatment?
Intubation with positive pressure ventilation and PEEP prn (let ribs heal on their own)

Cardiac Tamponade

What is it?
Bleeding into the pericardial sac, resulting in constriction of heart, decreasing inflow and resulting in decreased cardiac output

What are the signs and symptoms?
Tachycardia/shock with **Beck's triad,** pulsus paradoxus, Kussmaul's sign

Define the following:

Beck's triad
1. Hypotension
2. Muffled heart sounds
3. JVD

Kussmaul's sign
JVD with inspiration

How is cardiac tamponade definitely diagnosed?
Ultrasound (echocardiogram)

What is the treatment?
Immediate IV fluid bolus; with pericardiocentesis, subsequent surgical exploration is mandatory

Massive Hemothorax

How is it diagnosed?
Hypotension; unilaterally decreased or absent breath sounds; dullness to percussion; obvious appearance on CXR if massive (but remember, on upright CXR the diaphragm can hide up to 500 ml of blood)

What is the treatment?

Volume replacement
Tube thoracostomy (chest tube)
Use of cell saver, if available
Removal of the blood (which will allow apposition of the parietal and visceral pleura, sealing the defect and slowing the bleeding)

What are indications for emergent thoracotomy for hemothorax?

Massive hemothorax =
1. > 1500 cc of blood on initial placement of chest tube
2. Persistent > 200 cc of bleeding via chest tube per hour

CIRCULATION

What are the goals in assessing circulation?

Securing adequate tissue perfusion; treatment of external bleeding

What is the initial test for adequate circulation?

Palpation of pulses:
As a rough guide, if a radial pulse is palpable, then systolic pressure is at least 80 mm Hg; if a femoral or carotid pulse is palpable, then systolic pressure is at least 60 mm Hg.

What comprises adequate assessment of circulation?

Heart rate, blood pressure, peripheral perfusion, urinary output, mental status, capillary refill (normal < 2 seconds), exam of skin: cold, clammy = hypovolemia

Who can be hypovolemic with normal blood pressure?

The young; autonomic tone can maintain blood pressure until cardiovascular collapse is imminent

Which patients may not mount a tachycardic response to hypovolemic shock?

Those with concomitant spinal cord injuries
Those on β-blockers
Well-conditioned athletes

How are sites of external bleeding treated?

By direct pressure; avoid tourniquets and blind clamping of bleeding sites (both lead to increased limb loss)

What is the best and preferred intravenous (IV) access in the trauma patient?

"Two large-bore IV's" (14–16 gauge), IV catheters in the upper extremities (peripheral IV access)

What are alternate sites of IV access?

Percutaneous and cutdown catheters in the lower leg saphenous (cutdown) and femoral veins (percutaneous); avoid subclavian and jugular lines if possible because of their increased morbidity in the trauma patient (e.g., PTX)

For a femoral vein catheter, how can the anatomy of the right groin be remembered?

Lateral to medial navel:
N—**n**erve
A—**a**rtery
V—**v**ein
E—**e**xtralymphatic material
L—**l**ymphatics
Thus, the vein is medial to the femoral artery pulse.

What is the resuscitation fluid of choice?

Lactated Ringer's (LR) solution (isotonic, and the lactate helps buffer the hypovolemia-induced metabolic acidosis)

What types of decompression must the trauma patient receive?

Gastric decompression with an NG tube and Foley catheter bladder decompression after **normal rectal exam**

What are the contraindications to placement of a Foley?

Signs of urethral injury:
Severe pelvic fracture in men
Blood at the urethral meatus (penile opening)
"High-riding" prostate (loss of urethral tethering)
Scrotal/perineal injury/ecchymosis

What test should be obtained prior to placing a Foley catheter if urethral injury is feared?

A retrograde urethrogram (RUG; dye in penis retrograde to the bladder and x-ray looking for extravasation of dye)

How is gastric decompression achieved with a maxillofacial fracture?

Not with an NG tube because the tube may perforate through the cribriform plate into the brain; place an **oral**-gastric tube (OGT), not an NG tube

DISABILITY

What are the goals in assessing disability?

Determination of neurologic injury (think: neurologic disability)

What comprises adequate assessment of disability?

Mental status—Glasgow Coma Scale (GCS)
Pupils—a blown pupil reflects ipsilateral brain mass (blood) as herniation of the brain compresses CN III
Motor/sensory—screening exam for lateralizing extremity movement, sensory deficits

Describe the GCS scoring system.

Eye opening (E)
4—Opens spontaneously
3—Opens to voice (command)
2—Opens to painful stimulus
1—Does not open eyes
(**think:** eyes = "four eyes")
Motor response (M)
6—Obeys commands
5—Localizes painful stimulus
4—Withdraws from pain
3—Decorticate posture
2—Decerebrate posture
1—No movement
(**think:** motor = 6 "cylinder motor")
Verbal response (V)
5—Appropriate and oriented
4—Confused
3—Inappropriate words
2—Incomprehensible sounds
1—No sounds
(**think:** verbal 5 = "Jackson 5")

What is the GCS score for a dead man?

GCS 3

What is the GCS score for a patient in a "coma"?

GCS < 8

How does scoring differ if the patient is intubated?

The verbal evaluation is omitted and replaced with a "T"; thus, the highest score for an intubated patient is 10T.

EXPOSURE AND ENVIRONMENT

What are the goals in obtaining adequate exposure?

Complete disrobing to allow a thorough visual inspection and digital palpation of the patient during the secondary survey

What is the "environment" of the E?	Keep a warm **E**nvironment (i.e., keep the patient warm; a hypothermic patient can become acidotic, dysrhythmic, and coagulopathic).

SECONDARY SURVEY

What principle is followed in completing the secondary survey?	Complete physical exam, including all orifices: ears, nose, mouth, vagina, rectum
Why look in the ears?	Hemotympanum is a sign of basilar skull fracture; otorrhea is a sign of basilar skull fracture.
Examination of what part of the trauma patient's body is often forgotten?	The patient's back (logroll the patient and examine!)
What are typical signs of basilar skull fracture?	Raccoon eyes, Battle's sign, clear otorrhea or rhinorrhea, hemotympanum
What diagnosis in the anterior chamber must not be missed on the eye exam?	Traumatic hyphema = blood in the anterior chamber of the eye
What potentially destructive lesion must not be missed on the nasal exam?	Nasal septal hematoma; the hematoma must be evacuated; if not, it can result in pressure necrosis of the septum!
What is the best indication of a mandibular fracture?	Dental malocclusion, tell the patient to "bite down" and ask: "Does that feel normal to you?"
What signs of thoracic trauma are often found on the neck exam?	Crepitus or subcutaneous emphysema from tracheobronchial disruption/PTX; tracheal deviation from tension pneumothorax; jugular venous distention from cardiac tamponade; carotid bruit heard with seatbelt neck injury, resulting in carotid artery injury
What is the best exam for broken ribs or sternum?	Lateral and anterior-posterior compression of the thorax to elicit pain/instability

What physical signs are diagnostic for thoracic great vessel injury?

None; diagnosis of great vessel injury requires a high index of suspicion based on the mechanism of injury, associated injuries, and CXR/radiographic findings (e.g., widened mediastinum)

What must be considered in every penetrating injury of the thorax at or below the level of the nipple?

Concomitant injury to the abdomen; remember, the diaphragm extends to the level of the nipples in the male on full expiration

What is the significance of subcutaneous air?

Indicates PTX, until proven otherwise

What is the proper technique for examining the thoracic and lumbar spine?

Logrolling the patient to allow complete visualization of the back and palpation of the spine to elicit pain over fractures

What conditions must exist to pronounce an abdominal physical exam negative?

An alert patient without any evidence of head/spinal cord injury or drug/ETOH intoxication (even then, the abdominal exam is not 100% accurate)

What physical signs may indicate intra-abdominal injury?

Tenderness; guarding, plus rebound tenderness and other signs of peritoneal irritation; progressive distention (always use a gastric tube for decompression of air); seatbelt sign

What is the seatbelt sign?

Ecchymosis on lower abdomen from wearing a seatbelt (up to 20% of patients with this sign have a small bowel perforation!)

What must be documented from the rectal exam?

Sphincter tone (as an indication of spinal cord injury); presence of blood (as an indication of colon or rectal injury); prostate position (as an indication of urethral injury)

What is the best physical exam technique to test for pelvic fractures?

Lateral compression of the iliac crests and greater trochanters and anterior-posterior compression of the symphysis pubis to elicit pain/instability

What physical signs indicate possible urethral injury, thus contraindicating placement of a Foley catheter?

High-riding ballotable prostate on rectal exam; presence of blood at the meatus; scrotal or perineal ecchymosis

What must be documented from the extremity exam?

Any fractures or joint injuries; any open wounds; motor and sensory exam, particularly distal to any fractures; distal pulses; peripheral perfusion

What complication after prolonged ischemia to the lower extremity must be treated immediately?

Compartment syndrome

What is the treatment for this condition?

Fasciotomy (four-compartment below the knee)

What injuries must be suspected in a trauma patient with a progressive decline in mental status?

Epidural hematoma, subdural hematoma, brain swelling with rising intracranial pressure
But **hypoxia/hypotension must be ruled out!**

TRAUMA STUDIES

During evaluation of blunt trauma, radiographic films are usually obtained sometime during the primary survey in the ER. What films are required?

The trauma triple:
1. Lateral cervical spine film
2. AP (anterior-to-posterior) chest film
3. AP pelvis film

Also during the primary survey, specimens are sent for laboratory analysis. Which specimens are usually sent?

Blood for complete blood count, chemistries, amylase, liver function tests, lactic acid, coagulation studies, and **type and crossmatch;** urine for urinalysis

Will the hematocrit be low after an acute massive hemorrhage?

No (no time to equilibrate)

How can a c-spine be cleared?

1. Clinically by physical exam
2. Radiographically

What patients can have their C-spines cleared by PE?
No neck pain on palpation or with full range of motion (FROM) with no neurologic injury (GCS 15), no ETOH/ drugs, no distracting injury, no pain meds

How can you clear the C-spine radiographically?
Hot area of controversy/study! But all would agree if the three-view plain films (AP, odontoid, lateral) views are negative and flexion-extension lateral views are all negative in an awake patient, the C-spine is cleared radiographically.

What films are required to evaluate for possible cervical spinal injury?
Lateral C-spine, AP C-spine, and open-mouth odontoid

What vertebral bodies must be seen to adequately evaluate a lateral cervical spine film?
C1 to T1

What view is used for seeing these vertebrae beyond the normal lateral spine film?
Swimmer's view can help visualize C7 to T1

What if you cannot see C7-T1 with the swimmer's view?
CT scan the area

Which x-rays are used for evaluation of cervical spine LIGAMENTOUS injury?
Lateral flexion and extension C-spine films

What findings on chest film are suggestive of thoracic great vessel injury?
Widened mediastinum (most common finding), apical pleural capping, loss of aortic contour/KNOB/a-p window, depression of left main stem bronchus, nasogastric tube/tracheal deviation, pleural fluid, elevation of right mainstem bronchus

What study is used to rule out thoracic great vessel injury?
Thoracic arch aortogram (gold standard)
Spiral CT of mediastinum looking for mediastinal hematoma

What percentage of thoracic aortograms will reveal an aortic injury?
Only about 10% of studies are positive

What studies are available to evaluate for intra-abdominal injury?

FAST, CT, DPL

What is a FAST exam?

Ultrasound: Focused Assessment with Sonography for Trauma = FAST

What does the FAST exam look for?

Blood in the peritoneal cavity looking at Morison's pouch, bladder, spleen, and pericardial sac

What does DPL stand for?

Diagnostic peritoneal lavage

What diagnostic test is rapidly replacing DPL for evaluation of the unstable patient with blunt abdominal trauma?

FAST

What is the indication for abdominal CT in blunt trauma?

Stable vital signs with abdominal pain/tenderness

What is the indication for DPL or FAST in blunt trauma?

Unstable vital signs

How is a DPL performed?

Place a catheter below the umbilicus (in patients without a pelvic fracture) into peritoneal cavity.

Aspirate for blood and if less than 10 cc are aspirated, infuse 1 L of saline or LR.

Drain the fluid (by gravity) and analyze.

Where should the DPL catheter be placed in a patient with a pelvic fracture?

Above the umbilicus

A common error—if you go below the umbilicus, you may get into a pelvic hematoma tracking between the fascia layers and thus obtain a false-positive DPL.

What constitutes a positive peritoneal tap?

Prior to starting a peritoneal lavage, the DPL catheter should be aspirated. If more than 10 ml of blood or enteric contents are aspirated, then this constitutes a positive tap and requires laparotomy.

What are the indicators of a positive peritoneal lavage?

Classic: inability to read newsprint through lavaged fluid
RBC ≥ 100,000/mm^3
WBC ≥ 500/mm^3 (Note: mm^3, not mm^2)
Lavage fluid (LR/NS) drained from chest tube, Foley, NG tube
Less common:
- Bile present
- Bacteria present
- Feces present
- Vegetable matter present
- Elevated amylase level

What must be in place before a DPL is performed?

NG tube and Foley catheter (to remove the stomach and bladder from the firing line!)

What injuries does CT miss?

Small bowel injuries and diaphragm injuries

What injuries does DPL miss?

Retroperitoneal injuries

What study is used to evaluate the urethra in cases of possible disruption due to blunt trauma?

Retrograde urethrogram (RUG)

What are the most emergent orthopaedic injuries?

1. Hip dislocation—must be reduced immediately (on the x-ray table or during resuscitation in the ER)
2. Exsanguinating pelvic fracture (external fixator)

What findings would require a celiotomy in a blunt trauma victim?

Peritoneal signs, free air on AXR/CT, unstable patient with positive FAST exam or positive DPL results

What is the treatment of a gunshot wound to the belly?

Exploratory laparotomy

What is the treatment of a stab wound to the belly?

If there are peritoneal signs, heavy bleeding, shock, omentum or bowel sticking out the wound, unstable vital signs, perform exploratory laparotomy. Otherwise, many surgeons observe the asymptomatic stab wound patient closely.

PENETRATING NECK INJURIES

What depth of neck injury must be further evaluated?
Penetrating injury through the platysma

Define the anatomy of the neck by trauma zones:

Zone III
Angle of the mandible and up

Zone II
Angle of the mandible to the cricoid cartilage

Zone I
Below the cricoid cartilage
Note: the zones are in the same anatomic order as the LeFort facial fractures (III, II, I).

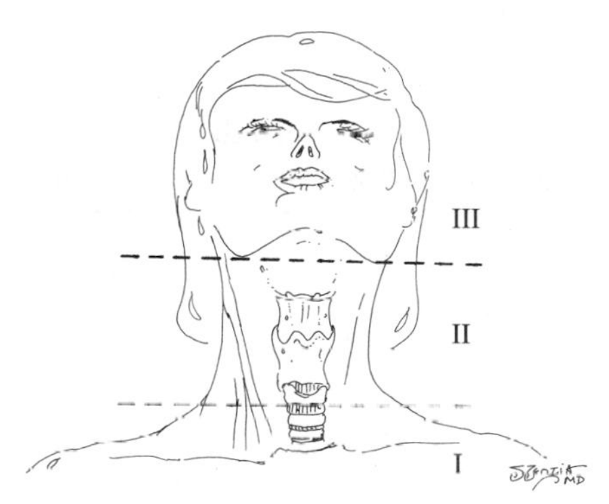

How do most surgeons treat penetrating neck injuries (those that penetrate the platysma) by neck zone:

Zone III
Selective exploration

Zone II
Surgical exploration

Zone I
Selective exploration

What is selective exploration?
Selective exploration is based on diagnostic studies that include A-Gram (carotid), bronchoscopy (trachea), esophagoscopy, and esophagography (esophagus). Explore surgically as indicated by study results.

What are the indications for surgical exploration in all penetrating neck wounds (Zones I, II, III)?

"**Hard** signs" of significant neck damage: **shock,** exsanguinating hemorrhage, expanding hematoma, pulsatile hematoma, neurologic injury, SUBQ emphysema

MISCELLANEOUS TRAUMA FACTS

What is the "3-for-1" rule?

The trauma patient in hypovolemic shock acutely requires 3 L of crystalloid (LR) for every 1 L of blood loss.

What is the minimal urine output for an adult trauma patient?

50 ml/hr

How much blood can be lost into the thigh with a closed femur fracture?

Up to 3 L of blood, or more than half the patient's blood volume!

Can an adult lose enough blood in the skull from a brain injury to cause hypovolemic shock?

Absolutely not! But infants can lose enough blood from a brain injury to cause shock.

What is the brief ATLS history?

An "AMPLE" history:
A—**A**llergies
M—**M**edications
P—**P**MH
L—**L**ast meal (when)
E—**E**vents (of injury, etc.)

In what population is a surgical cricothyroidotomy not recommended?

Any patient younger than 12 years; instead perform needle cricothyroidotomy

What are the signs of a laryngeal fracture?

Subcutaneous emphysema in neck
Altered voice
Palpable laryngeal fracture

What is the treatment of rectal penetrating injury?

Diverting proximal colostomy; closure of perforation (if easy, and definitely if intraperitoneal); and **presacral drainage**

What is the treatment of extraperitoneal minor bladder rupture?

Catheter bladder (Foley) drainage and observation; intraperitoneal or large bladder rupture requires operative closure in three layers

What intraabdominal injury is associated with seatbelt use?

Small bowel injuries (L2 fracture, pancreatic injury)

What is the treatment of a pelvic fracture?

± MAST trousers until the external fixator is placed; IVF/blood, supraumbilical DPL; and A-gram to embolize bleeding pelvic vessels

Do not enter pelvic hematoma in the OR for positive DPL unless there is major arterial injury.

Bleeding from pelvic fractures is most commonly caused by arterial or venous bleeding?

Venous

If a patient has a laceration through an eyebrow, should you shave the eyebrow prior to suturing it closed?

No—20% of the time, the eyebrow will not grow back if shaved!

What is the treatment of extensive irreparable duodenal and pancreatic head injury?

Trauma Whipple

What is the most common intra-abdominal organ injured with penetrating trauma?

Small bowel

How high up do the diaphragms go?

To the nipples (intercostal space # 4); thus, intra-abdominal injury with penetrating injury below the nipples must be ruled out

Classic trauma question: "If you have only one vial of blood from a trauma victim to send to the lab, what test should be ordered?"

Type and cross (for blood transfusion)

What is the treatment of penetrating injury to the colon?

If the patient is unstable, there is abundant fecal soilage, or both, resection and colostomy

If the patient is stable and there is minimal fecal soilage, the trend is primary anastomosis/repair ± resection

What is the treatment of small bowel injury?

Primary closure or resection and primary anastomosis

What is the treatment of minor pancreatic injury?

Drainage (e.g., JP drains)

What is the most commonly injured abdominal organ with blunt trauma?

Spleen

What is the treatment for significant duodenal injury?

Pyloric exclusion:

1. Close duodenal injury
2. Staple off pylorus
3. Gastrojejunostomy

What is the treatment for massive tail of pancreas injury?

Distal pancreatectomy (usually perform splenectomy also)

What is Damage control surgery?

Stop major hemorrhage and GI soilage. Pack and get out of the OR ASAP to bring the patient to the ICU to warm, correct coags, and resuscitate. Return patient to OR when more stable.

What is the "Lethal triad"?

1. Hypothermia
2. Coagulopathy
3. Acidosis

What comprises the workup/treatment of a stable parasternal chest gun shot/stab wound?

1. CXR
2. Chest tube, OR for subxiphoid window; if blood returns, then sternotomy to assess for cardiac injury

What is the diagnosis with NGT in chest on CXR?

Ruptured diaphragm with stomach in pleural cavity

What films are typically obtained to evaluate extremity fractures?

Complete views of the involved extremity, including the joints above and below the fracture

What is the only indication for MAST trousers?

Pelvic fracture

What is the treatment for human and dog bites?

Leave wound open

Outline basic work up for a victim of severe blunt trauma :

In E.R.: Airway, physical exam. IV X 2, 2 L LR, labs, spun HCT, type and cross, OGT/NGT, Foley, chest tube PRN
X-rays: CXR, Pelvis, cross-table C-spine, Femur (if femur fracture is suspected)

- +/- Blood transfusion → **Unstable** vital signs
  - + Pelvic fracture → FAST or supraumbilical DPL
    - (+)DPL/(+)FAST → OR Ex Lap → External pelvic fixator → Pelvic A-gram PRN, Thoracic A-gram PRN, Head CT → AP and lat C/T/L spine films, Ext films PRN → ICU → Flex/ext C-spine films
    - (-)DPL/(-)FAST → Ext fixator PRN → Pelvic A-gram PRN → Thoracic A-gram PRN → Head CT → AP and lat C/T/L spine films, Ext films PRN → ICU → Flex/ext C-spine films
  - - Pelvic fracture → FAST or DPL
    - (+)DPL/(+)FAST → OR Ex Lap → Thoracic A-gram PRN → Head CT → AP and lat C/T/L spine films, Ext films PRN → ICU → Flex/ext C-spine films
    - (-)DPL/(-)FAST → Thoracic A-gram PRN, Head CT → AP and lat C/T/L spine films, Ext films PRN → ICU → Flex/ext C-spine films
- **Stable** vital signs → +/- Thoracic aortogram, Head CT, abd/pelvis CT → AP and lat C/T/L spine films, Extremity films PRN → ICU → Flex/ext lat C-spine films

[Note: +/- = if indicated. A-gram = aortogram. AP = anteroposterior. DPL = diagnostic peritoneal lavage. Ex Lap = exploratory laparotomy. Ext = extremity. ICU = Intensive Care Unit. OGT = orogastric tube. FAST = Focused Abdominal (or Assessment) Sonogram for Trauma. lat = lateral. C = cervical. T = thoracic. L = lumbar. PRN = as needed.]

36 Burns

Are acid or alkali chemical burns more serious?

In general, **ALKALI** burns are more serious because the body cannot buffer the alkali, thus allowing them to burn for much longer.

Why are electrical burns so dangerous?

Most of the destruction from electrical burns is internal because the route of least electrical resistance follows nerves, blood vessels, and fascia. Injury is usually far worse than external burns at entrance and exit sites would indicate. **Cardiac dysrhythmias,** myoglobinuria, acidosis, and renal failure are common.

How is myoglobinuria treated?

To avoid renal injury:
HAM:
Hydration with IV fluids
Alkalization of urine with IV bicarbonate
Mannitol diuresis

Define level of burn injury:

First degree burns?

Epidermis only

Second degree burns?

Epidermis and varying levels of dermis

Third degree burns?

A.K.A. "full thickness"; all layers of the skin including the entire dermis (Think: "getting the third degree")

Fourth degree burns?

Burn injury into bone or muscle

How do first degree burns present?

Painful, dry, red areas that do not form blisters (think of sunburn)

How do second degree burns present?

Painful, hypersensitive, swollen, mottled areas with blisters and open weeping surfaces

How do third degree burns present?

Painless, insensate, swollen, dry, mottled white, and charred areas; often described as dried leather

What is the major clinical difference between second and third degree burns?

Third degree burns are painless, and second degree burns are very painful (laudable pain).

By which measure is burn severity determined?

Depth of burn and total body surface area (TBSA) affected by second and third degree burns

TBSA is calculated by the "rule of nines" in adults and by a modified rule in children to account for the disproportionate size of the head and trunk

What is the "rule of nines"?

In an adult, the total body surface area that is burned can be estimated by the following:

- Each upper limb = 9%
- Each lower limb = 18%
- Anterior and posterior trunk = 18% each
- Head and neck = 9%
- Perineum and genitalia = 1%

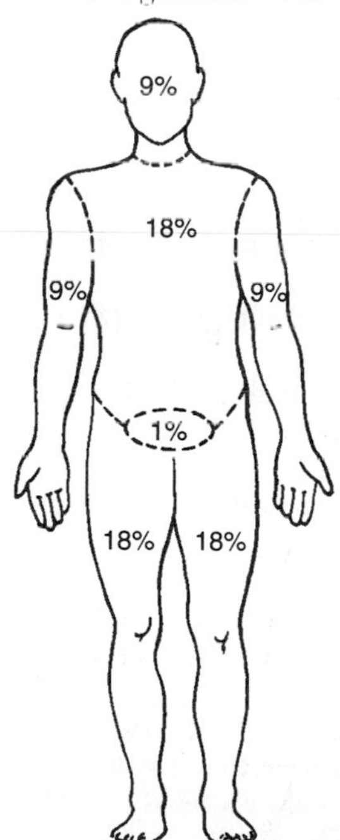

What is the "rule of the palm"?
The surface area of the patient's palm is approximately 1% of the TBSA used for estimating size of small burns

Burn center referral criteria?

Second degree burns
> 20% TBSA

Third degree burns
>5% TBSA
Second degree > 10% TBSA in children and the elderly
Any burns involving the face, hands, feet, or perineum
Any burns with inhalation injury
Any burns with associated trauma
Any electrical burns

What is the treatment of first degree burns?
Keep clean, ± Neosporin, pain meds

What is the treatment of second degree burns?
Remove blisters; apply antibiotic ointment (usually Silvadene) and dressing; pain meds. Most second degree burns do not require skin grafting (epidermis grows from hair follicles and from margins).

What is the treatment of third degree burns?
Early excision of eschar (within first week postburn) and split-thickness skin grafting (STSG)

How can you decrease bleeding during excision?
Tourniquets as possible, topical epinephrine, topical thrombin

What is an autograft STSG?
STSG from the patient's own skin

What is an allograft STSG?
STSG from a cadaver (temporary coverage)

What thickness is the STSG?
12/1000 to 15/1000 of an inch (down to the dermal layer)

What prophylaxis should the burn patient get in the ED?
Tetanus

What is used to evaluate the eyes after a third degree burn?
Fluorescein

What principles guide the initial assessment and resuscitation of the burn patient?

Airway, breathing, circulation, disability, and exposure (same as for the trauma patient)

What are the signs of smoke inhalation?

Smoke and soot in sputum/mouth/nose; nasal/facial hair burns, carboxyhemoglobin, throat/mouth erythema, history of loss of consciousness/explosion/fire in small enclosed area, dyspnea, low O_2 saturation, confusion, headache, coma

What lab value assesses smoke inhalation?

Carboxyhemoglobin level (a carboxyhemoglobin level of more than 60% is associated with a 50% mortality); treat with 100% O_2 and time

How should the airway be managed in the burn patient with an inhalational injury?

With a low threshold for **intubation;** oropharyngeal swelling may so occlude the airway that intubation is impossible, either very rapidly or slowly and progressively over 24 to 48 hours; 100% oxygen should be administered immediately and continued until significant carboxyhemoglobin is ruled out

What is "burn shock"?

Burn shock describes the loss of fluid from the intravascular space as a result of burn injury, which causes "leaking capillaries" that require huge crystalloid infusion.

What is the "Parkland formula"?

V = Total Body Surface Area (%) × Weight (kg) × 4

Formula widely used to estimate the volume (V) of crystalloid necessary for the initial resuscitation of the burn patient; half of the calculated volume is given in the **first 8 hours,** the rest in the next 16 hours

How is the crystalloid given?

Through two large-bore peripheral venous catheters introduced through unburned skin

Why is glucose-containing IVF contraindicated in burn patients in the first 24 hours postburn?

The patient's serum glucose will be elevated on its own because of the stress response

What fluid is used after the first 24 hrs postburn?

Colloid; use D5W **and** 5% albumin at 0.5 cc/kg/% burn surface area over 4 to 8 hours

Why should D5W IV be administered after 24 hours postburn?

Because of the massive sodium load in the first 24 hrs of LR infusion and because of the massive evaporation of H_2O from the burn injury, the patient will need free water; after 24 to 36 hours, the capillaries begin to work and then the patient can usually benefit from **albumin** IV (i.e., colloid).

What is the minimal urine output for burn patients?

Adults > 0.5 cc/kg/hr; children 1–2 cc/kg/hr

How is volume status monitored in the burn patient?

Blood pressure, heart rate, peripheral perfusion, mental status, and urinary output; Foley catheter is mandatory and may be supplemented by central venous pressure and pulmonary capillary wedge pressure monitoring

Why do most severely burned patients require nasogastric decompression?

Patients with greater than 20% TBSA burns usually develop a paralytic ileus → vomiting → aspiration risk → pneumonia

What stress prophylaxis must be given to the burn patient?

H_2 blocker to prevent burn stress ulcer (Curling's ulcer)

What are the clinical signs of burn wound infection?

Fever (possibly), increased WBC with left shift, **discoloration of burn eschar** (most common sign), green pigment, necrotic skin lesion in unburned skin, edema, ecchymosis tissue below eschar, second degree burns that turn into third degree burns

What are the common organisms found in burn wound infections?

Staphylococcus aureus, Pseudomonas, Streptococcus, Candida albicans

How is a burn wound infection diagnosed?

Send burned tissue in question to the laboratory for quantitative burn wound bacterial count. If the count is more than 105/g, infection is present and IV antibiotics should be administered.

How are minor burns dressed?

Gentle cleaning with nonionic detergent and debridement of loose skin and broken blisters; the burn is dressed with a topical antibacterial (e.g., neomycin) and covered with a sterile dressing

How are major burns dressed?

Cleansing and application of topical antibacterial agent

Why are systemic IV antibiotics contraindicated?

The bacteria live in the eschar, which is avascular (the systemic antibiotic will not be delivered to the eschar); thus, apply topical antimicrobial agents.

Note some advantages and disadvantages of the following topical antibiotic agents:

Silver sulfadiazine (Silvadene)

Painless, does not cause **electrolyte imbalances,** does not require occlusive dressing, but little eschar penetration, misses *Pseudomonas,* and has idiosyncratic **neutropenia;** agent of choice for small burns

Mafenide acetate (Sulfamylon)

Penetrates eschars, broad spectrum (but misses *Staphylococcus*), causes pain on application; triggers allergic reaction in 7% of patients; may cause **acid-base imbalances** (think: **M**afenide **AC**etate = **M**etabolic **AC**idosis); agent of choice in already-contaminated burn wounds

Polysporin

Polymyxin B sulfate; painless, clear, used for facial burns; does not have a wide antimicrobial spectrum

Are prophylactic systemic antibiotics administered to burn patients?

No. Prophylactic antibiotics have not been shown to reduce the incidence of sepsis, but rather have been shown to select for resistant organisms. IV antibiotics are reserved for established wound infections, pneumonia, urinary tract infections, etc.

Are prophylactic antibiotics administered for inhalational injury?

No

Circumferential, full-thickness burns to the extremities are at risk for what complication?
Distal neurovascular impairment, similar to compartment syndrome

How is it treated?
Escharotomy: full-thickness longitudinal incision through the eschar with scalpel or electrocautery; incision must extend into healthy fat

What is the major infection complication (other than wound infection) in burn patients?
Pneumonia, central line infection (change central lines prophylactically every 3 to 4 days)

What are the most common causes of postburn pneumonia?
1. *S. aureus*
2. *Pseudomonas*

Is tetanus prophylaxis required in the burn patient?
Yes, it is mandatory in all patients except those actively immunized within the past 12 months (with complete immunization: toxoid ×3).

From which burns is water evaporation highest?
Third degree

Can infection convert a partial-thickness injury into a full-thickness injury?
Yes!

How is carbon monoxide inhalation overdose treated?
100% O_2 (± hyperbaric O_2)

Which electrolyte must be closely followed acutely after a burn?
Na^+ (sodium)

When should central lines over a wire be changed in the burn patient?
Every 3 to 4 days (**only in the burn patient**)

What is the name of the gastric/duodenal ulcer associated with burn injury?
Curling's ulcer (think: curling iron burn = Curling's burn ulcer)

37 Upper GI Bleeding

What is it?
Bleeding into the lumen of the proximal GI tract, usually proximal to the ligament of Treitz

What are the signs/symptoms?
Hematemesis, melena, syncope, shock, fatigue, coffee-ground emesis, hematochezia, epigastric discomfort, epigastric tenderness, signs of hypovolemia, guaiac-positive stools

Why is it possible to have hematochezia?
Blood is a cathartic and hematochezia usually indicates a vigorous rate of bleeding from the UGI source.

Are stools melenic or melanotic?
Melenic (melanotic is incorrect)

How much blood do you need to have melena?
> 50 cc of blood

What are the risk factors?
Alcohol, cigarettes, liver disease, burn/trauma, aspirin/NSAIDs, vomiting, sepsis, steroids, previous UGI bleeding, history of peptic ulcer disease (PUD), esophageal varices, portal hypertension, splenic vein thrombosis, abdominal aortic aneurysm repair (aortoenteric fistula), burn injury, trauma

What is the most common cause of significant UGI bleeding?
PUD—duodenal and gastric ulcers (50%)

What are possible differential diagnoses of UGI bleeding?
Duodenal ulcer
Gastric ulcer
Acute gastritis
Esophageal varices

	Mallory-Weiss tear Also: gastric cancer, esophagitis, hemobilia, duodenal diverticula, gastric volvulus, Boerhaave's syndrome, aortoenteric fistula, paraesophageal hiatal hernia, epistaxis, NGT irritation, Dieulafoy's ulcer, angiodysplasia
Which diagnostic tests are useful?	History, NGT aspirate, abdominal x-ray, endoscopy (EGD)
What is the diagnostic test of choice with UGI bleeding?	EGD
What are the treatment options with the endoscope during an EGD?	Coagulation, injection of epinephrine (for vasoconstriction), injection of sclerosing agents (varices), variceal ligation (banding)
Which lab tests should be performed?	Chem-7, bilirubin, LFTs, CBC, **type & cross,** PT/PTT, amylase
Why is BUN elevated?	Because of absorption of blood by the GI tract
What is the initial treatment?	1. **IVFs** (16 G or larger peripheral IVS × 2), **Foley** catheter (monitor fluid status) 2. **NGT** suction (determine rate and amount of blood) 3. Water lavage (use warm H_2O—will remove clots, facilitating esophagogastroduodenoscopy) 4. **EGD:** Endoscopy (determine etiology/location of bleeding and possible treatment—coagulate bleeders)
What test may help identify the site of MASSIVE UGI bleeding when EGD fails to diagnose cause and blood continues per NGT?	Selective mesenteric angiography
What are the indications for surgical intervention in UGI bleeding?	Refractory or recurrent bleeding and site known, > 3 u PRBCS to stabilize or > 6 u PRBCs overall

What percentage of patients require surgery?	Approximately 10%
What percentage of patients spontaneously stop bleeding?	Approximately 80% to 85%
What is the mortality of acute UGI bleeding?	Overall 10%, 60–80 years of age 15%, older than 80 years of age 25%
What are the risk factors for death following UGI bleed?	Age older than 60 years Shock More than 5 units of PRBC transfusion Concomitant health problems

PEPTIC ULCER DISEASE (PUD)

What is it?	Includes gastric and duodenal ulcers
What is the incidence in the United States?	Approximately 10% of all Americans will suffer from PUD during their lifetime!
What are the possible consequences of PUD?	Pain, hemorrhage, perforation, obstruction
What percentage of patients with PUD develop bleeding from the ulcer?	Approximately 20%
Which bacteria are associated with PUD?	*Helicobacter pylori*
What is the treatment?	Treat *H. pylori* with MOC, AMO, or ACO antibiotic regimens: **MOC: M**etronidazole, **O**meprazole, **C**larithromycin (think, "**MOCK**") **AMO: A**mpicillin, **M**etronidazole, **O**meprazole or **ACO: A**mpicillin, **C**larithromycin, **O**meprazole
What is the name of the sign with RLQ pain/peritonitis as a result of succus collecting from a perforated peptic ulcer?	Valentino's sign

DUODENAL ULCERS

In which age group are these ulcers most common?	Between 40 and 65 years of age (younger than patients with gastric ulcer)
What is the ratio of male to female patients?	Men > women (3 to 1)
What is the most common location?	Most are within 2 cm of the pylorus in the duodenal bulb.
What is the classic pain response to food intake?	Food classically relieves duodenal ulcer pain (**think, D**uodenum = **D**ecreased with foo**D**).
What is the cause?	Increased production of gastric acid
What syndrome must you always think of with a duodenal ulcer?	Z-E syndrome (Zollinger-Ellison)
What are the associated risk factors?	Male gender, smoking, aspirin and other NSAIDs, uremia, Z-E syndrome, *H. pylori,* trauma, burn injury
What are the symptoms?	Epigastric pain—burning or aching, usually several hours after a meal (food, milk, or antacids initially relieve pain) Bleeding Back pain Nausea, vomiting, and anorexia ↓ appetite
What are the signs?	Tenderness in epigastric area (possibly), guaiac-positive stool, melena, hematochezia, hematemesis
What is the differential diagnosis?	Acute abdomen, pancreatitis, cholecystitis, **all causes of UGI bleeding,** Z-E syndrome, gastritis, MI, gastric ulcer
How is the diagnosis made?	History, PE, EGD, UGI series (**if patient is not actively bleeding**)
When is surgery indicated with a bleeding duodenal ulcer?	Most surgeons use: > 6 u PRBC transfusions, > 3 u PRBCs needed to stabilize, or significant rebleed

What EGD finding is associated with rebleeding?
Visible vessel in the ulcer crater, recent clot, active oozing

What is the medical treatment?
PPIs (proton pump inhibitors) or H_2 receptor antagonists—heal ulcers in 4 to 6 weeks in most cases
Treatment for *H. pylori*

When is surgery indicated?
The acronym **I HOP:**
I—**i**ntractability
H—**h**emorrhage (massive or relentless)
O—**o**bstruction (gastric outlet obstruction)
P—**p**erforation

How is a bleeding duodenal ulcer corrected?
Opening of the duodenum through the pylorus
Oversewing of the bleeding vessel

What are the common surgical options for the following conditions:

Vagotomy
Pyloroplasty

Treatment of duodenal perforation?
Graham patch (poor candidates, shock, prolonged perforation)
Truncal vagotomy and pyloroplasty incorporating ulcer
Graham patch and highly selective vagotomy
Truncal vagotomy and antrectomy (higher mortality rate, but lowest recurrence rate)

Treatment of duodenal obstruction resulting from duodenal ulcer scarring (gastric outlet obstruction)?
Truncal vagotomy, antrectomy, and gastroduodenostomy (BI or BII)
Truncal vagotomy and drainage procedure (gastrojejunostomy)

Duodenal ulcer intractability?
PGV (highly selective vagotomy)
Vagotomy and pyloroplasty
Vagotomy and antrectomy BI or BII (especially if there is a coexistent pyloric/prepyloric ulcer) but associated with a higher mortality

Which ulcer operation has the highest ulcer recurrence rate and the lowest dumping rate?
PGV (proximal gastric vagotomy)

Which ulcer operation has the lowest ulcer recurrence rate and the highest dumping rate?
Vagotomy and antrectomy

Which duodenal ulcer operation has the lowest mortality rate?
PGV (1/200 mortality), truncal vagotomy and pyloroplasty (1–2/200), vagotomy and antrectomy (1%—2% mortality)
Thus, PGV is the operation of choice for intractable duodenal ulcers with the cost of increased risk of ulcer recurrence.

What is a "kissing" ulcer?
Two ulcers are each on opposite sides of the lumen so that they can "kiss."

Why may a duodenal rupture be painless?
Fluid can be sterile, with a nonirritating pH of 7.0 initially.

Why may a perforated duodenal ulcer present as lower quadrant abdominal pain?
Fluid from stomach/bile drains down paracolic gutters to lower quadrants and causes localized irritation.

GASTRIC ULCERS

In which age group are these ulcers most common?
Between 40 and 70 years old (older than the duodenal ulcer population)
Rare in patients younger than 40 years

How does the incidence in men compare with that of women?
Men > women

Which is more common overall: gastric or duodenal ulcers?
Duodenal ulcers are more than twice as common as gastric ulcers.

What is the classic pain response to food?
Food classically increases gastric ulcer pain.

What is the cause?
Decreased cryoprotection or gastric protection (i.e., decreased bicarbonate/ mucous production)

Is gastric acid production high or low?
Gastric acid production is normal or low!

Which gastric ulcers are associated with increased gastric acid?

Prepyloric
Pyloric
Coexist with duodenal ulcers

What are the associated risk factors?

Smoking, alcohol, burns, trauma, CNS tumor/trauma, NSAIDs, steroids, shock, severe illness, male gender, advanced age

What are the symptoms?

Epigastric pain
Most often transiently relieved by food/antacids (but food can make pain worse in some cases)
Associated with vomiting, anorexia, and nausea

How is the diagnosis made?

History, PE, EGD with multiple biopsy (looking for gastric cancer)

What is the most common location?

Approximately 70% are on a lesser curvature; 5% are on a greater curvature.

When and why should biopsy be performed?

With all gastric ulcers, to rule out gastric cancer
If the ulcer does not heal in 6 weeks after medical treatment **rebiopsy** (biopsy in OR also) must be performed.

What is the medical treatment?

Similar to that of duodenal ulcer—PPIs or H_2 blockers

When do patients with gastric ulcers need to have an EGD?

1. For diagnosis with biopsies
2. 6 weeks postdiagnosis to confirm healing and rule out gastric cancer!

What are the indications for surgery?

The acronym **I CHOP**
I—intractability
C—**c**ancer (rule out)
H—**h**emorrhage (massive or relentless)
O—**o**bstruction (gastric outlet obstruction)
P—**p**erforation
(Surgery is indicated if gastric cancer cannot be ruled out.)

What is the common operation for hemorrhage, obstruction, and perforation?

Distal gastrectomy with excision of the ulcer **without** vagotomy unless there is duodenal disease (i.e., BI or BII)

What are the options for concomitant duodenal and gastric ulcers?
BI, BII, and **truncal vagotomy**

What is a common option for surgical treatment of a pyloric gastric ulcer?
Truncal vagotomy and antrectomy (i.e., BI or BII)

What is a common option for a poor operative candidate with a perforated gastric ulcer?
Graham patch

What must be performed in every operation for gastric ulcers?
Biopsy looking for gastric cancer

What is the recurrence rate?
~ up to two-thirds in 2 years with medical treatment alone (usually recur within 6 months of the first event)

Define the following terms:

Cushing's ulcer
PUD/gastritis associated with Neurologic trauma or tumor (**think,** Dr. **C**ushing = **n**euro**s**urgeon)

Curling's ulcer
PUD/gastritis associated with major burn injury (**think:** curling iron burn)

Marginal ulcer
Ulcer at the margin of a GI anastomosis

Dieulafoy's ulcer
Pinpoint gastric mucosal defect bleeding from an underlying vascular malformation

PERFORATED PEPTIC ULCER

What are the symptoms?
Acute onset of upper abdominal pain

What causes pain in the lower quadrants?
Passage of perforated fluid along colic gutters

What are the signs?
Decreased bowel sounds, tympanic sound over the liver (air), peritoneal signs, tender abdomen

What are the signs of posterior duodenal erosion/perforation?
Bleeding from gastroduodenal artery (and acute pancreatitis)

What sign indicates anterior duodenal perforation?
Free air (anterior perforation is more common than posterior)

What is the differential diagnosis?
Acute pancreatitis, acute cholecystitis, perforated acute appendicitis, colonic diverticulitis, MI, any perforated viscus

Which diagnostic tests are indicated?
X-ray: free air under diaphragm or in lesser sac in an upright CXR (if upright CXR is not possible, then left lateral decubitus can be performed because air can be seen over the liver and not confused with the gastric bubble)

What are the associated lab findings?
Leukocytosis, high amylase serum (secondary to absorption into the blood stream from the peritoneum)

What is the initial treatment?
NGT (↓ contamination of the peritoneal cavity)
IVF/Foley catheter
Antibiotics
Surgery

What is a Graham patch?
A piece of omentum incorporated into the suture closure of perforation

What are the surgical options for treatment of a duodenal perforation?
Graham patch
Truncal vagotomy and pyloroplasty incorporating ulcer
Graham patch and highly selective vagotomy

What are the surgical options for perforated gastric ulcer?
Antrectomy incorporating perforated ulcer, Graham patch or wedge resection in unstable/poor operative candidates

What is the significance of hemorrhage and perforation with duodenal ulcer?
May indicate two ulcers (kissing); posterior is bleeding and anterior is perforated with free air

What type of perforated ulcer may present just like acute pancreatitis?
Posterior perforated duodenal ulcer into the pancreas (i.e., epigastric pain radiating to the back; high serum amylase)

What is the classic difference between duodenal and gastric ulcer symptoms as related to food ingestion?

Duodenal = decreased pain
Gastric = increased pain
(**think, D**uodenal = **D**ecreased pain)

TYPES OF SURGERIES

Define the following terms:

Graham patch

For treatment of duodenal perforation in poor operative candidates/unstable patients
Place viable omentum over perforation and tack into place with sutures

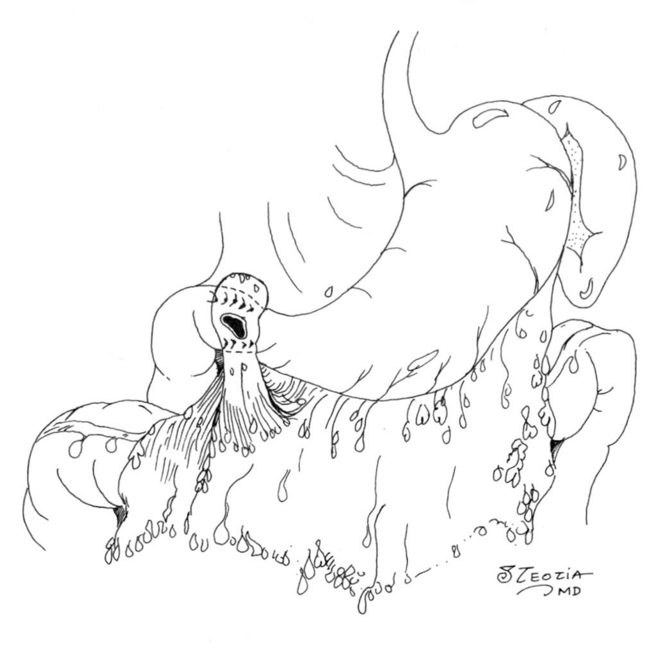

Truncal vagotomy

Resection of a 1- to 2-cm segment of each vagal **trunk** as it enters the abdomen on the distal esophagus, decreasing gastric acid secretion and gastric emptying; also selective vagotomies

What other procedure must be performed along with a truncal vagotomy?

A "drainage procedure" (pyloroplasty, antrectomy, or gastrojejunostomy), because vagal fibers provide relaxation of the pylorus and if you cut them the pylorus will not open

Vagotomy and pyloroplasty — Pyloroplasty performed with vagotomy to compensate for decreased gastric emptying

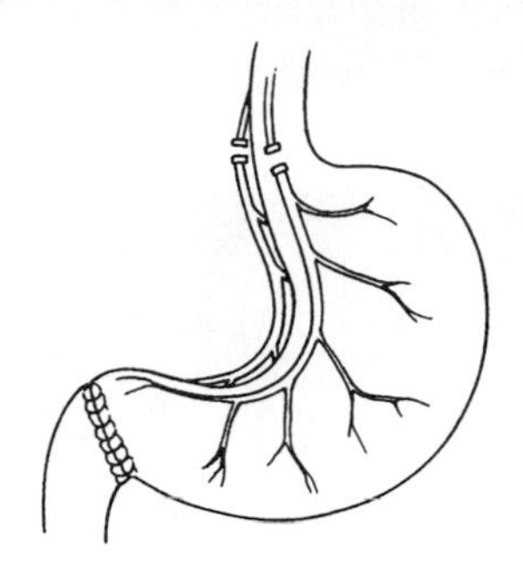

Vagotomy and antrectomy — Remove antrum in addition to vagotomy; reconstruct as a Billroth I or II

What is the goal of surgery? — Decrease gastric acid secretion and fix IHOP

What is the advantage of proximal gastric vagotomy (highly selective vagotomy)? — No drainage procedure is needed; vagal fibers to the pylorus are preserved; rate of dumping syndrome is low.

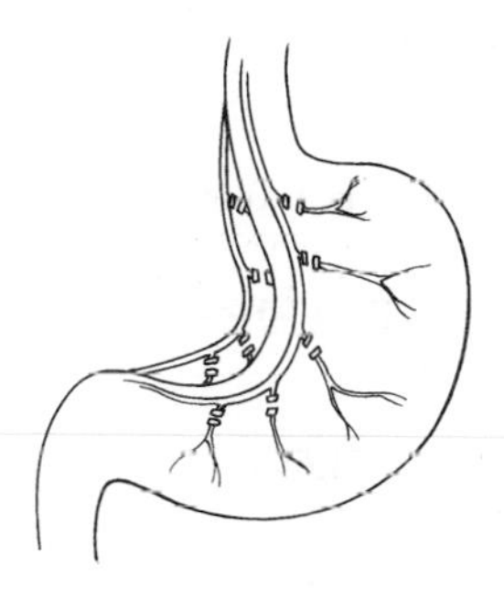

What is a Billroth I (BI)? — Truncal vagotomy, antrectomy, and gastroduodenostomy (**think:** BI = one limb off of the stomach remnant)

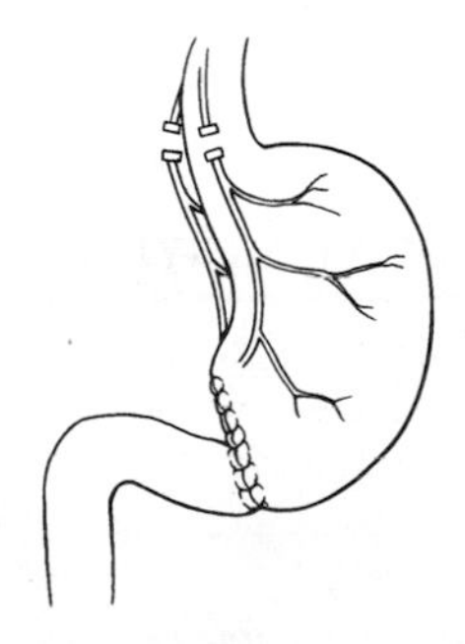

What is a Billroth II (BII)?

Truncal vagotomy, antrectomy, and gastrojejunostomy (**think:** BII = two limbs off of the stomach remnant)

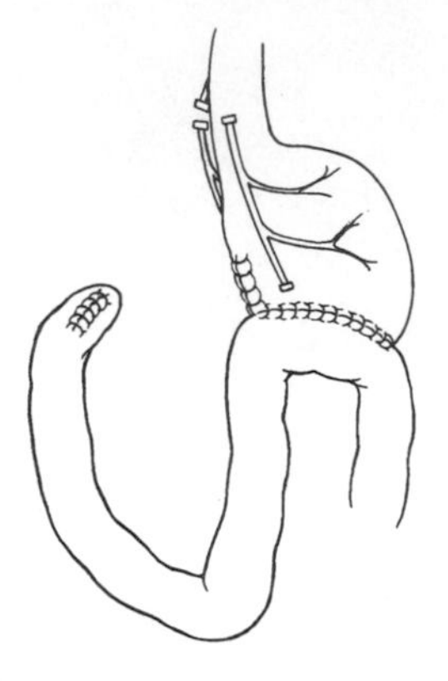

What is the Kocher maneuver?

Dissect the left lateral peritoneal attachments to the duodenum to allow visualization of posterior duodenum.

STRESS GASTRITIS

What is it?

Superficial mucosal erosions in the stressed patient

What are the risk factors?

Sepsis, intubation, trauma, shock

What is the prophylactic treatment?

H_2 blockers, antacids, sucralfate

What are the signs/ symptoms?

NGT blood (usually), painless (usually)

How is it diagnosed?

EGD, if bleeding is significant

What is the disadvantage of H_2 blockers and antacids in ICU patients?

Loss of acidic environment of stomach acid and bacterial overgrowth are associated with higher rates of pneumonia from aspiration of stomach contents.

MALLORY-WEISS SYNDROME

What is it?

Post-retching, postemesis longitudinal tear (submucosa and mucosa) of the stomach near the GE junction; approximately three-fourths are in the stomach

For what percentage of all upper GI bleeds does this syndrome account?
About 10%

What are the causes of a tear?
Increased gastric pressure, often aggravated by hiatal hernia

What are the risk factors?
Retching, alcoholism (50%), more than 50% of patients have hiatal hernia

What are the symptoms?
Epigastric pain, thoracic substernal pain, emesis, hematemesis

What percentage of patients will have hematemesis?
85%

How is the diagnosis made?
EGD

What is the "classic" history?
Alcoholic patient after binge drinking—first, vomit food and gastric contents, followed by forceful retching and bloody vomitus

What is the treatment?
Room temperature water lavage (90% of patients stop bleeding), electrocautery, arterial embolization, or surgery for refractory bleeding

When is surgery indicated?
When medical/endoscopic treatment fails (> 6 u PRBCs infused)

Can you use the Songstaken-Blakemore tamponade balloon for treatment of Mallory-Weiss tear bleeding?
No, it makes bleeding worse.
Use the balloon only for bleeding from esophageal varices.

ESOPHAGEAL VARICEAL BLEEDING

What is it?
Bleeding from formation of esophageal varices from back up of portal pressure via the coronary vein to the submucosal esophageal venous plexi secondary to portal hypertension from liver cirrhosis

What is the "rule of two-thirds" of esophageal variceal hemorrhage?
Two-thirds of patients with portal hypertension develop esophageal varices.
Two-thirds of patients with esophageal varices bleed.

What are the signs/ symptoms?

Liver disease, portal hypertension, hematemesis, caput medusa, ascites

How is the diagnosis made?

EGD (very important because only 50% of UGI bleeding in patients with known esophageal varices are bleeding from the varices; the other 50% have bleeding from ulcers, etc.)

What is the medical treatment?

Lower portal pressure with vasopressin or somatostatin

In the patient with CAD what must you give in addition to the vasopressin?

Nitroglycerin—otherwise you will have coronary artery vasoconstriction that may result in MI

What is the definitive treatment?

Sclerotherapy or ligation via endoscope
Sengstaken-Blakemore balloon tamponade, if bleeding is massive
Liver transplant

What is the Sengstaken-Blakemore balloon?

Tamponades with an esophageal balloon and a gastric balloon
Warren shunt (distal splenorenal shunting of portal blood to vena cava), other shunts

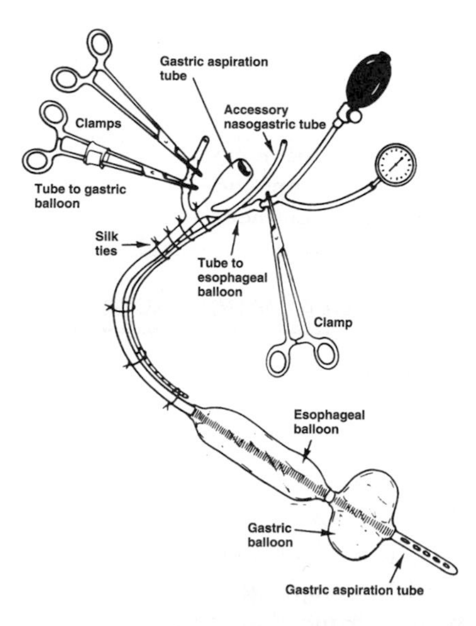

What is the problem with shunts?

Decreased portal pressure, but increased encephalopathy

BOERHAAVE'S SYNDROME

What is it?
Postemetic esophageal rupture (all layers), does not bleed profusely very frequently

Why is the esophagus susceptible to perforation and more likely to break down an anastomosis?
No serosa

What is the most common location?
Posterolateral aspect of the esophagus (on the left), 3 to 5 cm above the GE junction

What is the cause of rupture?
Increased intraluminal pressure, usually caused by violent retching and vomiting

What is the associated risk factor?
Esophageal reflux disease (50%)

What are the symptoms?
Pain postemesis (may radiate to the back, dysphagia)

What are the signs?
Left pneumothorax, Hamman's sign, left pleural effusion, subcutaneous/mediastinal emphysema, fever, tachypnea, tachycardia, signs of infection by 24 hours, neck crepitus, widened mediastinum on CXR

What is Mackler's triad?
1. Emesis
2. Lower chest pain
3. Cervical emphysema (sub Q air)

What is Hamman's sign?
"Mediastinal crunch or clicking" produced by the heart beating against air-filled tissues

How is the diagnosis made?
History, physical examination, CXR, esophagram with water-soluble contrast

What is the treatment?
Surgery within 24 hours to drain the mediastinum and surgically close the perforation and placement of pleural patch; broad-spectrum antibiotics

What is the mortality rate in less than 24 hours until surgery for perforated esophagus?
Approximately 15%

What is the mortality rate if more than 24 hours until surgery for perforated esophagus?

Approximately 33%

Overall, what is the most common cause of esophageal perforation?

Iatrogenic

38 The Stomach

ANATOMY

Identify the parts of the stomach:

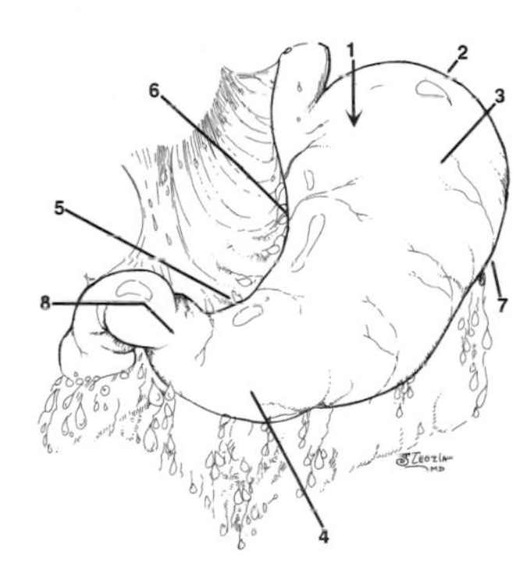

1. Cardia
2. Fundus
3. Body
4. Antrum
5. Incisura angularis
6. Lesser curvature
7. Greater curvature
8. Pylorus

Identify the blood supply to the stomach:

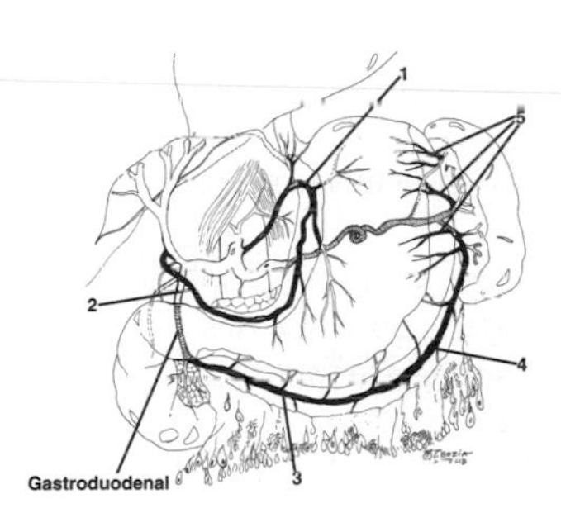

1. Left gastric artery
2. Right gastric artery
3. Right gastroepiploic artery
4. Left gastroepiploic artery
5. Short gastrics (from spleen)

What space lies behind the stomach?

The lesser sac; the pancreas lies behind the stomach

What is the opening into the lesser sac?

Foramen of Winslow

What are the folds of gastric mucosa called?	Rugae

GASTRIC PHYSIOLOGY

Define the products of the following stomach cells:	
Gastric parietal cells	HCl Intrinsic factor
Chief cells	Pepsinogen (think: "a peppy chief")
G cells	Gastrin (think: **G** cells = **G** astrin)
Where are G cells located?	Antrum
Mucous neck cells	Bicarbonate Mucus
What is pepsin?	A proteolytic enzyme that hydrolyzes peptide bonds
What is intrinsic factor?	A protein secreted by the parietal cells that combines with vitamin B_{12} and allows for absorption in the terminal ileum

GASTROESOPHAGEAL REFLUX DISEASE (GERD)

What is it?	Excessive reflux of gastric contents into the esophagus (everyone refluxes to a small degree); "heartburn"
What is pyrosis?	Medical term for heartburn
What are the causes?	Decreased lower esophageal sphincter (LES) tone (> 50% of cases) Decreased esophageal motility to clear refluxed fluid Gastric outlet obstruction Hiatal hernia
What are the signs/ symptoms?	Heartburn, regurgitation, respiratory problems/pneumonia from aspiration of refluxed gastric contents; substernal pain
What disease must be ruled out when the symptoms of GERD are present?	Coronary artery disease

What tests are included in the workup?

EGD
UGI contrast study with esophagogram
Twenty-four hour acid analysis (pH probe in esophagus)
Manometry

What is the medical treatment?

Small meals
Omeprazole or other PPIs (proton pump inhibitors)
Elevation of head at night and no meals prior to sleeping

What are the indications for surgery?

Intractability (failure of medical treatment)
Respiratory problems as a result of reflux and aspiration of gastric contents (e.g., pneumonia)
Severe esophageal injury (e.g., ulcers, hemorrhage, stricture, ± Barrett's esophagus)
Young age at onset

What is Barrett's esophagus?

Columnar metaplasia from the normal squamous epithelium as a result of chronic irritation from reflux

What is the major concern with Barrett's esophagus?

Developing cancer

What type of cancer develops in Barrett's esophagus?

Adenocarcinoma

What percentage of patients with GERD develop Barrett's esophagus?

7% (5 10%)

What percentage of patients with Barrett's esophagus will develop adenocarcinoma?

7% lifetime (5–10%)

Define the following surgical options for severe GERD:

LAP Nissen

360° fundoplication—2 cm long and loose (laparoscopically)

Belsey mark IV	240° to 270° fundoplication performed through a thoracic approach
Hill	Arcuate ligament repair (close large esophageal hiatus) and gastropexy to diaphragm (suture stomach to diaphragm)
Toupet	Incomplete (around 200°) posterior wrap (laparoscopic) often used with severe decreased esophageal motility
How does the Nissen wrap work?	Controversial but thought to work by: 1. Increasing LES muscular tone 2. Elongating LES 3. Restoring angle of His 4. Decreasing distal esophageal diameter Note: may have competent wrap intrathoracic!
Lap Nissen works in	
What percentage of patients?	90%
What are the postoperative complications?	1. Gas-bloat syndrome 2. Stricture 3. Dysphagia 4. Spleen injury requiring splenectomy 5. Esophageal perforation 6. Pneumothorax
What is gas bloat syndrome?	Inability to burp or vomit

GASTRIC CANCER

What is the incidence?	Low in United States (10/100,000); high in Japan (780/100,000)
What are the associated risk factors?	Diet—smoked meats, high nitrates, low fruits and vegetables, alcohol, tobacco Environment—raised in high-risk area, poor socioeconomic status, atrophic gastritis, male gender, blood type A, previous partial gastrectomy, pernicious anemia, polyps, *H. pylori*
What is the average age at the time of discovery?	Older than 60 years

What is the ratio of male to female patients?	3:2
Which blood type is associated with gastric cancer?	Blood type A (there is an "**A**" in gastric but no "O" or "B" = g**A**stric = type "**A**")
What are the symptoms?	Asymptomatic in early stages Epigastric pain Anorexia Weight loss Vomiting (also dysphagia, hematemesis, melena, dyspepsia, nausea)
What are the signs?	Anemia, melena, heme occult, epigastric mass (in advanced disease), hepatomegaly, coffee-ground emesis, Blumer's shelf, Virchow's node, enlarged ovaries, axillary adenopathy
What is a Blumer's shelf?	A solid peritoneal deposit anterior to the rectum, forming a "shelf," palpated on **rectal examination**
What is a Virchow's node?	Metastatic gastric cancer to the nodes in the left supraclavicular fossa
What is Sister Mary Joseph's sign?	Periumbilical lymph node gastric cancer metastases; presents as periumbilical mass
What is a Krukenberg's tumor?	Gastric cancer (or other adenocarcinoma) that has metastasized to the ovary
What is "Irish's" node?	Left axillary adenopathy from gastric cancer metastasis
What is a surveillance laboratory finding?	CEA elevated in 30% of cases (if + useful for surveillance)
Which diagnostic tests should be performed?	EGD with biopsy, endoscopic US to evaluate the level of invasion, CT of abdomen for metastasis
What is the histology?	Adenocarcinoma
What are the two histologic types?	1. Intestinal (glands) 2. Diffuse (no glands)

What is the morphology?	Ulcerative (25%) Polyploid (25%) Superficial spreading (10%) Linitis plastica (10%)
Are gastric cancers more common on the lesser or greater curvatures?	Lesser ("lesser is greater")
Which morphologic type is named after a "leather bottle"?	Linitis plastica—the entire stomach is involved and looks thickened
What is the treatment?	Surgical resection with wide (> 5 cm checked by frozen section) margins and lymph node dissection
What operation is performed for tumor in the:	
Antrum?	Distal subtotal gastrectomy
Midbody?	Total gastrectomy
Proximal?	Total gastrectomy
What is the difference between a subtotal gastrectomy and a hemigastrectomy?	Hemigastrectomy = 50% of stomach removed Subtotal gastrectomy = 75% of stomach removed
What type of anastomosis?	Billroth II or Roux-en-Y (never use a Billroth I)
When should splenectomy be performed?	When the tumor directly invades the spleen/splenic hilum or with splenic hilar adenopathy
Define "extended lymph node dissection."	Extensive lymph node dissection, usually one group past the lymph node group with positive metastases
What percentage of patients are inoperable at presentation?	Approximately 10–15%
What is the role of postoperative chemotherapy?	No clear benefit

What is the 5-year survival rate for gastric cancer?	10% of patients are alive 5 years after diagnosis in the United States (in Japan, 50% are alive at 5 years)
Why is it thought that the postoperative survival is so much higher in Japan?	Aggressive screening and capturing early cancers
What is the differential diagnosis for gastric tumors?	Adenocarcinoma, leiomyoma, leiomyosarcoma, lymphoma, carcinoid, ectopic pancreatic tissue, gastrinoma, benign gastric ulcer, polyp

39 Bariatric Surgery

What is it?

Weight reduction surgery for the morbidly obese

Define morbid obesity.

1. BMI > 40 (basically, > 100 pounds above ideal body weight) or
2. BMI > 35 with a medical problem related to morbid obesity

What is the BMI?

Body **M**ass **I**ndex

What is the formula for BMI?

Body weight in kg divided by height in meters squared

What medical conditions are associated with morbid obesity?

Coronary artery disease, pulmonary disease, diabetes mellitus, venous stasis ulcers, arthritis, infections, sex-hormone abnormalities

What are the current options for surgery?

Gastric bypass (malabsorptive)
Vertical-banded gastroplasty

Define gastric bypass.

Stapling off of small gastric pouch (restrictive)
Roux-en-Y limb to gastric pouch

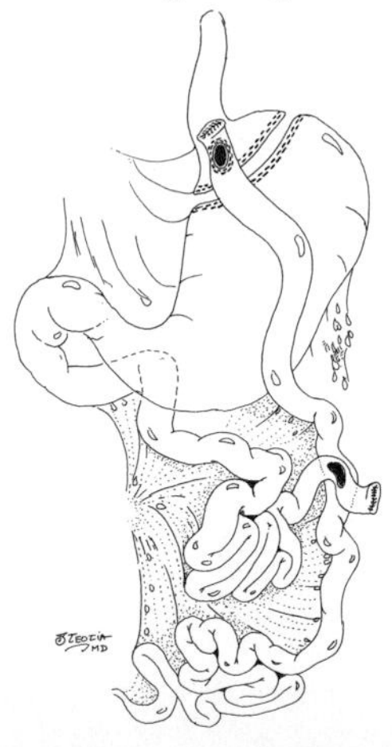

Define vertical-banded gastroplasty.

Vertical stapled small gastric pouch
Placement of silastic ring **band**

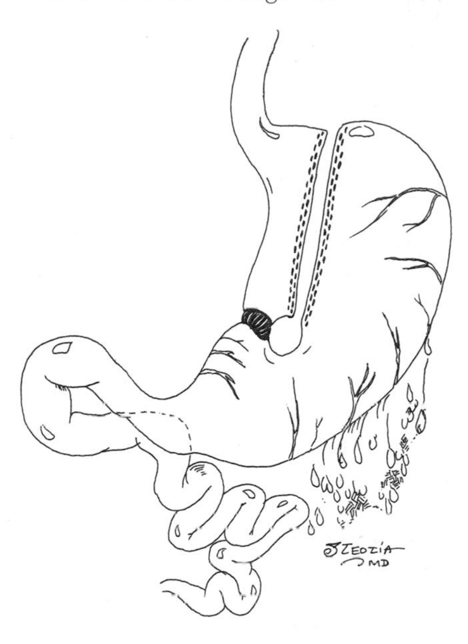

How does vertical-banded gastroplasty work?

Decreases the gastric reservoir and promotes early satiety

How can patients "beat" vertical-banded gastroplasty?

By eating sweets and high-calorie liquids

How does gastric bypass work?

1. Creates a small gastric reservoir
2. Causes dumping symptoms when a patient eats too much food or high-calorie foods; the food is "dumped" into the Roux-en-Y limb
3. Bypass of small bowel by Roux en Y limb

Which operation works best overall?

Gastric bypass (mean weight loss 50% of excess weight)

What are the possible postoperative complications after weight reduction surgery?

Gallstones (if gallbladder in situ), anastomotic leak, marginal ulcer, stenosis of pouch/anastomosis, malnutrition, incisional hernia, spleen injury (often resulting in bleeding or splenectomy)

40 Ostomies

Define the following terms:

Ostomy — An operation that connects the GI tract to abdominal wall skin or the lumen of another hollow organ; a man-made fistula

Stoma — The opening of the ostomy (Gr. "mouth")

Gastrostomy — G-tube through the abdominal wall to the stomach for drainage or feeding

Jejunostomy — J-tube through the abdominal wall to the jejunum for feeding

Kock pouch — "Continent ileostomy"
Pouch is made of several ileal loops.
Patient must access the pouch with a tube intermittently.

Colostomy — Connection of colon mucosa to the abdominal wall skin for stool drainage

End colostomy — Proximal end of colon brought to the skin for stool drainage

Mucus fistula — Distal end of transected colon brought to the skin for decompression; the mucosa produces mucus, a colostomy is a fistula, and, hence, the term **mucus fistula** (proximal colon brought up as a colostomy or, if the proximal colon is removed, an ileostomy)

Hartmann's pouch — Distal end of transected colon stapled and dropped back into the peritoneal cavity, resulting in a blind pouch; mucus is decompressed through the anus (proximal colon is brought up as an end colostomy or, if proximal colon is removed, an end ileostomy)

Double-barrel colostomy

End colostomy and a mucus fistula (i.e., two barrels brought up to the skin)

Loop colostomy

A loop of large bowel is brought up to the abdominal wall skin and a plastic rod is placed underneath the loop. The colon is then opened and sewn to the abdominal wall skin as a colostomy.

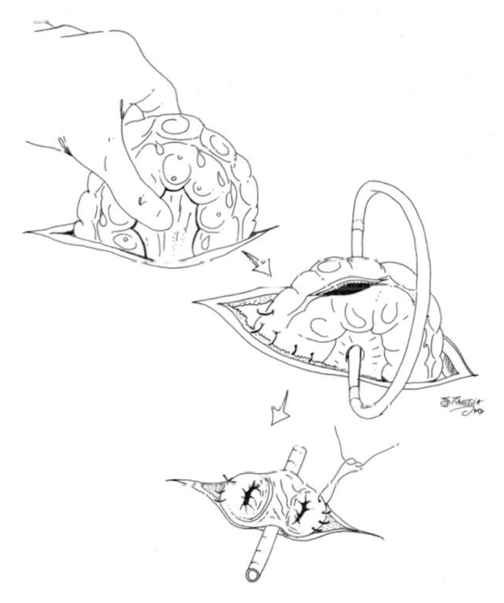

Ileal conduit

Loops of stapled-off ileum made into a pouch, anastomosed to the ureters, and then brought to the abdominal wall skin to allow drainage of urine in patients who undergo removal of the bladder (cystectomy)

Brooke ileostomy

Ileostomy folded over itself to provide clearance from skin

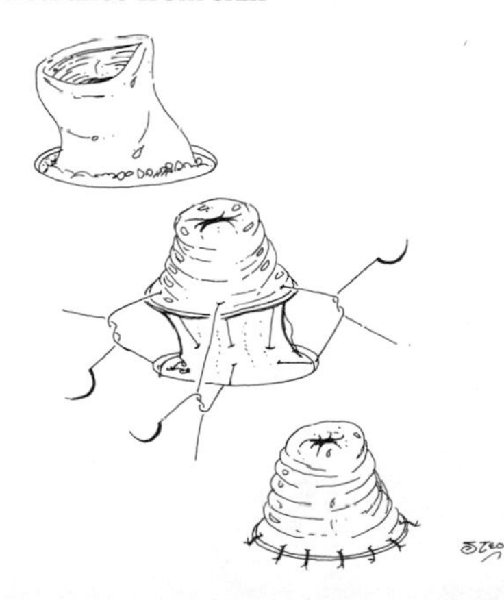

Why doesn't an ileostomy or colostomy close?

Epithelialization (mucosa to skin) from the acronym FRI**E**ND (see Fistula chapter)

Why doesn't a gastrostomy close?

Foreign body (the plastic tube) from the acronym **F**RIEND

If the plastic tube, G-tube, or J-tube is removed, how fast can the hole to the stomach or jejunum close?

In a matter of hours! (Thus, if it comes out inadvertently from a well-established tract, it must be replaced immediately.)

What is a "tube check"?

A Gastrografin contrast study to confirm that a G-tube or J-tube is within the lumen of the stomach or jejunum, respectively

41 Small Intestine

SMALL BOWEL

ANATOMY

What comprises the small bowel?
Duodenum, jejunum, and ileum

How long is the duodenum?
Approximately 12 inches—thus the name: duodenum!

What marks the end of the duodenum and the start of the jejunum?
Ligament of Treitz

What is the length of the entire small bowel?
Approximately 6 meters (20 feet)

What provides blood supply to the small bowel?
Branches of the superior mesenteric artery

What does the small bowel do?
Major site of digestion and absorption

What are the plicae circulares?
Plicae means folds, circulares means circular; thus, circular folds of mucosa (A.K.A., valvulae conniventes) in small bowel lumen

What are the major structural differences between the jejunum and the ileum?
Jejunum—long vasa rectae, large plicae circulares, thicker wall
Ileum—shorter vasa rectae, smaller plicae circulares, thinner wall
(think: **I**leum = **I**nferior vasa rectae, **I**nferior plicae circulares, and **I**nferior wall thickness in comparison to the jejunum)

What does the terminal ileum absorb? B_{12}, fatty acids, bile salts

SMALL BOWEL OBSTRUCTION

What is small bowel obstruction (SBO)? Mechanical obstruction to the passage of intraluminal contents

What are the signs/symptoms? Abdominal discomfort, cramping, nausea, abdominal distention, emesis, high-pitched bowel sounds

What lab tests are performed with SBO? Electrolytes, CBC, type and screen, urinalysis

What are classic electrolyte/acid-base findings with proximal obstruction? Hypovolemic hypochloremic hypokalemia alkalosis

What must be ruled out on physical exam in patients with SBO? Incarcerated hernia (also look for surgical scars)

What major AXR findings are associated with SBO? Distended loops of small bowel
Air-fluid levels on upright film

Define complete SBO. Complete obstruction of the lumen; usually paucity or no colon gas

What is the danger of complete SBO? Closed loop strangulation of the bowel leading to bowel necrosis

Define partial SBO. Incomplete SBO; some colon gas

What is initial management of all patients with SBO? NGT, IVF, Foley (to monitor urine output)

What tests can differentiate partial from complete bowel obstruction? CT with oral contrast, small bowel follow through

What are the ABCs of SBO? Causes of SBO:

1. **A**dhesions
2. **B**ulge (hernias)
3. **C**ancer and tumors

What are other causes of SBO?

Acronym: **"GIVES BAD CRAMPS":**

G-Gallstone ileus
I-Intussusception
V-Volvulus
E-External compression
S-SMA syndrome
B-Bezoars, bowel wall hematoma
A-Abscesses
D-Diverticulitis
C-Crohn's disease
R-Radiation enteritis
A-Annular pancreas
M-Meckel's diverticulum
P-Peritoneal adhesions
S-Stricture

What is SMA syndrome?

Seen with weight loss—SMA compresses duodenum, causing obstruction

What is the treatment of complete SBO?

Laparotomy and lysis of adhesions

What is LOA?

Lysis **O**f **A**dhesions

What is the treatment of incomplete SBO?

Initially, conservative treatment with close observation

Intraoperatively, how can the level of obstruction be determined in patients with SBO?

Transition from dilated bowel proximal to the decompressed bowel distal to the obstruction

What is the most common indication for abdominal surgery in patients with Crohn's disease?

SBO

Can a patient have complete SBO and bowel movements and flatus?

Yes; the bowel distal to the obstruction can clear out gas and stool.

After a small bowel resection, why should the mesenteric defect always be closed?

To prevent an internal hernia

What may cause SBO if patient is on coumadin?

Bowel wall hematoma

What is the #1 cause of SBO in adults?

Postoperative adhesions

What is the #1 cause of SBO around the world?

Hernias

What is the #1 cause of SBO in children?

Hernias

What are the signs of strangulated bowel with SBO?

Fever, severe/continuous pain, hematemesis, **shock,** gas in the bowel wall or portal vein, abdominal free air, **peritoneal signs, acidosis** (increased lactic acid)

What are the clinical parameters that will lower the threshold to operate on a partial SBO?

Increasing **WBC**
Fever
Tachycardia/tachypnea

What is an absolute indication for operation with partial SBO?

Peritoneal signs, free air on AXR

What classic saying is associated with complete SBO?

"Never let the sun set or rise on complete SBO."

What condition commonly mimics SBO?

Paralytic ileus (AXR reveals gas distention throughout, including the colon)

What is the differential diagnosis of paralytic (nonobstructive) ileus?

Postoperative ileus after abdominal surgery (normally resolves in 3–5 days)
Electrolyte abnormalities (hypokalemia is most common)
Medications (anticholinergic, narcotics)
Inflammatory intra-abdominal process
Sepsis/shock
Spine injury/spinal cord injury
Retroperitoneal hemorrhage

SMALL BOWEL TUMORS

What is the differential diagnosis of benign tumors of the small intestine?

Leiomyoma, lipoma, lymphangioma, fibroma, adenomas, hemangiomas

What is the most common benign small bowel tumor?

Leiomyoma

What is the most common malignant small bowel tumor?

Adenocarcinoma

What is the differential diagnosis of malignant tumors of the small intestine?

1. Adenocarcinoma (50%)
2. Carcinoid (25%)
3. Lymphoma (20%)
4. Sarcomas

What malignancy is classically associated with metastasis to small bowel?

Melanoma

MECKEL'S DIVERTICULUM

What is it?

Remnant of the omphalomesenteric duct/vitelline duct, which connects the yolk sac with the primitive midgut in the embryo

What is its claim to fame?

Most common small bowel congenital abnormality

What is the usual location?

Within approximately 2 feet of the ileocecal valve on the **antimesenteric** border of the bowel

What is the major differential diagnosis?

Appendicitis

Is it a true diverticulum?

Yes; all layers of the intestine are found in the wall

What is the incidence?

Approximately 2% of the population at autopsy

What is the gender ratio?

Two times more common in **men**

What is the average age at onset of symptoms?

Most frequently in the first **2 years of life,** but can occur at any age

What are the possible complications?

Intestinal hemorrhage (painless)—50%; accounts for half of all lower GI bleeding in patients younger than 2 years

Bleeding results from ectopic gastric mucosa secreting acid → ulcer → bleeding
Intestinal obstruction—25%; most common complication in adults; includes volvulus and intussusception
Inflammation (± perforations)—20%

What are the signs/ symptoms?
Painless lower GI bleeding, with or without abdominal pain or SBO

What is the most common complication of Meckel's diverticulum in adults?
Intestinal obstruction

In what percentage of cases is heterotopic tissue found in the diverticulum?
More than 50%

What heterotopic tissue type is most often found?
Gastric mucosa (60%), but duodenal, pancreatic, and colonic mucosa are also found

What is the "rule of 2s"?
2% of patients are **symptomatic**
Found approximately **2 feet** from the ileocecal valve
Found in **2%** of the population
Most symptoms occur before age **2** years
Ectopic tissue found in 1 of **2** patients
Most diverticula are approximately **2** inches long
2 to 1 male : female ratio

What is the role of incidental Meckel's diverticulectomy (surgical removal upon finding asymptomatic diverticulum)?
Most experts would remove in children (very controversial in adults).

What is a Meckel's scan?
Scan for ectopic gastric mucosa in Meckel's diverticulum; uses **technetium pertechnetate** IV, which is preferentially taken up by gastric mucosa

What is the treatment of a Meckel's diverticulum that is causing bleeding and obstruction?
Surgical resection, with small bowel resection as the actual ulcer is usually on the mesenteric wall opposite the diverticulum!

What is the name of the hernia associated with incarcerated Meckel's diverticulum?	Littre's hernia
In patients with guaiac-positive stools and a negative upper- and lower-GI workup, what must be ruled out?	A small bowel tumor; evaluate with enteroclysis (small bowel contrast study)
What is the most common cause of small bowel bleeding?	Small bowel angiodysplasia

42 The Appendix

What vessel provides blood supply to the appendix?	Appendiceal artery
Name the mesentery of the appendix.	Mesoappendix (contains the appendiceal artery)
How can the appendix be located if the cecum has been identified?	Follow the taenia coli down to the appendix. The taeniae converge on the appendix.

APPENDICITIS

What is it?	Inflammation of the appendix caused by **obstruction** of the appendiceal lumen, producing a closed loop with resultant inflammation that can lead to necrosis and perforation
What are the causes?	**Fecalith** 35% (A.K.A. appendicolith); **lymphoid hyperplasia** 65% Rare—parasite, foreign body, tumor (e.g., carcinoid)
What is the lifetime incidence of acute appendicitis in the United States?	Approximately 7%!
What is the most common cause of emergent abdominal surgery in the United States?	Acute appendicitis
How does it present?	Onset of referred **periumbilical pain** followed by **anorexia,** nausea, and vomiting

(**Note:** Unlike gastroenteritis, pain precedes vomiting.) Pain then migrates to the RLQ, where it becomes more intense and localized because of local peritoneal irritation. The presentation may vary, depending on the anatomic location of the appendix. Anorexia is almost always present; if the patient is hungry and can eat, seriously question the diagnosis of appendicitis.)

Why does periumbilical pain occur?

Referred pain

Why does RLQ pain occur?

Peritoneal irritation

How is the diagnosis made?

History and physical examination

What are the signs/ symptoms?

Signs of peritoneal irritation may be present: guarding, muscle spasm, rebound tenderness, obturator and psoas signs, low-grade fever (high-grade if perforation occurs), RLQ hyperesthesia

Define the following terms:

Obturator sign

Pain upon internal rotation of the leg with the hip and knee flexed; seen in patients with appendicitis/pelvic abscess

Psoas sign

Pain elicited by extending the hip with the knee in full extension or by flexing the hip against resistance; seen with appendicitis and psoas inflammation

Rovsing's sign

Palpation or rebound pressure of the LLQ results in pain in the RLQ; seen in appendicitis

Valentino's sign

RLQ pain/peritonitis from succus draining down to the RLQ from a perforated gastric or duodenal ulcer

McBurney's point

Point one-third from the anterior iliac spine to the umbilicus (often the point of maximal tenderness)

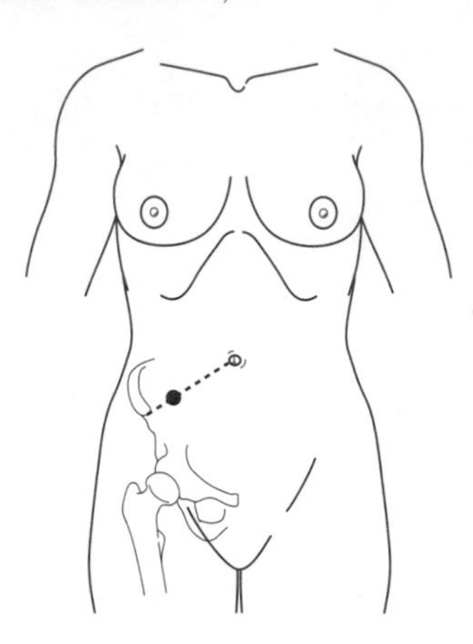

What is the differential diagnosis?

Meckel's diverticulum; Crohn's disease; ovarian torsion, cyst, or tumor; perforated ulcer; pancreatitis; pelvic inflammatory disease; ruptured ectopic pregnancy; mesenteric lymphadenitis; mittelschmerz; constipation; gastroenteritis; intussusception; volvulus; tumors; UTI (e.g., cystitis); pyelonephritis

What lab tests should be performed?

CBC: increased WBC (> 10,000 per mm^3 in > 90% of cases), most often with a "left shift"

Urinalysis: to evaluate for pyelonephritis or renal calculus

(Note: Mild hematuria and pyuria are common in appendicitis with pelvic inflammation, resulting in inflammation of the ureter.)

What additional tests can be performed if the diagnosis is not clear?

AXR, spiral CT, US (may see a large, noncompressible appendix or fecalith)

In acute appendicitis, what classically precedes vomiting?

Pain (in gastroenteritis, the pain classically follows vomiting)

Does a positive urinalysis rule out appendicitis?

No; ureteral inflammation resulting from the periappendiceal inflammation can cause abnormal urinalysis.

What radiographic studies are often performed?

CXR: to rule out RML or RLL pneumonia
AXR: abdominal films are usually nonspecific, but calcified fecaliths present in about 5% of cases

What are the radiographic signs of appendicitis on AXR?

Fecalith, sentinel loops, **scoliosis** away from the right because of pain, mass effect (abscess), loss of psoas shadow, loss of preperitoneal fat stripe, and (very rarely) a small amount of free air if perforated

With acute appendicitis, in what percentage of cases will a radiopaque fecalith be on AXR?

Only approximately 5% of the time!

What are the CT findings with acute appendicitis?

Periappendiceal fat stranding, appendiceal diameter > 6 mm, periappendiceal fluid

What are the preoperative medications/preparation?

1. Rehydration with **IV fluids** (LR)
2. Preoperative **antibiotics** with anaerobic coverage (appendix is considered part of the colon); cefoxitin (Mefoxin) most often used

What is a lap appy?

Laparoscopic appendectomy; used in most cases in women (can see adnexa) or if patient has a need to quickly return to physical activity

How does treatment differ for nonperforated and perforated appendicitis?

Nonperforated—prompt appendectomy (prevents perforation), 24 hours of antibiotics, discharge home usually on postoperative day 1
Perforated—IV fluid resuscitation and prompt appendectomy; all pus is drained and cultures obtained, with postoperative antibiotics continued for 3 to 7 days; wound is left open in most cases of perforation after closing the fascia (heals by secondary intention or delayed primary closure)

How is an appendiceal abscess treated?

Usually by **percutaneous** drainage of the abscess, antibiotic administration, and elective appendectomy approximately 6 to 8 weeks later (A.K.A. interval appendectomy)

If a normal appendix is found upon exploration, should you take out the normal appendix?
Yes

How long after removal of a NONRUPTURED appendix should antibiotics continue postoperatively?
For 24 hours

Which antibiotic is used for nonperforated appendicitis?
Anaerobic coverage: Cefoxitin®, Cefotetan®, or Unasyn®

What antibiotic is used for a PERFORATED appendix?
Usually triple antibiotics (e.g., Amp/Gent/Clinda)

How long do you give antibiotics for perforated appendicitis?
Until the patient has a normal WBC count and is afebrile, ambulating, and eating a regular diet (usually 3–7 days)

What is the risk of perforation?
Approximately 25% by 24 hours from onset of symptoms, approximately 50% by 36 hours, and approximately 75% by 48 hours

What is the most common general surgical abdominal emergency in pregnancy?
Appendicitis (about 1/1750; **appendix may be in the RUQ because of the enlarged uterus)**

What are the possible complications of appendicitis?
Pelvic abscess, liver abscess, free perforation, portal pylethrombophlebitis (very rare)

What percentage of the population has a retrocecal, retroperitoneal appendix?
Approximately 15%

What percentage of negative appendectomies is acceptable?
Up to 20%; taking out some normal appendixes is better than missing a case of acute appendicitis that eventually ruptures.

Who is at risk of dying from acute appendicitis?
Very old and very young patients

What bacteria are associated with "mesenteric adenitis" that can closely mimic acute appendicitis?
Yersinia enterolytica

What is an "incidental appendectomy"?

Removal of normal appendix during abdominal operation for different procedure

What are complications of an appendectomy?

SBO, enterocutaneous fistula, wound infection, infertility with perforation in women, increased incidence of right inguinal hernia, stump abscess

What is the most common postoperative complication?

Wound infection

INTRAOPERATIVE QUESTIONS

What is the difference between a McBurney's incision and a Rocky-Davis incision?

McBurney's is angled down (follows ext oblique fibers) and Rocky-Davis is straight across (transverse).

What are the layers of the abdominal wall during a McBurney incision?

1. Skin
2. Subcutaneous fat
3. Scarpa's fascia
4. External oblique
5. Internal oblique
6. Transversus muscle
7. Transversalis fascia
8. Preperitoneal fat
9. Peritoneum

What are the steps in laparoscopic appendectomy (lap appy)?

1. Identify the appendix.
2. Staple the mesoappendix (or coagulate).
3. Staple and transect the appendix at the base (or use Endoloop® and cut between).
4. Remove the appendix from the abdomen.
5. Irrigate and aspirate until clear.

Do you routinely get peritoneal cultures for acute appendicitis (nonperforated)?

No

How can you find the appendix after identifying the cecum?

Follow the taenia down to where they converge on the appendix.

Which way should your finger sweep trying to find the appendix?
Lateral to medial along the lateral peritoneum—this way you will not tear the mesoappendix that lies medially!

How to get to a retrocecal and retroperitoneal appendix?
Divide the lateral peritoneal attachments of the cecum.

Why use electrocautery on the exposed mucosa on the appendiceal stump?
To kill the mucosal cells so they do not form a mucocele

If you find Crohn's disease in the terminal ileum, will you remove the appendix?
Yes, if the cecal/appendiceal base is not involved

If the appendix is normal what do you inspect intraoperatively?
Terminal ileum: Meckel's diverticulum, Crohn's disease, intussusception
Gynecologic: Cysts, torsion, etc.
Groin: hernia, rectus sheath hematoma, adenopathy (adenitis)

Who performed the first appendectomy?
Harry Hancock in 1848 (McBurney popularized the procedure in 1880s)

Who performed the first lap appy?
Dr. Semm (GYN) 1983

APPENDICEAL TUMORS

What is the most common appendiceal tumor?
Carcinoid tumor

What is the treatment of appendiceal carcinoid less than 2 cm?
Appendectomy (if not through the bowel wall)

What is the treatment of appendiceal carcinoid larger than 2 cm?
Right hemicolectomy

What percentage of appendiceal carcinoids are malignant?
Less than 5%

What are the differential diagnoses of appendiceal tumor?
Carcinoid, adenocarcinoma, malignant mucoid adenocarcinoma

What type of appendiceal tumor can cause the dreaded pseudomyxoma peritonei if the appendix ruptures?

Malignant mucoid adenocarcinoma

43 Carcinoid Tumors

What is a carcinoid tumor?

A tumor arising from neuroendocrine cells (APUDomas), A.K.A. **Kulchitsky cells;** basically, a tumor that secretes **serotonin**

How can one remember that Kulchitsky cells are found in carcinoid tumors?

Think: "COOL CAR" or **KUL**chitsky **CAR**cinoid

What is the incidence?

Between 0.2 and 1.0% and about 25% of all small bowel tumors

What are the common sites of occurrence?

1. Appendix (most common)
2. Ileum
3. Rectum
4. Bronchus

Other sites: jejunum, stomach, duodenum, colon, ovary, testicle, pancreas, thymus

What are the signs/ symptoms?

Depends on location; most cases are asymptomatic; also SBO, abdominal pain, bleeding, weight loss, diaphoresis, **pellagra skin changes,** intussusception, or carcinoid syndrome

What are the pellagra-like symptoms?

3-Ds:

Dermatitis
Diarrhea
Dementia

What is carcinoid syndrome?

Syndrome of symptoms caused by release of substances from a carcinoid tumor

What are the symptoms of carcinoid syndrome?

Acronym **B FDR:**

Bronchospasm
Flushing (skin)
Diarrhea
Right-sided heart failure (from valve failure)

What is a complete memory aid for carcinoid?	"Be FDR in a cool car."
Why does right-sided heart failure develop but not left-sided heart failure?	The lungs act as a filter (just like the liver); thus, the left heart doesn't see all the vasoactive compounds.
What is the incidence of carcinoid SYNDROME in patients who have a carcinoid TUMOR?	Approximately 10%
What released substances cause carcinoid syndrome?	**Serotonin** and vasoactive peptides
What is medical treatment for carcinoid syndrome?	Octreotide IV
How does the liver prevent carcinoid syndrome?	By degradation of serotonin and the other vasoactive peptides when the **tumor drains into the portal vein**
Why does carcinoid syndrome occur in some tumors and not in others?	It occurs when **venous drainage from the tumor gains access to the systemic circulation** by avoiding hepatic degradation of the vasoactive substances.
What tumors can produce carcinoid syndrome?	**Liver metastases** Retroperitoneal disease draining into paravertebral veins Primary tumor outside the GI tract, portal venous drainage (e.g., ovary, **testicular,** bronchus), or both
To what does the liver break down the serotonin?	5-hydroxyindoleacetic acid (**5-HIAA**)
What are the associated diagnostic lab findings?	**Elevated urine 5-HIAA,** as well as urine and blood **serotonin** levels
What stimulation test can often elevate serotonin levels and cause symptoms of carcinoid syndrome?	Pentagastrin stimulation
What are special radiologic localization tests?	111In-Octreotide/111In-labeled Pentetreotide scintigraphy and 131-MIBG (Metaiodobenzylguanidine), which is less sensitive

What radiologic studies should be performed?	Barium enema, upper GI series with small bowel follow-through, colonoscopy, abdominal CT
Is abdominal CT helpful for finding primary tumors?	Abdominal CT is usually not helpful because these tumors are small and slow growing.
What is the surgical treatment?	Excision of the primary tumor and single or feasible metastasis in the liver (liver transplant is an option with unresectable liver metastasis); chemotherapy for advanced disease
What is the medical treatment?	Medical therapy for palliation of the carcinoid syndrome (serotonin antagonists, somatostatin analogue [**octreotide**])
How effective is octreotide?	It relieves diarrhea and flushing in more than 85% of cases and may shrink tumor in 10% to 20% of cases.
What is a common antiserotonin drug?	**Cyproheptadine**
What is the overall prognosis?	Two-thirds of patients are alive at 5 years.
What is the prognosis of patients with liver metastasis or carcinoid syndrome?	50% are alive at 3 years.
What does carcinoid tumor look like?	Usually intramural bowel mass; appears as **yellowish** tumor upon incision
For appendiceal carcinoid, when is a right hemicolectomy indicated versus an appendectomy?	If the tumor is **more than 2 cm,** right **hemicolectomy** is indicated; if there are no signs of serosal involvement and tumor is less than **2 cm, appendectomy** should be performed (controversial; some experts state 1.5 cm).
Which primary site has the highest rate of metastasis?	Ileal primary tumor

Can a carcinoid tumor be confirmed malignant by looking at the histology?

No; metastasis must be present to diagnose malignancy.

What is the correlation between tumor size and malignancy potential?

The vast majority of tumors less than 2 cm are benign. In tumors more than 2 cm, malignancy potential is significant.

44 Fistulas

What is a fistula?

An abnormal **communication** between two hollow organs or a hollow organ and the exterior (i.e., two epithelial cell layers)

What are the predisposing factors and conditions that maintain patency of a fistula?

The acronym **HIS FRIEND:**
High output fistula (> 500 cc/day)
Intestinal destruction (> 50% of circumference)
Short segment fistula < 2.5 cm

Foreign body (e.g., G-tube)
Radiation
Infection
Epithelization (e.g., colostomy)
Neoplasm
Distal obstruction

SPECIFIC TYPES OF FISTULAS

ENTEROCUTANEOUS

What is it?

A fistula from GI tract to skin (entero—cutaneous = **bowel to skin)**

What are the causes?

Anastomotic leak, trauma/injury to the bowel/colon, Crohn's disease, abscess, diverticulitis, inflammation/infection, inadvertent suture through bowel

How is diagnosis confirmed?

P.O. charcoal and look for black output on dressings

What is the work up?

CT to rule out abscess/inflammatory process

What are the possible complications?

High-output fistulas, malnutrition, skin breakdown

What is the treatment?

NPO; TPN; rule out and correct underlying causes, may feed distally (or if fistula is distal, feed elemental diet proximally)
Half will close spontaneously, but the other half require operation and resection of the involved bowel segment

Which enterocutaneous fistula closes faster: short or long?

A long fistula (may be counterintuitive—but true)

What is the overall mortality of an enterocutaneous fistula?

Up to 20%!

COLONIC FISTULAS

What are they?

Include colovesical, colocutaneous, colovaginal, and coloenteric fistulas

What are the most common causes?

Diverticulitis (most common cause), cancer, IBD, foreign body, and irradiation

What is the most common type?

Colovesical fistula, which often presents with recurrent urinary tract infections
Other signs include pneumaturia, dysuria, and fecaluria

How is the diagnosis made?

Via BE and cystoscopy

What is the treatment?

Surgery: segmental colon resection and primary anastomosis; repair/resection of the involved organ (may require temporary colostomy)

What is a cholecystenteric fistula?

Connection between gallbladder and duodenum or other loop of small bowel due to large gallstone erosion, often resulting in SBO as the gallstone lodges in the ileocecal valve (gallstone ileus)

What are the common causes of a gastrocolic fistula?

Penetrating ulcers, **gastric** or **colonic cancer,** and Crohn's disease

What are the possible complications of gastrocolic fistula?

Malnutrition and severe **enteritis** due to reflux of colonic contents into the stomach and small bowel with subsequent bacterial overgrowth

FISTULA IN ANO

What is it?

Anal fistula, from rectum to perianal skin

What are the causes?

Usually anal crypt/gland infection (usually perianal abscess)

What are the signs/ symptoms?

Perianal drainage, perirectal abscess, recurrent perirectal abscess, "diaper rash," itching

What disease should be considered with fistula in ano?

Crohn's disease

How is the diagnosis made?

Exam, proctoscope

What is Goodsall's rule?

Fistulas originating **anterior** to a transverse line through the anus will course **straight** ahead and exit anteriorly, whereas those exiting **posteriorly** have a **curved** tract.

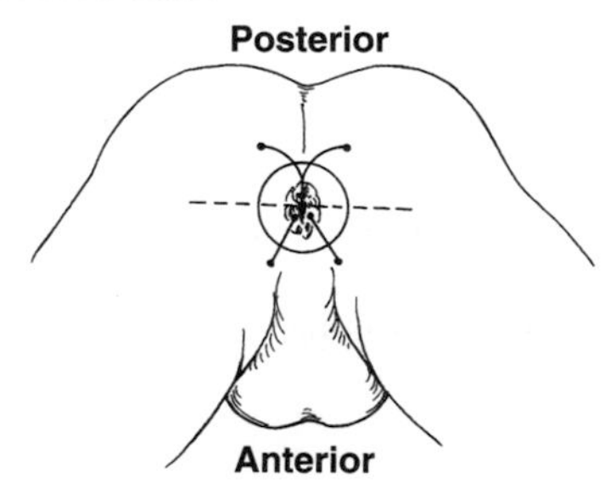

How can Goodsall's rule be remembered?

Think of a dog with a **straight** nose (anterior) and **curved** tail (posterior)

What is the management of anorectal fistulas?

Define the pathoanatomy
Marsupialization of fistula tract (i.e., fillet tract open)
Wound care: routine Sitz baths and dressing changes
Seton placement if fistula is through the sphincter muscle

What is a Seton?

A thick suture placed through fistula tract to allow slow transection of sphincter muscle; scar tissue formed will hold the sphincter muscle in place and allow for continence after transection

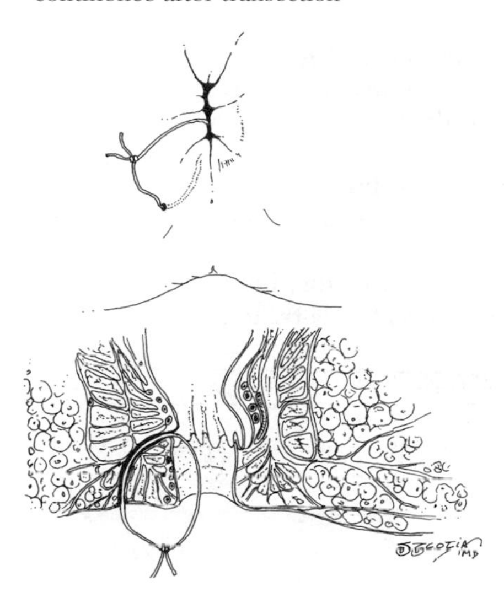

What percentage of patients with a perirectal abscess develop a fistula in ano after drainage?

Approximately 50%

How to find the internal rectal opening of an anorectal fistula?

Inject H_2O_2 or methylene blue in external opening—then look for bubbles coming out of internal opening!

PANCREATIC ENTERIC FISTULA

What is it?

Decompression of a **pseudocyst** or **abscess** into an adjacent organ (a **rare** complication); usually done surgically or endoscopically to treat a pancreatic pseudocyst

EXTERNAL PANCREATIC FISTULA

What is it?

Pancreaticocutaneous fistula; drainage of pancreatic exocrine secretions through to abdominal skin (usually through drain tract/wound)

What is the treatment?
NPO, TPN, skin protection, **octreotide**

What is a "refractory" pancreatic fistula?
Pancreaticocutaneous fistula that does not resolve with conservative medical management (the minority of cases)

What is the diagnostic test for "refractory" pancreatic fistulas?
ERCP to define site of fistula tract (i.e., tail versus head of pancreas)

How is refractory tail of a pancreas fistula treated?
Resection of the tail of the pancreas and the fistula

How is refractory head of a pancreas fistula treated?
Pancreaticojejunostomy

BLADDER FISTULAS

What are the specific types?
Vesicoenteric (50% due to sigmoid diverticulitis)
Vesicovaginal (most are secondary to gynecologic procedures; signs include urinary leak through vagina, and diagnosis is by IVP or instilling bladder with methylene blue and monitoring vagina for the appearance of dye)

45 Colon and Rectum

ANATOMY

Identify the arterial blood supply to the colon:

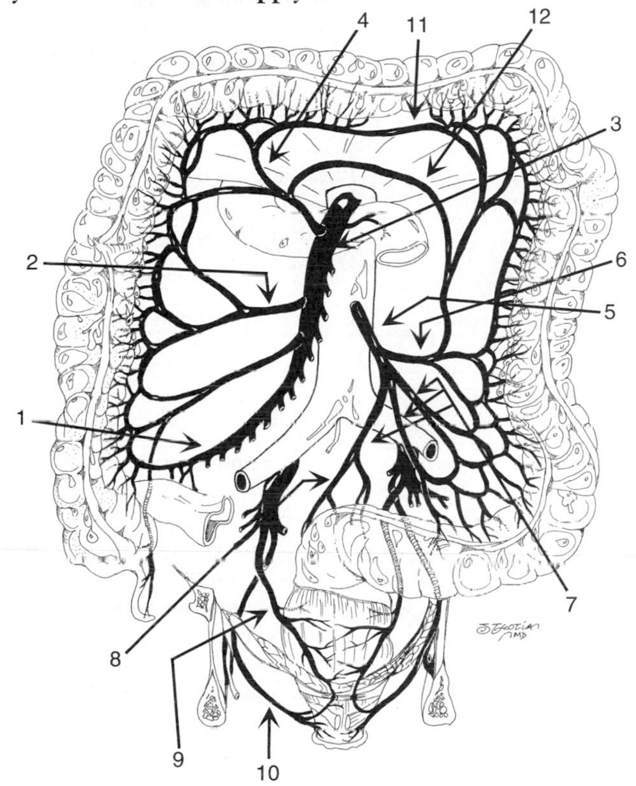

1. Ileocolic artery
2. Right colic artery
3. Superior mesenteric artery (SMA)
4. Middle colic artery
5. Inferior mesenteric artery (IMA)
6. Left colic artery
7. Sigmoidal artery
8. Superior hemorrhoidal artery (superior rectal)
9. Middle hemorrhoidal artery
10. Inferior hemorrhoidal artery
11. Marginal artery of Drummond
12. Meandering artery of Gonzalez

What are the white lines of Toldt?
The lateral peritoneal reflections of the ascending and descending colon

What part of the GI tract does not have a serosa?
Esophagus, middle and distal **rectum**

What are the major anatomic differences between the colon and the small bowel?
The colon has taenia coli, haustra, and appendices epiploicae (fat appendages), whereas the small intestine is smooth.

What is the blood supply to the rectum?
Proximal: superior hemorrhoidal (or superior rectal) from the IMA
Middle: middle hemorrhoidal (or middle rectal) from the hypogastric (int. iliac)
Distal: inferior hemorrhoidal (or inferior rectal) from the pudendal artery (a branch of the hypogastric artery)

What is the venous drainage of the rectum?
Proximal: via the IMV to the splenic vein, then **to the portal vein**
Middle: via the iliac vein to the **IVC**
Distal: via the iliac vein to the **IVC**

What is the main purpose of the colon?
H_2O absorption and stool storage

COLORECTAL CARCINOMA

What is it?
Adenocarcinoma of the colon or rectum

What is the incidence?
Most common GI cancer
Second most common cancer in the United States
Incidence increases with age starting at 40 and peaks at 70 to 80 years.

How common is it as a cause of cancer deaths?
Second most common cause of cancer deaths

What is the male to female ratio?
Approximately 1:1

What are the risk factors?
Dietary: Low-fiber, high-fat diets correlate with increased rates.
Genetic: Family history is important when taking history.
FAP, Lynch's syndrome
IBD: ulcerative colitis > Crohn's disease
Age, previous colon cancer

What is Lynch's syndrome?

HNPCC = **H**ereditary **n**on**p**olyposis **c**olon **c**ancer—autosomal-dominant inheritance of high risk for development of colon cancer

What are current ACS recommendations for colorectal screening without family (first-degree) history of colorectal cancer?

Annual digital rectal exam starting at age 40 (remember that approximately 10% of tumors are palpable by rectal exam!)
Annual test for fecal occult blood starting at age 40
Flex sig or colonoscopy at age 50, repeated every 3 to 5 years thereafter

What is a flex sig?

Flexible sigmoidoscopy (limited scope up to splenic flexure)

What are the current recommendations for colorectal cancer screening if there is a history of colorectal cancer in a first-degree relative?

Patients with a family history of colorectal cancer need a more aggressive approach: colonoscopy or air contrast barium enema (ACBE) at age 40.

What percentage of adults will have a guaiac-positive stool test?

Approximately 2%

What percentage of patients with a guaiac-positive stool test will have colon cancer?

Approximately 10%

What signs/symptoms are associated with the following conditions:

Right-sided lesions?

Right side of bowel has a large luminal diameter, so a tumor may attain a large size before causing problems.
Microcytic anemia, occult/melena > hematochezia PR, postprandial discomfort, fatigue

Left-sided lesions?

Left side of bowel has smaller lumen and semisolid contents.
Change in bowel habits (small-caliber stools), colicky pain, signs of obstruction, abdominal mass, heme(+) or gross red blood
Nausea, vomiting, constipation

From which site is melena more common?
Right-sided colon cancer

From which site is hematochezia more common?
Left-sided colon cancer

What is the incidence of rectal cancer?
Comprises 20% to 30% of all colorectal cancer

What are the signs/ symptoms of rectal cancer?
Most common symptom is hematochezia (passage of red blood ± stool) or mucus; also tenesmus, feeling of incomplete evacuation of stool (because of the mass), and rectal mass.

What is the differential diagnosis of a colon tumor/ mass?
Adenocarcinoma, carcinoid tumor, lipoma, liposarcoma, leiomyoma, leiomyosarcoma, lymphoma, diverticular disease, ulcerative colitis, Crohn's disease, polyps

Which diagnostic tests are helpful?
History and physical exam (**Note: approximately 10% of cancers are palpable on rectal exam**), heme occult, CBC, barium enema, sigmoid/ colonoscopy

What disease does microcytic anemia signify until proven otherwise in a man or postmenopausal woman?
Colon cancer

What tests help find metastases?
CXR (lung metastases), LFTs (liver metastases), abdominal CT (liver metastases), other tests based on history and physical exam (e.g., head CT for left arm weakness looking for brain metastasis)

What is the preoperative workup for colorectal cancer?
History, physical exam, LFTs, CEA, CBC, Chem 10, PT/PTT, type and cross 2 u PRBCs, CXR, U/A, abdominopelvic CT

What are the means by which the cancer spreads?
Direct extension: circumferentially and then through bowel wall to later invade other abdominoperineal organs

	Hematogenous: portal circulation to liver; lumbar/vertebral veins to lungs Lymphogenous: regionally Transperitoneal Intraluminal
Is CEA useful?	Not for screening but for baseline and recurrence surveillance (but offers no proven survival benefit)
What unique diagnostic test is helpful in patients with rectal cancer?	Endorectal ultrasound (probe is placed transanally and depth of invasion and nodes are evaluated)
How are tumors staged?	Astler-Coller modified Dukes, and the TMN staging system
The Duke stages were first described for what disease?	Rectal cancer (not colon cancer!) in 1932
Give the Astler-Coller modified Dukes stages:	
A	Invasion of submucosa
B1	Invasion of muscularis propria
B2	Invasion of subserosa
C	Positive nodal metastasis
D	Distant metastasis (D = Distant)
Give the TNM stages:	
Stage I	Invades submucosa or muscularis propria (T1–2,N0,M0)
Stage II	Invades through muscularis propria or surrounding structures but with negative nodes (T3–4, N0, M0)
Stage III	Positive nodes, no distant metastasis (any T, N1–3, M0)
Stage IV	Positive distant metastasis (any T, any N, M1)

What is the approximate 5-year survival by stage:	
Stage I?	**90%**
Stage II?	**75%**
Stage III?	**50%**
Stage IV?	**5%**
Define the preoperative "bowel prep."	Preoperative preparation for colon/rectal resection: 1. Golytely colonic lavage or Fleets Phospho-Soda until clear effluent per rectum 2. PO antibiotics (1 gm neomycin and 1 gm erythromycin × 3 doses) Patient should also receive preoperative and 24-hr IV antibiotics.
What are the common preoperative IV antibiotics?	Cefoxitin, cefotetan, Unasyn
What are the treatment options?	Resection: wide surgical resection of lesion and its regional lymphatic drainage
What decides low anterior resection (LAR) versus abdominal perineal resection (APR)?	**Distance from the anal verge, pelvis size**
What is the lowest LAR possible?	Coloanal anastomosis (anastomosis normal colon directly to anus)
What do you need with any anastomosis less than 5 cm from the anus?	Temporary ileostomy
What surgical margins are needed for colon cancer?	Traditionally more than 5 cm; margins must be at least 2 cm
What is the minimal surgical margin for rectal cancer?	2 cm
What is the adjuvant treatment of Dukes' C colon cancer?	5-FU and levamisole (or leucovorin) chemotherapy if there is nodal metastasis

What is the adjuvant treatment for T3-T4 rectal cancer?	**Preop radiation therapy** and 5-FU chemotherapy as a "radiosensitizer"
What is the most common site of distant (hematogenous) metastasis from colorectal cancer?	Liver
What is the treatment of liver metastases from colorectal cancer?	Resect with 1 to 2 cm margins and administer chemotherapy.
What is the 5-year survival rate after resection of liver colorectal metastases?	Approximately 25% if resected with 1 to 2 cm margins (0% survive 5 years without resection)
What is the appropriate postoperative follow-up at 3 months?	Physical exam, stool guaiac, CEA (every 3 months for 3 years, then every 6 months for 2 years)
Why is follow-up so important the first 3 postoperative years?	Approximately 90% of colorectal recurrences are within 3 years of surgery.
What is the most common cause of colonic obstruction in the adult population?	Colon cancer (number two is diverticular disease, number three is colonic volvulus)
What is the 5-year survival rate after liver resection with clean margins for colon cancer liver metastasis?	Approximately 25%
What is the 5-year survival rate after diagnosis of unresectable colon cancer liver metastasis?	0%

POLYPS

POLYPS OF THE COLON AND RECTUM

What are they?	Tissue growth into bowel lumen, usually consisting of mucosa, submucosa, or both
How are they anatomically classified?	*Sessile* (flat) *Pedunculated* (on a stalk)

What are the histologic classifications of the following types:

Inflammatory (pseudopolyp)? As in Crohn's disease or ulcerative colitis

Hamartomatous? Normal tissue in abnormal configuration

Hyperplastic? Benign—normal cells—no malignant potential

Neoplastic? Proliferation of undifferentiated cells; premalignant or malignant cells

What are the subtypes of neoplastic polyps?
Tubular adenomas (usually pedunculated)
Tubulovillous adenomas
Villous adenomas (usually sessile and look like broccoli heads)

What determines malignant potential of an adenomatous polyp?
Size
Histologic type
Atypia of cells

What is the most common type of adenomatous polyp? Tubular 85%

What is the correlation between size and malignancy? Polyps larger than 2 cm have a high risk of carcinoma (33%–55%).

What about histology and cancer potential of an adenomatous polyp? Villous polyps have a higher risk of carcinoma than tubulovillous, which have a higher risk than tubular (**think: VILL**ous = **VILL**ain).

What is the approximate percentage of carcinomas found in the following polyps overall:

Tubular adenoma? 5%

Tubulovillous adenoma? 20%

Villous adenoma? 40%

Where are most polyps found? Rectosigmoid (30%)

What are signs/symptoms?
Bleeding (red or dark blood), change in bowel habits, mucus per rectum, electrolyte loss, totally asymptomatic

What are the diagnostic tests?
Fecal occult blood, CBC, BE, endoscopy—all suspect tissue should be biopsied or excised (snare) and sent to pathology

What is the treatment?
Endoscopic resection (snared) if polyps are small; large sessile villous adenomas should be removed with bowel resection

POLYPOSIS SYNDROMES

FAMILIAL POLYPOSIS

What is another name for this condition?
Familial adenomatous polyposis (FAP)

What are the characteristics?
Hundreds of adenomatous polyps within the rectum and colon that begin developing at puberty; all undiagnosed; untreated patients develop cancer by ages 40 to 50

What is the inheritance pattern?
Autosomal dominant (i.e., 50% of offspring)

What is the genetic defect?
APC (adenomatous polyposis coli) gene

What is the treatment?
Total proctocolectomy and ileostomy
Total colectomy and rectal mucosal removal (mucosal proctectomy) and ileoanal anastomosis

GARDNER'S SYNDROME

What are the characteristics?
Neoplastic polyps of the **small bowel** and **colon;** cancer by age 40 in 100% of undiagnosed patients, as in FAP

What are the other associated findings?
Desmoid tumors (in abdominal wall or cavity), **osteomas** of skull (seen on x-ray), **sebaceous** cysts, adrenal and thyroid tumors, retroperitoneal fibrosis, duodenal and periampullary tumors

How can the findings associated with Gardner's syndrome be remembered?

Think of a gardener planting **SOD:**
S = **S**ebaceous cysts
O = **O**steomas
D = **D**esmoid tumors

What is a desmoid tumor?

Tumor of the musculoaponeurotic sheath, usually of the abdominal wall; benign, but grows locally; treated by wide resection

What is the inheritance pattern?

Varying degree of penetrance from an autosomal-dominant gene

What is the treatment of colon polyps in patients with Gardner's syndrome?

Total proctocolectomy and ileostomy
Total colectomy and rectal mucosal removal (mucosal proctectomy) and ileoanal anastomosis

PEUTZ-JEGHERS SYNDROME

What are the characteristics?

Hamartomas throughout the GI tract (jejunum/ileum > colon > stomach)

What is the associated cancer risk from polyps?

Increased

What is the associated cancer risk for women with Peutz-Jeghers?

Ovarian cancer (granulosa cell tumor is most common)

What is the inheritance pattern?

Autosomal dominant

What are the other signs?

Melanotic pigmentation (black/brown) of buccal mucosa (mouth), lips, digits, palms, feet (soles)
(Think: **P**eutz = **P**igmented)

What is the treatment?

Removal of polyps, if symptomatic (i.e., bleeding, intussusception, or obstruction) or large (> 1.5 cm)

What are juvenile polyps?

Benign hamartomas in the small bowel and colon; not premalignant; also known as "retention polyps"

What is Cronkhite-Canada syndrome?

Diffuse GI hamartoma polyps (i.e., no cancer potential) associated with malabsorption/weight loss, diarrhea, and **loss of electrolytes/protein;** signs include alopecia, nail atrophy, skin pigmentation

What is Turcot's syndrome?

Colon polyps with malignant CNS tumors (glioblastoma multiforme)

DIVERTICULAR DISEASE OF THE COLON

DIVERTICULOSIS

What is diverticulosis?

A condition in which diverticula can be found within the colon, especially the sigmoid; diverticula are actually **false diverticula** in that only mucosa and submucosa herniate through the bowel musculature; true diverticula involve all layers of the bowel wall and are rare in the colon

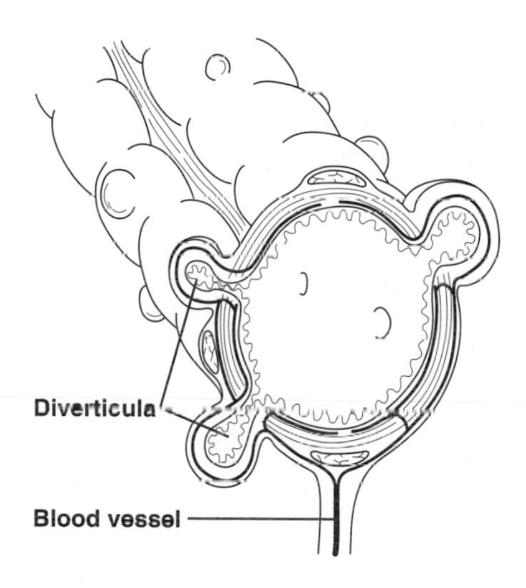

Describe the pathophysiology

Weakness in the bowel wall develops at points where nutrient **blood vessels** enter between antimesenteric and mesenteric taenia; increased intraluminal pressures then cause herniation through these areas.

What is the incidence?

Approximately 50% to 60% in the United States by age 60, with only 10% to 20% becoming symptomatic

What is the most common site?	95% of people with diverticulosis have **sigmoid** colon involvement.
Who is at risk?	People with **low-fiber diets,** chronic constipation, and a positive family history; incidence increases with age
What are the symptoms/ complications?	**Bleeding:** may be massive Diverticulitis asymptomatic (80% of cases)
What is the diagnostic approach:	
Bleeding?	Without signs of inflammation: colonoscopy
Pain and signs of inflammation?	Abdominal or pelvic CT; BE or colonoscopy may be done 6 to 8 weeks after inflammation resolves
What is the treatment of diverticulosis?	High-fiber diet is recommended.
What are the indications for operation with diverticulosis?	Complications of diverticulitis (e.g., abscess, fistula, obstruction, stricture); recurrent episodes; hemorrhage; suspected carcinoma; prolonged symptoms

DIVERTICULITIS

What is it?	Infection or perforation of a diverticulum
What is the pathophysiology?	**Obstruction** of diverticulum by a fecalith leading to inflammation and microperforation
What are the signs/ symptoms?	LLQ pain (cramping or steady), change in bowel habits (**diarrhea**), fever, chills, anorexia, LLQ mass, nausea/vomiting, dysuria
What are the associated lab findings?	Increased WBCs
What are the associated radiographic findings?	On x-ray: ileus; partially obstructed colon; air-fluid levels; free air if perforated On abdominal/pelvic CT: swollen, edematous bowel wall; particularly helpful in diagnosing an abscess

What are the associated barium enema findings?
Barium enema should be avoided in acute cases.

What are the associated colonoscopic findings?
Also should be avoided in acute cases

What are the possible complications?
Abscess, peritonitis, fistula (e.g., colovesicular), obstruction

What is the initial therapy?
IV fluids, NPO, broad-spectrum antibiotics with anaerobic coverage, NG suction (as needed)

When is surgery warranted?
Obstruction, fistula, free perforation, abscess not amenable to percutaneous drainage, sepsis

What is the lifelong risk of recurrence after first episode?
33% (50% recurrence after second episode)

What are the indications for elective resection?
Two episodes of diverticulitis or after the **first** episode in a young, diabetic, or immunosuppressed patient

What surgery is usually performed ELECTIVELY for recurrent bouts?
A one-stage operation: resection of involved segment and primary anastomosis (with preoperative bowel prep)

What type of surgery is usually performed for an acute case of diverticulitis with a complication (e.g., perforation, obstruction)?
Hartmann's procedure: resection of involved segment with an end colostomy and stapled rectal stump (will need subsequent reanastomosis of colon usually after 2–3 postoperative months)

What is the treatment of diverticular abscess?
Percutaneous drainage, if abscess is not amenable to percutaneous drainage, then surgical approach for drainage is necessary, IV antibiotics, bowel rest

How common is massive lower GI bleeding with diverticulitis?
Very **rare**! Massive lower GI bleeding is seen with diverticulosis, not diverticulitis.

What are the most common causes of massive lower GI bleeding in adults?
Diverticulosis (especially right-sided), vascular ectasia

What must you rule out in any patient with diverticulitis/diverticulosis?
Colon cancer

COLONIC VOLVULUS

What is it?
Twisting of colon on itself about its mesentery, resulting in obstruction and, if complete, vascular compromise with potential necrosis, perforation, or both

What is the most common type of colonic volvulus?
Sigmoid volvulus (makes sense because the sigmoid is a redundant/"floppy" structure!)

SIGMOID VOLVULUS

What is it?
Volvulus or "twist" in the sigmoid colon

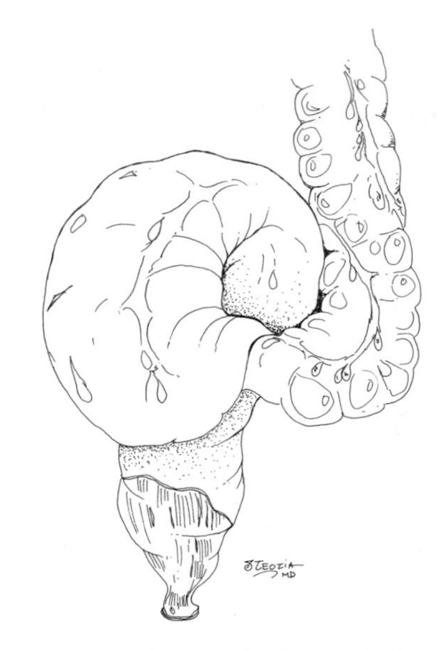

What is the incidence?
Approximately 75% of colonic volvulus cases

What are the etiologic factors?
High-residue diet resulting in bulky stools and tortuous, elongated colon; chronic constipation; laxative abuse; pregnancy; seen most commonly in bedridden elderly or institutionalized patients, many of whom have history of prior abdominal surgery or distal colonic obstruction

What are the signs/ symptoms?
Acute abdominal pain, progressive abdominal distention, anorexia, obstipation, cramps, nausea/vomiting

What findings are evident on abdominal plain film?
Distended loop of sigmoid colon, often in the classic "bent inner tube" or "omega" sign with the loop aiming toward the RUQ

What are the signs of necrotic bowel in colonic volvulus?
Free air, pneumatosis (air in bowel wall)

How is the diagnosis made?
Sigmoidoscopy or radiographic exam with gastrografin enema

Under what conditions is gastrografin enema useful?
If sigmoidoscopy and plain films fail to confirm the diagnosis; "**bird's beak**" is pathognomonic seen on enema contrast study as the contrast comes to a sharp end

What are the signs of strangulation?
Discolored or hemorrhagic mucosa on sigmoidoscopy, bloody fluid in the rectum, frank ulceration or necrosis at the point of the twist, peritoneal signs, fever, hypovolemia, ↑ WBCs

What is the initial treatment?
Nonoperative: If there is no strangulation, sigmoidoscopic reduction is successful in approximately 85% of cases; enema study will occasionally reduce (5%).

What is the percentage of recurrence after nonoperative reduction of a sigmoid volvulus?
Approximately 50%!

What are the indications for surgery?
Emergently if strangulation is suspected or nonoperative reduction unsuccessful (Hartmann's procedure); most patients should undergo resection during same hospitalization of redundant sigmoid after successful nonoperative reduction because of high recurrence rate (50%)

CECAL VOLVULUS

What is it?
Twisting of the cecum upon itself and the mesentery

What is a cecal "bascule" volvulus?	Instead of the more common axial twist, the cecum folds upward (lies on the ascending colon).
What is the incidence?	Approximately 25% of colonic volvulus (i.e., much less common than sigmoid volvulus)
What is the etiology?	Idiopathic poor fixation of the right colon; many patients have history of abdominal surgery
What are the signs/ symptoms?	Acute onset of abdominal or colicky pain beginning in the RLQ and progressing to a constant pain, vomiting, obstipation, abdominal distention, and SBO; many patients will have had previous similar episodes
How is the diagnosis made?	Abdominal plain film; dilated, ovoid colon with large air/fluid level in the RLQ often forming the classic "**coffee bean**" sign with the apex aiming toward the epigastrium or LUQ (must rule out gastric dilation with NG aspiration)
What diagnostic studies should be performed?	Colonoscopy or water-soluble contrast study (gastrografin), if diagnosis cannot be made by AXR
What is the treatment?	Emergent surgery: if cecum is viable, **cecopexy** (tack cecum down to abdominal wall) is performed; if cecum has infarcted or perforated, right colectomy with primary anastomosis or ileostomy and mucus fistula (primary anastomosis may be performed in stable patients)
What are the major differences in the EMERGENT management of cecal volvulus versus sigmoid?	Patients with cecal volvulus require surgical reduction, whereas the vast majority of patients with sigmoid volvulus undergo initial endoscopic reduction of the twist.

46 The Anus

ANATOMY

Identify the following:

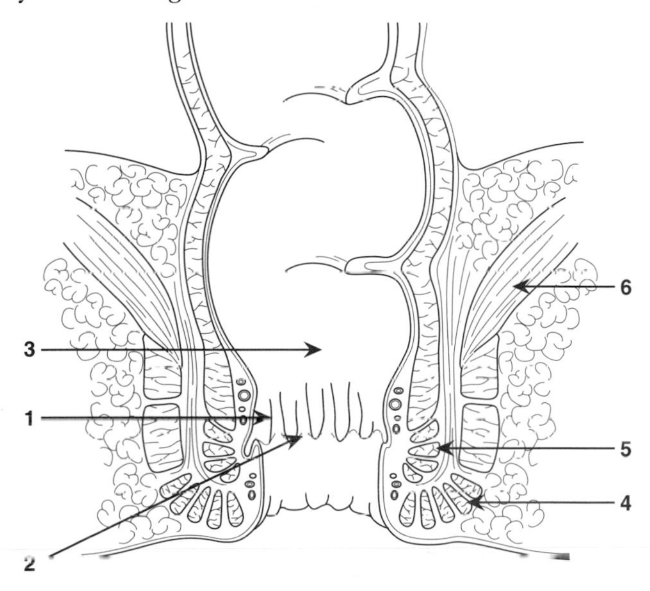

1. Anal columns
2. Dentate line
3. Rectum
4. External sphincter
5. Internal sphincter
6. Levator ani muscle

ANAL CANCER

What is the most common carcinoma of the anus?

Squamous cell carcinoma

What cell types are found in carcinomas of the anus?

1. Squamous cell carcinoma (accounts for two-thirds)
2. Cloacogenic (transitional cell)
3. Adenocarcinoma/melanoma/mucoepidermal

What is the incidence of anal carcinoma?
Rare (1% of colon cancers incidence)

What is anal Bowen's disease?
Squamous cell carcinoma in situ (think B.S.)

How is Bowen's disease treated?
With local wide excision

What is Paget's disease of the anus?
Adenocarcinoma in situ of the anus

How is Paget's disease treated?
With local wide excision

What are the risk factors for anal cancer?
Any chronic inflammatory process: fistula, abscess, infections (e.g., condyloma), Crohn's disease
Also, higher incidence in homosexual men, renal transplant patients, patients with herpes, and smokers

What is the most common symptom of anal carcinoma?
Anal bleeding

What are the other signs/ symptoms of anal carcinoma?
Pain, mass, mucus per rectum, pruritus

What percentage of patients with anal cancer are asymptomatic?
Approximately 25%

To what locations do anal cancers metastasize?
Lymph nodes, liver, bone, lung

Are most patients with anal cancer diagnosed early or late?
Late (diagnosis is often missed)

What is the workup of a patient with suspected anal carcinoma?
History
Physical exam: digital rectal exam, proctoscopic exam, and colonoscopy
Biopsy of mass
Abdominal/pelvic CT scan, with or without pelvic MRI or transanal U/S
CXR
LFTs

What are the epidermal cancers?	Squamous cell carcinoma, cloacogenic carcinoma, mucoepidermal carcinoma
How is an anal canal epidermal carcinoma treated?	NIGRO protocol: 1. Chemotherapy (5-FU and Mitomycin C) 2. Radiation 3. Postradiation therapy scar biopsy (6–8 weeks post XRT)
What percentage of patients have a "complete" response with the NIGRO protocol?	90%
What is the 5-year survival with the NIGRO protocol?	85%
How is a small (< 5 cm) anal margin cancer treated?	Usually by surgical excision with 1 cm margins
What is the treatment of anal basal cell carcinoma?	Local excision
What is the treatment of anal melanoma?	Wide excision or APR (especially if tumor is large)
What percentage of patients with anal melanoma have an amelanotic anal tumor?	Approximately one-third, thus making diagnosis difficult without pathology
What is the prognosis of anal melanoma?	Less than 5% 5-year survival rate

FISTULA IN ANO

What is it?	Anal fistula from rectum to perianal skin
What are the causes?	Usually anal crypt/gland (at dentate line) infection with extension/abscess formation
What are the signs/symptoms?	Perianal drainage, perirectal abscess, recurrent perirectal abscess, "diaper rash" from drainage (i.e., excoriation), itching

What disease should be considered with fistula in ano?
Crohn's disease (also consider ulcerative colitis, pilonidal abscess)

How is the diagnosis made?
Exam, proctoscope

What is Goodsall's rule?
Fistulas originating **anterior** to a transverse line through the anus will course **straight** ahead and exit anteriorly, whereas those exiting **posteriorly** have a **curved** tract.

How can Goodsall's rule be remembered?
Think of a dog with a straight nose (anterior) and a curved tail (posterior)

What is the management of anorectal fistulas?
1. Definition of the pathoanatomy
2. Marsupialization of fistula tract (i.e., fillet tract open)
3. Wound care—routine Sitz baths and dressing changes, stool softeners
4. Seton placement, if fistula is through the sphincter muscle

What is a Sitz bath?
Sitting in a warm bath (usually done after bowel movement and TID)

What percentage of patients with a perirectal abscess develop a fistula in ano?
Approximately 50%

PERIRECTAL ABSCESS

What is it?
Abscess formation around the anus/rectum

What are the signs/ symptoms?
Rectal pain, drainage of pus, fever, perianal mass

How is the diagnosis made?
Physical/digital exam reveals perianal/rectal submucosal mass/fluctuance

What is the cause?
Crypt abscess in dentate line with spread

What is the treatment?
As with all abscesses (except simple liver amebic abscess) **drainage,** with or without antibiotics against colonic flora (antibiotics are absolutely indicated with diabetes, artificial or prosthetic heart

	valve, spreading infection, or immunocompromised patients), Sitz bath, anal hygiene, stool softeners
What percentage of patients develop a fistula in ano during the 6 months after surgery?	Approximately 50%

ANAL FISSURE

What is it?	Tear or fissure in the anal epithelium
What is the most common site?	Posterior midline (comparatively low blood flow)
What is the cause?	Hard stool passage (constipation), hyperactive sphincter, disease process (e.g., Crohn's disease)
What are the signs/ symptoms?	Pain in the anus, painful (can be excruciating) bowel movement, rectal bleeding, blood on toilet tissue after bowel movement, sentinel tag, tear in the anal skin, extremely painful rectal exam, sentinel pile, hypertrophic papilla
What is a sentinel pile?	Thickened mucosa/skin at the distal end of an anal fissure that looks like a small hemorrhoid
What is the conservative treatment?	Sitz baths, stool softeners, high fiber diet, excellent anal hygiene, nitro paste, bot. toxin
What disease processes must be considered with a chronic anal fissure?	Crohn's disease, anal cancer, sexually transmitted disease, ulcerative colitis, AIDS
What are the indications for surgery?	Chronic fissure refractory to conservative treatment
What is one surgical option?	Lateral internal sphincterotomy (LIS) cut the integral sphincter to release it from spasm)

PERIANAL WARTS

What are they?	Warts around the anus/perineum

What is the cause? Condyloma acuminatum (human papilloma virus)

What is the major risk? Squamous cell carcinoma

What is the treatment if warts are small? Topical podophyllin, Aldara®

What is the treatment if warts are large? Surgical resection or laser ablation

HEMORRHOIDS

What are they? Engorgement of the venous plexi of the rectum, anus, or both; with protrusion of the mucosa, anal margin, or both

What are the signs/symptoms? Anal mass/prolapse, bleeding, itching, pain

Which type, internal or external, is painful? External, below the dentate line

If a patient has excruciating anal pain and history of hemorrhoids, what is the likely diagnosis? Thrombosed external hemorrhoid

What are the causes of hemorrhoids? Constipation/straining, portal hypertension, pregnancy

What is an internal hemorrhoid? Hemorrhoid above the (proximal) dentate line

What is an external hemorrhoid? Hemorrhoid below the dentate line

What are the three "hemorrhoid quadrants"?

1. Left lateral
2. Right posterior
3. Right anterior

Classification By Degrees

Define the following terms for internal hemorrhoids:

First-degree hemorrhoid Hemorrhoid that does not prolapse

Second-degree hemorrhoid Prolapses with defecation, but returns on its own

Third-degree hemorrhoid	Prolapses with defecation or any type of Valsalva maneuver and requires active manual reduction (eat fiber!)
Fourth-degree hemorrhoid	Prolapsed hemorrhoid that cannot be reduced
What is the treatment?	High-fiber diet, anal hygiene, topical steroids, Sitz baths Rubber band ligation (in most cases anesthetic is not necessary for internal hemorrhoids) Surgical resection for large refractory hemorrhoids
What are the dreaded complications of hemorrhoidectomy?	Exsanguination (bleeding may pool proximally in lumen of colon without any signs of external bleeding) Pelvic infection (may be extensive and potentially fatal) Incontinence (injury to sphincter complex) Anal stricture
What condition is a contraindication for hemorrhoidectomy?	Crohn's disease
What must be ruled out with lower GI bleeding believed to be caused by hemorrhoids?	Colon cancer (colonoscopy or proctoscopy followed up with a barium enema)

47 Lower GI Bleeding

What is the definition of lower GI bleeding?

Bleeding distal to the ligament of Treitz; vast majority occurs in the colon

What are the symptoms?

Hematochezia (bright red blood per rectum [BRBPR]), with or without abdominal pain, melena, anorexia, fatigue, syncope, shortness of breath, shock

What are the signs?

BRBPR, positive hemoccult, abdominal tenderness, hypovolemic shock, orthostasis

What are the causes?

Diverticulosis (usually **right**-sided in severe hemorrhage), vascular ectasia, colon cancer, hemorrhoids, trauma, hereditary hemorrhagic telangiectasia, intussusception, volvulus, ischemic colitis, IBD (especially ulcerative colitis), anticoagulation, rectal cancer, Meckel's diverticulum (with ectopic gastric mucosa), stercoral ulcer (ulcer from hard stool), infectious colitis, aortoenteric fistula chemotherapy, irradiation injury, infarcted bowel, strangulated hernia, anal fissure

What are the most common causes of massive lower GI bleeding?

1. **Diverticulosis**
2. Vascular ectasia

What lab tests should be performed?

CBC, Chem-7, PT/PTT, type and cross

What is the initial treatment?

IVFs: lactated Ringer's; packed red blood cells as needed, IV × 2, Foley catheter to follow urine output, d/c aspirin, NGT

What diagnostic tests should be performed for all lower GI bleeds?

History, physical exam, NGT aspiration (to rule out UGI bleeding; bile or blood must be seen; otherwise, perform EGD), anoscopy/proctoscopic exam

What must be ruled out in patients with lower GI bleeding?

Upper GI bleeding! Remember, NGT aspiration is not 100% accurate (even if you get bile without blood).

How can you have a UGI bleed with only clear succus back in the NGT?

A duodenal bleeding ulcer can bleed distal to the pylorus with the NGT sucking normal nonbloody gastric secretions! **If there is any question, perform EGD.**

What would an algorithm for diagnosing and treating lower GI bleeding look like?

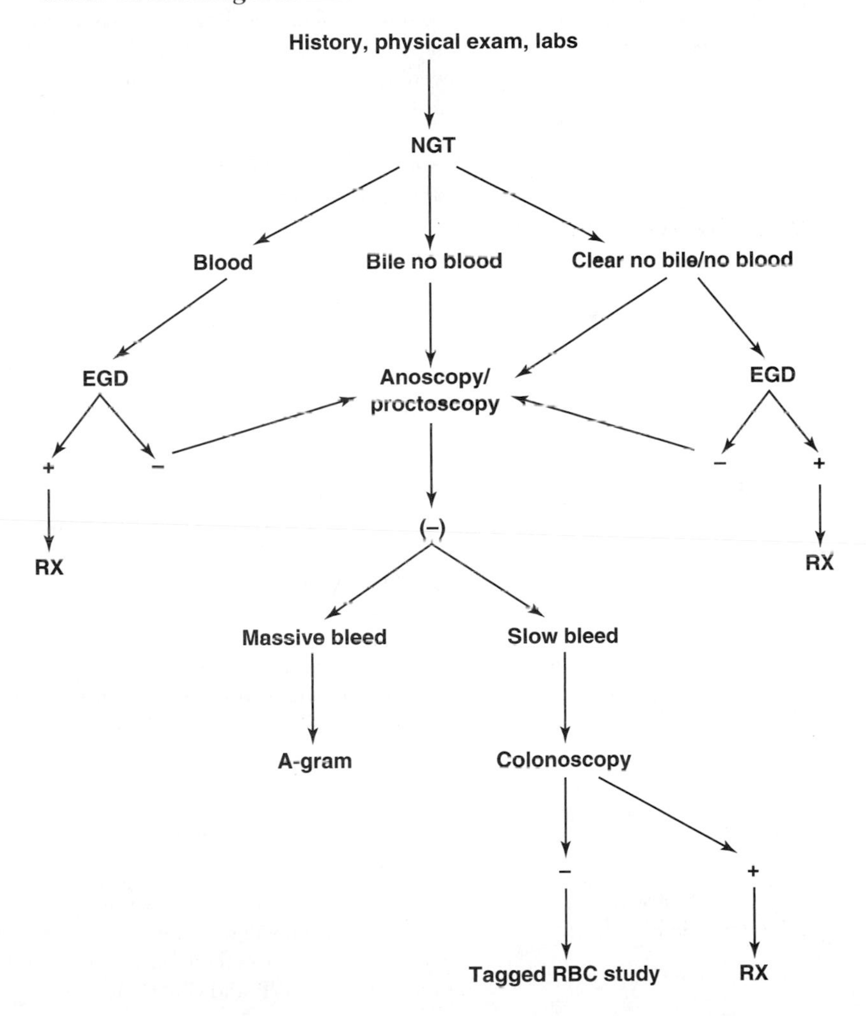

What is the diagnostic test of choice for localizing a slow to moderate lower GI bleeding source?
Colonoscopy

What test is performed to localize bleeding if there is too much active bleeding to see the source with a colonoscope?
A-gram

What is more sensitive for a slow, intermittent amount of blood loss: A-gram or tagged RBC study?
Radiolabeled RBC scan is more sensitive for blood loss at a rate of 0.1 ml/min or intermittent blood loss because it has a longer half life (for arteriography, bleeding rate must be greater than 0.5–1.0 ml/min).

What is the colonoscopic treatment option for bleeding vascular ectasia or polyp?
Laser or electrocoagulation; local epinephrine injection

What is the treatment if bleeding site is KNOWN and massive or recurrent lower GI bleeding continues?
Segmental resection of the bowel

What is the surgical treatment of massive lower GI bleeding WITHOUT localization?
Exploratory laparotomy with or without small intestine enteroscopy and total abdominal colectomy with primary anastomosis of ileum to rectum (ileorectostomy) as last resort

What percentage of cases spontaneously stop bleeding?
Between 80% and 90% stop bleeding with resuscitative measures only (at least temporarily).

What percentage of patients require emergent surgery for lower GI bleeding?
Only about 10%

Does melena always signify active colonic bleeding?
NO—the colon is very good at storing material and often will store melena/ maroon stools and pass them days later (follow patient, HCT, and vital signs).

What is the therapeutic advantage of doing a colonoscopy?

The options of injecting substance (epinephrine) or coagulating vessels is an option with C-scope to control bleeding

What is the therapeutic advantage of doing an A-gram?

Can inject vasopressin (control of bleeding from vasoconstriction in about 50%)

48

Inflammatory Bowel Disease (IBD): Crohn's Disease and Ulcerative Colitis

What is IBD?	Inflammatory disease of the GI tract
What are the two inflammatory bowel diseases?	Crohn's disease and ulcerative colitis
What is another name for Crohn's disease?	Regional enteritis
What is ulcerative colitis often called?	U.C.
What is the cause of IBD?	No one knows, but probably an autoimmune process with environmental factors contributing
What is the differential diagnosis?	Crohn's versus ulcerative colitis, infectious colitis (e.g., *C. difficile*, amebiasis, shigellosis), ischemic colitis, irritable bowel syndrome, diverticulitis, Zollinger-Ellison (Z-E) syndrome, colon cancer, carcinoid, ischemic bowel
What are the extraintestinal manifestations seen in both types of IBD?	Ankylosing spondylitis, aphthous (oral) ulcers, iritis, pyoderma gangrenosum, erythema nodosum, clubbing of fingers, sclerosing cholangitis, arthritis, kidney disease (nephrotic syndrome, amyloid deposits)
How can these manifestations be remembered?	Think of the acronym "A PIE SACK" **A:** Aphthous ulcers

P: Pyoderma gangrenosum
I: Iritis
E: Erythema nodosum

S: Sclerosing cholangitis
A: Arthritis, ankylosis spondylitis
C: Clubbing of fingers
K: Kidney (amyloid deposits, nephrotic syndrome)

COMPARISON OF CROHN'S DISEASE AND ULCERATIVE COLITIS

INCIDENCE

Crohn's disease?

3–6/100,000.
High in the Jewish population, low in the African black population, similar rates between African-Americans and U.S. white population
Female > male
Bimodal distribution (i.e., two peaks in incidence): peak incidence at 25 to 40 years of age; second bimodal distribution peak at 50 to 65 years of age

Ulcerative colitis?

10/100,000
High in the Jewish population, low in the African-American population
Positive family history in 20% of cases
Seen in families
Male > female
Bimodal distribution at 20 to 35 and 50 to 65 years of age

INITIAL SYMPTOMS

Crohn's disease?

Abdominal pain, diarrhea, fever, weight loss, anal disease

Ulcerative colitis?

Bloody diarrhea (hallmark), fever, weight loss

ANATOMIC DISTRIBUTION

Crohn's disease?

Classically said to involve **"mouth to anus"**
Small bowel alone—20%

Small bowel and colon—40%
Colon alone—30%

Ulcerative colitis? Colon alone (can have "backwash ileitis")

ROUTE OF SPREAD

Crohn's disease? Small bowel, colon, or both **with "skip areas"** of normal bowel; hence, the name "regional enteritis"

Ulcerative colitis? Almost always involves the rectum and spreads proximally always in a continuous route without "skip areas"

What is "backwash" ileitis? Mild inflammation of the terminal ileum in ulcerative colitis; thought to be "backwash" of inflammatory mediators from the colon into the terminal ileum

BOWEL WALL INVOLVEMENT

Crohn's disease? Full thickness (transmural involvement)

Ulcerative colitis? Mucosa/submucosa only

ANAL INVOLVEMENT

Crohn's disease? Common (fistulae, abscesses, fissures, ulcers)

Ulcerative colitis? Uncommon

RECTAL INVOLVEMENT

Crohn's disease? Rare

Ulcerative colitis? 100%

MUCOSAL FINDINGS

Crohn's disease (6)?

1. Aphthoid ulcers
2. Granulomas
3. Linear ulcers
4. Transverse fissures
5. Swollen mucosa
6. **Full-thickness wall involvement**

Ulcerative colitis (5)?

1. Granular, flat mucosa
2. Ulcers
3. **Crypt abscess**
4. Dilated mucosal vessels
5. **Pseudopolyps**

DIAGNOSTIC TESTS

Crohn's disease?

Colonoscopy with biopsy, barium enema, UGI with small bowel follow-through, stool cultures

Ulcerative colitis?

Colonoscopy, barium enema, UGI with small bowel follow-through (to look for Crohn's disease), stool cultures

COMPLICATIONS

Crohn's disease?

Anal fistula/abscess, **fistula,** stricture, perforation, **abscesses,** toxic megacolon, colovesical fistula, enterovaginal fistula, hemorrhage, **obstruction,** cancer

Ulcerative colitis?

Cancer, toxic megacolon, colonic perforation, hemorrhage, strictures, obstruction, complications of surgery

Why are fistulae and abscesses more often Crohn's disease versus ulcerative colitis?

Crohn's disease involves the entire bowel wall (transmural), whereas ulcerative colitis involves only the mucosa/ submucosa.

CANCER RISK

Crohn's disease?

High risk in areas surgically bypassed from the fecal stream; overall increased risk, but much less than that of ulcerative colitis

Ulcerative colitis?

Approximately 1% to 2% risk of developing colon cancer at 10 years; then, risk increases approximately 1% per year; thus, an incidence of about 20% after 20 years of the disease (30% at 35 years)

INCIDENCE OF TOXIC MEGACOLON

Crohn's disease?

Approximately 5%

Ulcerative colitis?
Approximately 10%

INDICATIONS FOR SURGERY

Crohn's disease?
Obstruction, massive bleeding, fistula, perforation, suspicion of cancer, abscess refractory to medical treatment, toxic megacolon (refractory to medical treatment), strictures, dysplasia

Ulcerative colitis?
Toxic megacolon (refractory to medical treatment); cancer prophylaxis; massive bleeding; failure of child to mature because of disease and steroids; perforation; suspicion of or documented cancer; acute severe symptoms refractory to medical treatment; inability to wean off of chronic steroids; obstruction; dysplasia; stricture

What are the common surgical options for ulcerative colitis?
1. Total proctocolectomy, distal rectal mucosectomy, and ileoanal pull through
2. Total proctocolectomy and Brooke ileostomy

What is "toxic megacolon"?
Toxic patient: sepsis, febrile, abdominal pain
Megacolon: acutely and massively distended colon

What are the medication options for treating IBD?
Sulfasalazine, mesalamine (5-aminosalicylic acid)
Steroids, metronidazole (Flagyl), azathioprine, mercaptopurine

What is the active metabolite of sulfasalazine?
5'-aminosalicylate (5'-ASA), which is released in the colon

What is the medical treatment of choice for perianal Crohn's disease?
PO metronidazole (Flagyl)

What are the treatment options for long-term remission of IBD?
6-Mercaptopurine (6-MP), azathioprine, mesalamine

What medication is used for IBD "flare-ups"?
Steroids

What is the medication route option for U.C.?	Enemas
Which disease has "cobblestoning" more often on endoscopic exam?	Crohn's disease (think: **C**rohn's = **C**obblestoning)
Which disease has pseudopolyps on colonoscopic exam?	Ulcerative colitis; pseudopolyps are polyps of hypertrophied mucosa surrounded by mucosal atrophy
Which disease has a "lead pipe" appearance on barium enema?	Chronic ulcerative colitis
Rectal bleeding/bloody diarrhea is a hallmark of which disease?	Ulcerative colitis (rare in Crohn's disease)
What is the most common indication for surgery in patients with Crohn's disease?	Small bowel obstruction (SBO)
What are the intraoperative findings of Crohn's disease?	Mesenteric "**fat creeping**" onto the antimesenteric border of the small bowel Shortened (and thick) mesentery Thick bowel wall Fistula(e) Abscess(es)
Why do you see fistulas and abscesses with Crohn's and not U.C.?	Crohn's disease is **transmural**.
What is the operation for short strictures of the small bowel in Crohn's disease?	Stricturoplasty; basically a Heineke-Mikulicz pyloroplasty on the strictured segment (i.e., opened longitudinally and sewn closed in a transverse direction)
Should the appendix be removed during a laparotomy for abdominal pain if Crohn's disease is discovered?	Yes, if the cecum is not involved with active Crohn's disease

What is pouchitis?

Inflammation of the pouch of an ileoanal pull through; treat with metronidazole (Flagyl)

Do you need a frozen section for margins during a bowel resection for Crohn's disease?

No, you need only grossly negative margins.

What do you call it when the entire colon is involved?

Pancolitis

49 Liver

ANATOMY

What is the name of the liver capsule?

Glisson's capsule

What is the "BARE" area?

The posterior section of the liver against the diaphragm that is "bare" without peritoneal covering

What is Cantle's line?

A line drawn between the gallbladder to just left of the inferior vena cava that transects the liver into the right and left lobes

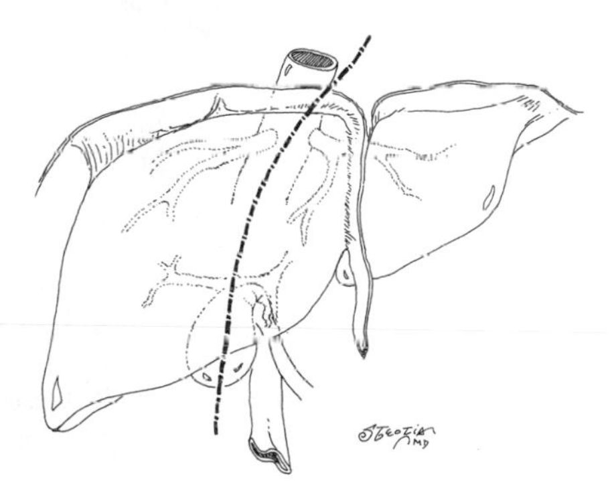

Which ligament goes from the anterior abdominal wall to the liver?

Falciform ligament (contains the ligament teres, which is the obliterated umbilical vein)

What is the coronary ligament?

The peritoneal reflection on top of the liver that crowns (hence "coronary") the liver and attaches it to the diaphragm

What are the triangular ligaments of the liver?

The right and left lateral extents of the coronary ligament, which form triangles

What is the origin of the hepatic arterial supply?

From the proper hepatic artery off of the celiac trunk (celiac trunk to common hepatic artery to proper hepatic artery)

Identify the arterial branches of the celiac trunk.

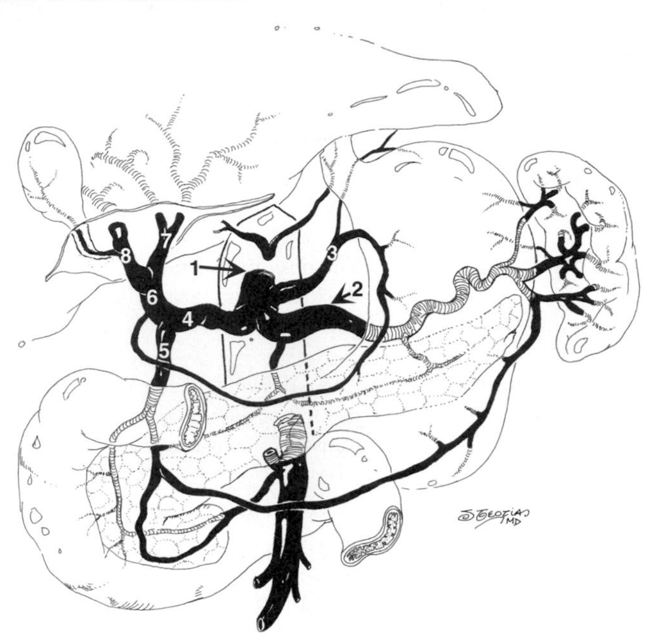

1. Celiac trunk
2. Splenic artery
3. Left gastric artery
4. Common hepatic artery
5. Gastroduodenal artery
6. Proper hepatic artery
7. Left hepatic artery
8. Right hepatic artery

What is the venous supply?

Portal vein (formed from the splenic vein and the superior mesenteric vein)

What is the hepatic venous drainage?

Via the hepatic veins, which drain into the IVC (three veins: left, middle, and right)

What sources provide oxygen to the liver?

Portal vein blood—50%
Hepatic artery blood—50%

From what sources does the liver receive blood?

Portal system—75%
Hepatic artery system—25%

What is the maximum amount of liver that can be resected while retaining adequate liver function?

More than 80%; if given adequate recovery time, the original mass can be **regenerated.**

What are the signs/ symptoms of liver disease?

Hepatomegaly, splenomegaly, icterus, pruritus (from bile salts in skin), blanching spider telangiectasia, gynecomastia, testicular atrophy, caput medusae, dark urine, clay-colored stools, bradycardia, edema, ascites, fever, fetor hepaticus (sweet musty smell), hemorrhoids, variceal bleeding, anemia, body hair loss, liver tenderness, palmar erythema

Which liver enzymes are made by hepatocytes?

AST and ALT (aspartate aminotransferase and alanine aminotransferase)

What is the source of alkaline phosphatase?

Ductal epithelium (thus, elevated with ductal obstruction)

What is Child's class?

A classification system that estimates hepatic reserve in patients with hepatic failure

What comprises the Child's classification?

Laboratory: bilirubin, albumin
Clinical: nutrition, encephalopathy, ascites

How can the criteria comprising the Child's classification be remembered?

Acronym: "A BEAN":
A: Ascites

B: Bilirubin
E: Encephalopathy
A: Albumin
N: Nutrition

Define Child's classification
A?
B?
C?

	Bili	ALB	Nutrit	Enceph	Ascites
A?	< 2	> 3.5	excellent	none	none
B?	2–3	3.–3.5	good	minimal	easily controlled
C?	> 3	< 3	poor	severe	poorly controlled

Think, as in a letter grading system, A is better than B, B is better than C

What is the operative mortality for a portocaval shunt in the following Child's classes:	
A?	Less than 5%
B?	Less than 15%
C?	Approximately 33%

TUMORS OF THE LIVER

What is the most common liver cancer?	**Metastatic disease** outnumbers primary tumors 20:1. Primary site is usually the GI tract.
What is the most common primary malignant liver tumor?	Hepatocellular carcinoma (hepatoma)
What is the most common primary benign liver tumor?	Hemangioma
What lab tests comprise the workup for liver metastasis?	LFTs (AST and alkaline phosphatase are most useful), CEA for suspected primary colon cancer
What are the associated imaging studies?	CT, ultrasound, A-gram
What is a right hepatic lobectomy?	Removal of the right lobe of the liver (i.e., all tissue to the right of Cantle's line is removed)
What is a left hepatic lobectomy?	Removal of the left lobe of the liver (i.e., removal of all the liver tissue to the left of Cantle's line)
What is a right trisegmentectomy?	Removal of all the liver tissue to the right of the falciform ligament
What are the three common types of primary benign liver tumors?	1. Hemangioma 2. Hepatocellular adenoma 3. Focal nodular hyperplasia

What are the four common types of primary malignant liver tumors?

1. Hepatocellular carcinoma (hepatoma)
2. Cholangiocarcinoma (when intrahepatic)
3. Angiosarcoma (associated with vinyl chloride, arsenic, or thorotrast contrast exposure)
4. Hepatoblastoma (most common in infants and children)

What is a "hepatoma"?

Hepatocellular carcinoma

What are the other benign liver masses?

Benign liver cyst, bile duct hamartomas, bile duct adenoma

What is a liver "HAMARTOMA"?

White hard nodule made up of normal liver cells in a nodular arrangement

HEPATOCELLULAR ADENOMA

What is it?

Benign liver tumor

Describe the histology.

Normal hepatocytes without bile ducts

What are the associated risk factors?

Women, birth control pills (think: **ABC** = **A**denoma **B**irth **C**ontrol), anabolic steroids (e.g., misguided athletes), glycogen storage disease

What is the female:male ratio?

9:1

What is the average age of occurrence?

Between 30 and 35 years of age

What are the signs/ symptoms?

Right upper quadrant pain/mass, right upper quadrant fullness, bleeding (rare)

What are the possible complications?

Rupture with bleeding, necrosis, pain, risk of hepatocellular carcinoma

How is the diagnosis made?

CT, U/S, +/− biopsy

What is the treatment?

Surgical resection, discontinuation of birth control pills/steroids, avoidance of pregnancy

FOCAL NODULAR HYPERPLASIA

What is it?
Benign liver tumor

Describe the histology.
Normal hepatocytes and **bile ducts (adenoma has no bile ducts)**

What is the average age of occurrence?
Approximately 40 years

What are the associated risk factors?
Women

Are the tumors associated with birth control pills?
Yes, but not as clearly associated as with adenoma

How is the diagnosis made?
Nuclear technetium 99 study, U/S, CT, A-gram, biopsy

What is the classic CT finding?
Liver mass with "central scar"

What are the possible complications?
Pain (no risk of cancer, very rarely hemorrhage)

What is the treatment?
Resection, if patient is symptomatic; otherwise, follow if diagnosis is confirmed

What study helps to differentiate focal nodular hyperplasia and hepatic adenoma?
Nuclear technetium 99 study (focal nodular hyperplasia will show up on the study and adenoma usually will not—THINK: **N**odular = **N**uclear)

HEPATIC HEMANGIOMA

What is it?
Benign vascular tumor of the liver

What is its claim to fame?
Most common primary benign liver tumor

What are the signs/symptoms?
Right upper quadrant pain/mass, bruits, shock with bleeding, congestive heart failure

What are the possible complications?
Hemorrhage, congestive heart failure, coagulopathy, obstructive jaundice, gastric outlet obstruction

How is the diagnosis made?	CT with IV contrast, ultrasound, tagged red blood scan, MRI
Should biopsy be performed?	No (risk of hemorrhage with biopsy)
What is the treatment?	**Observation** Resection, if the patient is symptomatic (or if easy removal is possible)

HEPATOCELLULAR CARCINOMA

What is it?	Most common primary malignancy of the liver
By what name is it also known?	Hepatoma
What is its incidence?	Accounts for 80% of all primary malignant liver tumors
What are the geographic high-risk areas?	Africa and Asia
What are the associated risk factors?	**Hepatitis B virus, cirrhosis, aflatoxin** (fungi toxin of *Aspergillus flavus*); Other risk factors: α-1-antitrypsin deficiency, hemochromatosis, liver fluke, *Clonorchis sinensis,* anabolic steroids, polyvinylchloride, glycogen storage disease (type I)
What percentage of patients with cirrhosis will develop hepatocellular carcinoma?	Approximately 5%
What are the signs/ symptoms?	Dull right upper quadrant pain, hepatomegaly (classic presentation: **painful hepatomegaly**), abdominal mass, weight loss, paraneoplastic syndromes, signs of portal hypertension, ascites, jaundice, fever, anemia, splenomegaly
What tests should be ordered?	Ultrasound, CT, angiography, tumor marker elevation

What is the tumor marker? Elevated α-fetoprotein

What is the most common way to get a tissue diagnosis? Needle biopsy with CT, ultrasound, or laparoscopic guidance

What is the most common site of metastasis? Lungs

What is the treatment of hepatocellular carcinoma? Surgical resection, if possible (e.g., lobectomy); liver transplant, percutaneous ethanol tumor injection, liquid nitrogen cryotherapy, and intra-arterial chemotherapy are other options.

What is the prognosis under the following conditions:

Unresectable? Almost none survive a year

Resectable? Approximately 25% are alive at 5 years

Which subtype has the best prognosis? Fibrolamellar hepatoma (young adults)

LIVER ABSCESSES

What is a liver abscess? Abscess (collection of pus) in the liver parenchyma

What are the types of liver abscess? Pyogenic (bacterial), parasitic (amebic), fungal

What is the most common location of abscess in the liver? Right lobe > left lobe

What are the sources?

Direct spread from biliary tract infection
or
Portal spread from GI infection (e.g., appendicitis, diverticulitis)
Systemic source (bacteremia)
Liver trauma (e.g., liver gunshot wound)
Cryptogenic (unknown source)

What are the two most common types? **Bacterial** (most common in the United States) and amebic (most common worldwide)

Define pyogenic.	Caused by bacteria

BACTERIAL LIVER ABSCESS

What are the three most common bacterial organisms affecting the liver?	Gram negatives: *E. coli, Klebsiella,* and *Proteus*
What are the most common sources/causes of bacterial liver abscesses?	Cholangitis, diverticulitis, liver cancer, liver metastasis
What are the signs/ symptoms?	**Fever, chills,** leukocytosis, **right upper quadrant pain,** increased liver function tests (LFTs), jaundice, sepsis, weight loss
What is the treatment?	IV antibiotics (triple antibiotics with metronidazole), percutaneous drainage with CT or U/S guidance
What are the indications for operative drainage?	Surgical drainage of multiple/loculated abscesses or if multiple percutaneous attempts have failed

AMEBIC LIVER ABSCESS

What is the etiology?	*Entamoeba histolytica* (typically reaches liver via portal vein from intestinal amebiasis)
How does it spread?	Fecal-oral transmission
What are the risk factors?	Patients from countries below the U.S.–Mexican border, institutionalized patients, homosexual men, alcoholic patients
What are the signs/ symptoms?	Right upper quadrant pain, fever, hepatomegaly, diarrhea *Note:* chills are much less common with amebic abscesses than with pyogenic abscesses.
Which lobe is most commonly involved?	The right lobe of the liver
Classic description of abscess contents?	"Anchovy paste" pus

How is the diagnosis made? Lab tests, ultrasound, CT

What lab tests should be performed? Indirect hemagglutination titers for *Entamoeba* antibodies elevated in more than 95% of cases, elevated LFTs

What is the treatment? Metronidazole IV; surgical drainage if refractory to metronidazole, if bacterial co-infection is present, or peritoneal rupture

What are the possible complications of large left lobe liver amebic abscess? Erosion into the pericardial sac (potentially fatal!)

HYDATID LIVER CYSTS

What is it? Usually a right lobe cyst filled with *Echinococcus granulosus*

What are the risk factors? Travel, exposure to dogs, sheep, and cattle (carriers)

What are the signs/symptoms? Right upper quadrant abdominal pain, jaundice, right upper quadrant mass

How is the diagnosis made? Indirect hemagglutination antibody test (serologic testing), Casoni skin test, ultrasound, CT, radiographic imaging

What are the findings on AXR? Possible calcified outline of cyst

What are the major risks? Erosion into the pleural cavity, pericardial sac, or biliary tree
Rupture into the peritoneal cavity causing fatal anaphylaxis

What is the risk of surgical removal of echinococcal (hydatid) cysts? Rupture or leakage of cyst contents into the abdomen may cause a fatal **anaphylactic** reaction

When should percutaneous drainage be performed? Never; may cause leaking into the peritoneal cavity and anaphylaxis

What is the treatment? **Mebendazole, followed by surgical resection;** large cysts can be drained and then injected with toxic irrigant

	(scoliocide) into the cyst unless aspirate is bilious (which means there is a biliary connection) followed by cyst removal
Which toxic irrigations are used?	Hypertonic saline, ethanol

HEMOBILIA

What is it?	Blood draining via the common bile duct into the duodenum
What are the signs/ symptoms of hemobilia?	Triad: 1. Right upper quadrant pain 2. Guaiac positive/upper GI bleeding 3. Jaundice
What are the causes?	Trauma, percutaneous transhepatic cholangiography (PTC), tumors
How is the diagnosis made?	EGD (blood out of the ampulla of Vater), A-gram
What is the treatment?	A-Gram with embolization of the bleeding vessel

50 Portal Hypertension

Define the anatomy of the portal venous system.

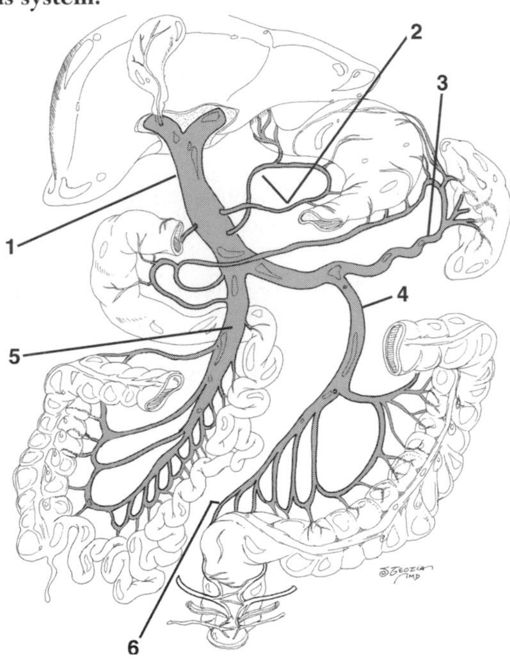

1. Portal vein
2. Coronary vein
3. Splenic vein
4. IMV (inferior mesenteric vein)
5. SMV (superior mesenteric vein)
6. Superior hemorrhoidal vein

Describe drainage of blood from the superior hemorrhoidal vein.

To the IMV, the splenic vein, and then the portal vein

Where does blood drain to from the IMV?

Into the splenic vein

Where does the portal vein begin?

At the confluence of the splenic vein and the SMV

What are the (6) potential routes of portal-systemic collateral blood flow (as seen with portal hypertension)?

1. Umbilical vein
2. Coronary vein to esophageal venous plexi
3. Retroperitoneal veins (veins of Retzius)
4. Diaphragm veins (veins of Sappey)
5. Superior hemorrhoidal vein to middle and inferior hemorrhoidal veins and then to the iliac vein
6. Splenic veins to the short gastric veins

What is the pathophysiology of portal hypertension?

Elevated portal pressure resulting from resistance to portal flow

What level of portal pressure is normal?

About 6 mm Hg (> 10 mm Hg)

>What is the etiology?

Prehepatic—Thrombosis of portal vein
Hepatic—**Cirrhosis** (distortion of normal parenchyma by regenerating hepatic nodules), hepatocellular carcinoma, etc.
Posthepatic—Budd Chiari syndrome: thrombosis of hepatic veins

What is the most common cause of portal hypertension in the United States?

Cirrhosis (> 90% of cases)

What percentage of patients with alcoholism develop cirrhosis?

Surprisingly, less than 1 in 5

What percentage of patients with cirrhosis develop esophageal varices?

Approximately 40%

What percentage of patients with cirrhosis develop portal hypertension?

Approximately two-thirds

What is the most common physical finding in patients with portal hypertension?

Splenomegaly

What are the associated CLINICAL findings in portal hypertension (4)?

1. Caput medusa (engorgement of periumbilical veins)
2. Hemorrhoids
3. Splenomegaly
4. Esophageal varices

What other physical findings are associated with cirrhosis and portal hypertension?

Spider angioma, palmar erythema, ascites, truncal obesity and peripheral wasting, encephalopathy, asterixis (liver flap), gynecomastia, jaundice

What is the name of the periumbilical bruit heard with caput medusa?

Cruveilhier-Baumgarten bruit

How is portal pressure measured?

Indirect hepatic vein wedge pressure

What constitutes the portal-systemic collateral circulation in portal hypertension in the following conditions:

Esophageal varices?

Coronary vein backing up into the azygous system

Caput medusa?

Umbilical vein (via falciform ligament) draining into the epigastric veins

Retroperitoneal varices?

Small mesenteric veins (veins of Retzius) draining retroperitoneally into lumbar veins

Hemorrhoids?

Superior hemorrhoidal vein (which normally drains into the inferior mesenteric vein) backing up into the middle and inferior hemorrhoidal veins

What is the etiology?

Cirrhosis (90%), schistosomiasis, hepatitis, Budd-Chiari syndrome, hemochromatosis, Wilson's disease, portal vein thrombosis, tumors, splenic vein thrombosis

What is the most common cause of portal hypertension outside North America?

Schistosomiasis

What is Budd-Chiari syndrome?	Thrombosis of the hepatic veins
What is the most feared complication of portal hypertension?	Bleeding from esophageal varices (up to 50% mortality!)
What are esophageal varices?	Engorgement of the esophageal venous plexi secondary to increased collateral blood flow from the portal system as a result of portal hypertension
What is the "rule of two-thirds" of portal hypertension?	Two-thirds of patients with cirrhosis will develop portal hypertension. Two-thirds of patients with portal hypertension will develop esophageal varices. Two-thirds of patients with esophageal varices will bleed from the varices.
In patients with cirrhosis and known varices who are suffering from upper GI bleeding, how often does that bleeding result from varices?	Only about 50% of the time
What are the signs/symptoms?	Hematemesis, melena, hematochezia
What is the mortality rate from an acute esophageal variceal bleed?	Approximately 50%
What is the initial treatment of variceal bleeding?	As with all upper GI bleeding: large bore IVS × 2, IV fluid, Foley catheter, NG tube, type and cross blood, send labs, correct coagulopathy (vitamin K, fresh frozen plasma)
What is the diagnostic test of choice?	**EGD (upper GI endoscopy)** Remember, bleeding is the result of varices only half the time; must rule out ulcers, etc.
If esophageal varices cause bleeding, what is the initial treatment?	**Emergent endoscopic sclerotherapy:** a sclerosing substance is injected into the esophageal varices under direct endoscopic vision

What is the next step if the patient continues to bleed after the initial treatment?

IV vasopressin (and nitroglycerin, to avoid MI) or somatostatin (Octreotide) to achieve vasoconstriction of the mesenteric vessels; if bleeding continues, consider balloon (**Sengstaken-Blakemore tube**) tamponade of the varices

What is a Sengstaken-Blakemore tube?

A tube with a gastric and esophageal balloon for tamponading an esophageal bleed (see Chapter 37 "Upper GI Bleeding")

What is the next therapy after the bleeding is controlled?

Repeat endoscopic sclerotherapy

What are the options if sclerotherapy and conservative methods fail to stop the variceal bleeding or bleeding recurs?

Repeat sclerotherapy and treat conservatively
TIPS
Surgical shunt
Liver transplantation

What is the preferred shunt in the following cases:

Patient who is a candidate for liver transplant or a very poor operative candidate?

TIPS procedure

Nonalcoholic patient who is not a transplant candidate?

Warren selective shunt (distal splenorenal shunt)

Patient who is an alcoholic and a good operative candidate, but not a liver transplant candidate?

Partial shunt: portocaval synthetic H-graft

What does the acronym TIPS stand for?

Transjugular **I**ntrahepatic **P**ortosystemic **S**hunt

What is a TIPS procedure?

An angiographic radiologist places a small tube stent intrahepatically between the hepatic vein and a branch of the portal vein via a percutaneous-jugular vein route.

What is a Warren shunt?

Distal splenorenal shunt with ligation of the coronary vein—elective shunt procedure associated with low incidence of encephalopathy in nonalcoholic patients postoperatively because only the splenic flow is diverted to decompress the varices

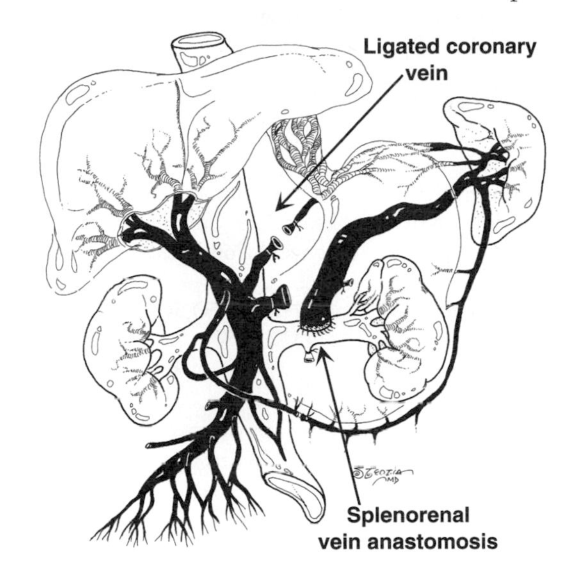

Define the following shunts:

End-to-side portocaval shunt

"Total shunt"—portal vein (end) to IVC (side)

Side-to-side portocaval shunt

Side of portal vein anastomosed to side of IVC—partially preserves portal flow ("partial shunt")

Synthetic portocaval H-graft

"Partial shunt"—synthetic tube graft from the portal vein to the IVC (good option for patients with alcoholism; associated with lower incidence of encephalopathy and easier transplantation later)

Synthetic mesocaval H-graft

Synthetic graft from the SMV to the IVC

What is the most common perioperative cause of death following shunt procedure?

Hepatic failure, secondary to decreased blood flow (accounts for two-thirds of deaths)

What is the major postoperative morbidity after a shunt procedure?

Increased incidence of hepatic encephalopathy because of decreased portal blood flow to the liver and decreased clearance of toxins/metabolites from the blood

What medication can be infused to counteract the coronary artery vasoconstriction of IV vasopressin?

Nitroglycerin IV drip

What lab value roughly correlates with degree of encephalopathy?

Serum ammonia level (Note: Thought to correlate with but not cause encephalopathy)

What medications are used to treat hepatic encephalopathy?

Lactulose PO, with or without neomycin PO

51 Biliary Tract

ANATOMY

Name structures 1 through 8 (below) of the biliary tract.

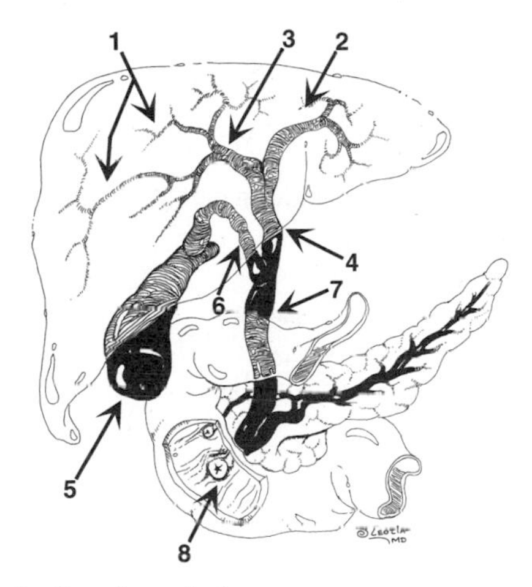

1. Intrahepatic ducts
2. Left hepatic duct
3. Right hepatic duct
4. Common hepatic duct
5. Gallbladder
6. Cystic duct
7. Common bile duct
8. Ampulla of Vater

Which is the proximal and which is the distal bile duct?

Proximal is close to the liver. (Bile and the liver is analogous to blood and the heart; they both flow distally.)

What is the name of the node in Calot's triangle?

Calot's node

What are the small ducts that drain bile directly into the gallbladder from the liver?

Ducts of Luschka

Which artery is susceptible to injury during cholecystectomy?
Right hepatic artery, because of its proximity to the cystic artery and Calot's triangle

What is the name of the valves of the gallbladder?
Spiral valves of Heister

Where is the infundibulum of the gallbladder?
Near the cystic duct

Where is the fundus of the gallbladder?
At the end of the gallbladder

What is "Hartmann's pouch"?
The gallbladder infundibulum

What are the boundaries of the triangle of Calot?
The 3 C's:
1. **C**ystic duct
2. **C**ommon hepatic duct
3. **C**ystic artery

some books say
1. inf. border liver
2. cystic duct
3. common hepatic duct

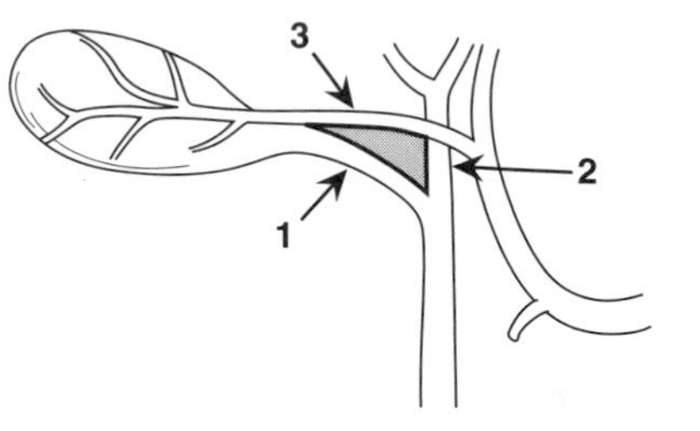

PHYSIOLOGY

What is the source of alkaline phosphatase?
Bile duct epithelium; expect alkaline phosphatase to be elevated in bile duct obstruction

What is in bile?
Cholesterol, lecithin (phospholipid), bile acids, and bilirubin

What does bile do?
Emulsify fats

What is the enterohepatic circulation?
Circulation of bile acids from liver to gut and back to the liver

Where are most of the bile acids absorbed?
In the terminal ileum

What stimulates gallbladder emptying?
Cholecystokinin and vagal input

What is the source of cholecystokinin?
Duodenal mucosal cells

What stimulates the release of cholecystokinin?
Fat, protein, amino acids, and HCl

What inhibits its release?
Trypsin and chymotrypsin

What are its actions?
Gallbladder emptying
Opening of ampulla of Vater
Slowing of gastric emptying
Pancreas acinar cell growth and release of exocrine products

PATHOPHYSIOLOGY

At what level of serum total bilirubin does one start to get jaundiced?
Greater than 2.5

Classically, what is thought to be the anatomic location where one first finds evidence of jaundice?
Under the tongue

With good renal function, how high can the serum total bilirubin go?
Very rarely, greater than 20

What are the signs and symptoms of obstructive jaundice?
Jaundice
Dark urine
Clay-colored stools (acholic stools)
Pruritus (itching)
Loss of appetite
Nausea

What causes the itching in obstructive jaundice?
Bile salts in the dermis (not bilirubin!)

Define the following terms:

Cholelithiasis
Gallstones in gallbladder

Choledocholithiasis
Gallstone in common bile duct

Cholecystitis	Inflammation of gallbladder
Cholangitis	Infection of biliary tract
Cholangiocarcinoma	Adenocarcinoma of bile ducts
Klatskin's tumor	Cholangiocarcinoma of bile duct at the junction of the right and left hepatic ducts
Biliary colic	It is pain from gallstones, usually from a stone at cystic duct. The pain is located in the RUQ, epigastrium, or right subscapular region of the back. It usually lasts minutes to hours but eventually goes away. It is often postprandial, especially after fatty foods.
Biloma	Intraperitoneal bile fluid collection
Choledochojejunostomy	Anastomosis between common bile duct and jejunum
Hepaticojejunostomy	Anastomosis of hepatic ducts or common hepatic duct to jejunum

DIAGNOSTIC STUDIES

What is the initial diagnostic study of choice for evaluation of the biliary tract/gallbladder/ cholelithiasis?	Ultrasound!
Define the following diagnostic studies:	
ERCP	**E**ndoscopic **R**etrograde **C**holangio**P**ancreatography
PTC	**P**ercutaneous **T**ranshepatic **C**holangiogram
IOC	**I**ntra**O**perative **C**holangiogram (done laparoscopically or open to rule out choledocholithiasis)
HIDA/PRIDA scan	Radioisotope study; isotope concentrated in liver and secreted into bile; will

demonstrate cholecystitis, bile leak, or CBD obstruction

How does the HIDA scan reveal cholecystitis?

Non-opacification of the gallbladder from obstruction of the cystic duct

How often will plain x-ray films see gallstones?

10% to 15%

BILIARY SURGERY

What is a cholecystectomy?

Removal of the gallbladder done laparoscopically or through standard Kocher incision

What is the Kocher incision?

Right subcostal incision

What is a sphincterotomy?

Cut through sphincter of Oddi to allow passage of gallstones from the common bile duct; most often done at ERCP; also known as papillotomy

How should postoperative biloma be treated after a lap chole?

1. Percutaneous drain bile collection
2. ERCP with placement of biliary stent past leak (usually cystic duct remnant)

What is the treatment of major CBD injury after a lap chole?

Choledochojejunostomy

OBSTRUCTIVE JAUNDICE

What is it?

Jaundice (hyperbilirubinemia > 2.5) from obstruction of bile flow to the duodenum

What is the differential diagnosis of *proximal* bile duct obstruction?

Cholangiocarcinoma
Lymphadenopathy
Metastatic tumor
Gallbladder carcinoma
Sclerosing cholangitis
Gallstones
Tumor embolus
Parasites
Postsurgical stricture
Hepatoma
Benign bile duct tumor

What is the differential diagnosis of *distal* bile duct obstruction?
Choledocholithiasis (**gallstones**)
Pancreatic carcinoma
Pancreatitis
Ampullary carcinoma
Lymphadenopathy
Pseudocyst
Postsurgical stricture
Ampulla of Vater dysfunction
Lymphoma
Benign bile duct tumor
Parasites

What is the initial study of choice for obstructive jaundice?
Ultrasound

What lab results are associated with obstructive jaundice?
Elevated alkaline phosphatase, elevated bilirubin with or without elevated LFTs

CHOLELITHIASIS

What is it?
The formation of gallstones

What is the incidence?
About 10% of U.S. population will develop gallstones.

What are the "Big 4" risk factors?
The "four Fs": **F**emale, **F**at, **F**orty, **F**ertile (multiparity)

What are other less common risk factors for gallstones?
Oral contraceptives
Bile stasis
Chronic hemolysis (pigment stones)
Cirrhosis
Infection
Native American heritage
Rapid weight loss
Obesity
Inflammatory bowel disease (IBD)
Terminal ileal resection
Total parenteral nutrition (TPN)
Vagotomy
Advanced age
Hyperlipidemia
Somatostatin therapy

What are the types of stones?
Cholesterol stones (75% of all stones) and pigment stones (25% of all stones)

What are the types of pigmented stones?
Black stones (contain calcium bilirubinate) and brown stones (associated with biliary tract infection)

What are the causes of black-pigmented stones?	Cirrhosis, hemolysis
What is the pathogenesis of cholesterol stones?	Secretion of bile **supersaturated** with cholesterol (relatively decreased amounts of lecithin and bile salts); then, cholesterol precipitates out and forms solid crystals, then gallstones
Is hypercholesterolemia a risk factor for gallstone formation?	No (but hyperlipidemia is)
What are the signs and symptoms?	Signs and symptoms of biliary colic: RUQ pain, usually postprandially (i.e., after eating a fatty meal) Referred right subscapular pain Epigastric pain Nausea Vomiting (Signs and symptoms usually last for hours; therefore, colic is a misnomer!)
What percentage of patients with gallstones are asymptomatic?	Eighty percent of patients with cholelithiasis are asymptomatic!
What is thought to cause biliary colic?	Gallbladder contraction against a stone temporarily at the gallbladder/cystic duct junction; a stone in the cystic duct; or a stone passing through the cystic duct
What is Boas' sign?	The referred right subscapular pain of biliary colic
What are the complications of gallstones?	Acute cholecystitis Choledocholithiasis Gallstone pancreatitis Gallstone ileus, cholangitis
How is cholelithiasis diagnosed?	History Physical examination **Ultrasound** Laboratory tests
How often does ultrasound detect cholelithiasis?	More than 98% of the time!

How often does ultrasound detect choledocholithiasis?
About 33% of the time . . . not a very good study for choledocholithiasis!

How are symptomatic or complicated cases of cholelithiasis treated?
By cholecystectomy (most by laparoscopic cholecystectomy—"lap chole")

What are the possible complications of a lap chole?
Common bile duct injury; right hepatic duct/artery injury; cystic duct leak; biloma (collection of bile)

What are the indications for cholecystectomy in the asymptomatic patient?
Sickle-cell disease
Calcified gallbladder (porcelain gallbladder)
The patient is a child.

Define IOC.
Intra**O**perative **C**holangiogram (dye in bile duct by way of the cystic duct with fluoro/x-ray)

What are the indications for an IOC?
Should be performed if there is any evidence of choledocholithiasis or question about anatomy:
1. Jaundice
2. Hyperbilirubinemia
3. Gallstone pancreatitis (resolved)
4. Elevated alkaline phosphatase
5. Choledocholithiasis on ultrasound
6. To define anatomy

What is choledocholithiasis?
Gallstones in the bile ducts

What is the management of choledocholithiasis?
1. ERCP with papillotomy and basket/balloon retrieval of stones
2. Laparoscopic transcystic duct or trans common bile duct retrieval
3. Open common bile duct exploration

What medication may dissolve a cholesterol gallstone?
Chenodeoxycholic acid, ursodeoxycholic acid (Actigall®); but if medication is stopped, gallstones recur

ACUTE CHOLECYSTITIS

What is the pathogenesis of acute cholecystitis?
Obstruction of cystic duct leads to inflammation of the gallbladder; about 95% of cases result from calculi, and about 5% from acalculous obstruction.

What are the risk factors?

Gallstones

What are the signs and symptoms?

Unrelenting RUQ pain or tenderness
Fever
Nausea/vomiting
Painful palpable gallbladder in 33%
Positive Murphy's sign
Right subscapular pain (referred)
Epigastric discomfort (referred)

What is Murphy's sign?

Acute pain and **inspiratory arrest** elicited by palpation of the RUQ during inspiration

What are the complications of acute cholecystitis?

Abscess
Perforation
Choledocholithiasis
Cholecystenteric fistula formation
Gallstone ileus

What lab results are associated with acute cholecystitis?

Increased WBC
Slight elevation in alkaline phosphatase, LFTs
Slight elevation in amylase, T. Bili

What is the diagnostic test of choice for acute cholecystitis?

Ultrasound

What are the signs of acute cholecystitis on ultrasound?

Thickened gallbladder wall (thicker than 3 mm)
Pericholecystic fluid
Distended gallbladder
Gallstones present/cystic duct stone
Sonographic Murphy's sign (pain on inspiration after placement of ultrasound probe over gallbladder)

What is the difference between acute cholecystitis and biliary colic?

Biliary colic has temporary pain. Acute cholecystitis has pain that does not resolve, usually with elevated WBCs, fever, and signs of acute inflammation on US.

What is the treatment of acute cholecystitis?

IVFs, antibiotics, and cholecystectomy early

What are the steps in lap chole?

1. Dissection of peritoneum overlying the cystic duct and artery

2. Clipping of cystic artery and cannulation of cystic duct
3. Intraoperative cholangiogram, if necessary
4. Division of cystic duct between clips
5. Dissection of gallbladder from the liver bed
6. Cauterization; irrigation; suction, to obtain hemostasis of the liver bed
7. Removal of the gallbladder through the umbilical trocar site

Why should the gallbladder specimen be opened in the operating room?

Looking for gallbladder cancer (and it's position—liver side or peritoneal side)

ACUTE ACALCULUS CHOLECYSTITIS

What is it?

Acute cholecystitis without evidence of stones

What is the pathogenesis?

It is believed to result from sludge and gallbladder disuse and **biliary stasis,** perhaps secondary to absence of cholecystokinin stimulation (decreased contraction of gallbladder).

What are the risk factors?

Prolonged fasting
TPN
Trauma
Multiple transfusions
Dehydration
Often occurs in prolonged postop or ICU setting

What is the diagnostic test of choice?

Ultrasound; sludge and inflammation usually present with acute acalculous cholecystitis

What is the management of acute acalculous cholecystitis?

Cholecystectomy, or cholecystostomy tube if the patient is unstable (placed percutaneously by radiology or open surgery)

CHOLANGITIS

What is it?

Bacterial infection of the biliary tract from obstruction (either partial or complete); potentially life-threatening

What are the common causes of obstruction?

Choledocholithiasis
Stricture (usually postoperative)
Neoplasm (usually ampullary carcinoma)
Extrinsic compression (pancreatic pseudocyst/pancreatitis)
Instrumentation of the bile ducts (e.g., PTC/ERCP)
Biliary stent

What is the most common cause of cholangitis?

Gallstones in common bile duct (choledocholithiasis)

What are the signs and symptoms?

Charcot's triad: fever/chills, RUQ pain, and jaundice
Reynold's pentad: Charcot's triad plus altered mental status and shock

What lab results are associated with cholangitis?

Increased WBC, bilirubin, and alkaline phosphatase; ± blood cultures

Which organisms are most commonly isolated with cholangitis?

Gram-negative organisms (*E. coli, Klebsiella, Pseudomonas, Enterobacter, Proteus, Serratia*) are the most common.
Enterococci are the most common gram-positive bacteria.
Anaerobes are less common (*B. fragilis* most frequent).
Fungi are even less common (*Candida*).

What are the diagnostic tests of choice?

Ultrasound and contrast study (i.e., PTC or ERCP) after patient has "cooled off" with IV antibiotics

What is suppurative cholangitis?

Severe infection with sepsis—"pus under pressure"

What is the management of cholangitis?

Nonsuppurative: IVF and antibiotics, with definitive treatment later
Suppurative: IVF, antibiotics, and decompression; decompression can be obtained by ERCP with papillotomy, PTC with catheter drainage, or laparotomy with T-tube placement if refractory to ERCP/PTC

SCLEROSING CHOLANGITIS

What is it?

Multiple inflammatory fibrous thickenings of bile duct walls resulting in biliary strictures

What is its natural history?

Progressive obstruction possibly leading to cirrhosis and liver failure; 10% of patients will develop cholangiocarcinoma

What is the etiology?

Unknown, but probably autoimmune

What are the risk factors?

Inflammatory bowel disease (about 60%); pancreatitis (20%); diabetes (10%)

What are the signs and symptoms of sclerosing cholangitis?

The same as the signs of obstructive jaundice:
Jaundice
Itching (pruritus)
Dark urine
Clay-colored stools
Loss of energy
Weight loss
(Many patients are asymptomatic.)

What are the complications?

Cirrhosis
Cholangiocarcinoma (10%)
Cholangitis
Obstructive jaundice

How is it diagnosed?

Elevated alkaline phosphatase, and PTC or ERCP revealing "beads on a string" appearance on contrast study

What are the management options?

Hepatoenteric anastomosis (if primarily extrahepatic ducts are involved) and removal of extrahepatic bile ducts because of the risk of cholangiocarcinoma
Transplant (if primarily intrahepatic disease or cirrhosis)
Endoscopic balloon dilations

What percentage of patients with IBD develop sclerosing cholangitis?

Less than 5%

GALLSTONE ILEUS

What is it?	Small bowel obstruction from a large gallstone (>2.5 cm) that has eroded through the gallbladder and into the duodenum/small bowel
What is the classic site of obstruction?	The ileocecal valve (but may cause obstruction in the duodenum, sigmoid colon)
What is the population at risk?	Gallstone ileus is most commonly seen in **women older than 70 years.**
What are the signs/ symptoms?	Symptoms of SBO: distention, vomiting, hypovolemia, RUQ pain
What is the differential diagnosis?	Other causes of SBO (A, B, C: adhesions, bulge/hernia, cancer)
Gallstone ileus causes what percentage of cases of SBO?	Less than 1%
What are the diagnostic tests of choice?	**Abdominal x-ray:** occasionally reveals radiopaque gallstone in the bowel; **40% of patients show air in the biliary tract,** small bowel distention, and air fluid levels secondary to ileus UGI: used if diagnosis is in question; will show cholecystenteric fistula and the obstruction **Abdominal CT:** reveals air in biliary tract, SBO +/− gallstone in intestine
What is the management?	Surgery: enterotomy with removal of the stone ± cholecystectomy/closure of fistula

CARCINOMA OF THE GALLBLADDER

What is it?	Malignant neoplasm arising in the gallbladder; very low incidence, vast majority are **adenocarcinoma (90%)**
What are the risk factors?	**Gallstones** (approximately 100% of cases, especially large gallstones), cholecystenteric fistula, **porcelain gallbladder** (approximately 50% will have gallbladder cancer)

What is the incidence?	**About 1% of all patients with cholelithiasis over a lifetime!**
What are the symptoms?	Biliary colic, weight loss, anorexia; many patients are asymptomatic until late; may present as acute cholecystitis
What are the signs?	Jaundice (from invasion of the common duct or compression by involved pericholedochal lymph nodes), RUQ mass, palpable gallbladder (advanced disease)
What are the diagnostic tests of choice?	Ultrasound, abdominal CT, ERCP
What is the route of spread?	Contiguous spread to the liver is most common.
What is the management under the following conditions?	
Confined to mucosa	Cholecystectomy
Confined to muscularis/ serosa	Radical cholecystectomy: cholecystectomy and wedge resection of overlying liver, and lymph node dissection
What is the main complication of a lap chole for gallbladder cancer?	Trocar site tumor implants (so if known preoperatively, perform open cholecystectomy)

CHOLANGIOCARCINOMA

What is it?	Malignancy of the extrahepatic or intrahepatic ducts—**primary bile duct cancer**
What is the histology?	Almost all are adenocarcinomas
What is the average age of the patient?	About 65 years
What are the signs and symptoms?	The signs and symptoms of biliary obstruction: jaundice, **pruritus, dark urine, clay-colored stools**

What are the risk factors?

Choledochal cysts
Ulcerative colitis
Thorotrast contrast dye (used in 1950s)
Sclerosing cholangitis
Liver flukes (clonorchiasis)
Toxin exposures (e.g., agent orange?)

What is a Klatskin tumor?

Tumor that involves the junction of the right and left hepatic ducts

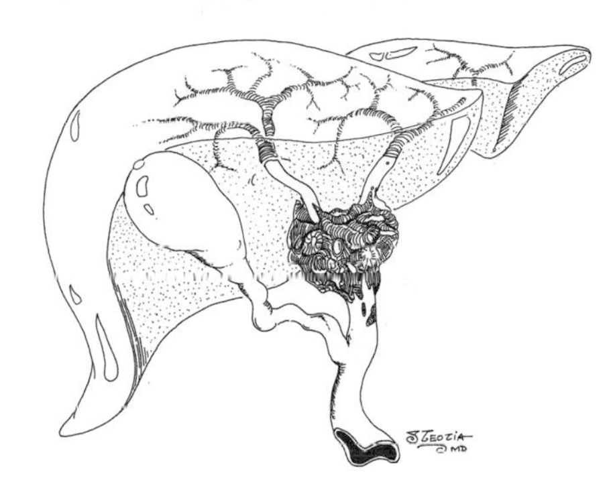

What are the diagnostic tests of choice?

Ultrasound, CT, ERCP/PTC with biopsy/brushings for cytology

What is the management of proximal bile duct cholangiocarcinoma?

Resection with Roux-en-Y hepaticojejunostomy (anastomose bile ducts to jejunum)

What is the management of distal common bile duct cholangiocarcinoma?

Whipple procedure

MISCELLANEOUS CONDITIONS

What is a porcelain gallbladder?

Calcified gallbladder seen on abdominal x-ray; results from chronic cholelithiasis/cholecystitis with calcified scar tissue in gallbladder wall; **cholecystectomy** required because of the strong association of **gallbladder carcinoma** with this condition

What is hydrops of the gallbladder?

Complete obstruction of the cystic duct by a gallstone, with filling of the gallbladder with fluid (not bile) from the gallbladder mucosa

What is Gilbert syndrome?	Inborn error in liver bilirubin uptake and glucuronyl transferase resulting in hyperbilirubinemia (Think **G**ilberts = **G**lucuronyl)
What is Courvoisier's gallbladder?	A palpable, **nontender** gallbladder (unlike acute cholecystitis) associated with cancer of the head of the pancreas; able to distend because it has not been "scarred down" by gallstones
What is Mirizzi's syndrome?	Common hepatic duct obstruction as a result of extrinsic obstruction from a gallstone impacted in the cystic duct

52 Pancreas

Identify the regions of the pancreas.

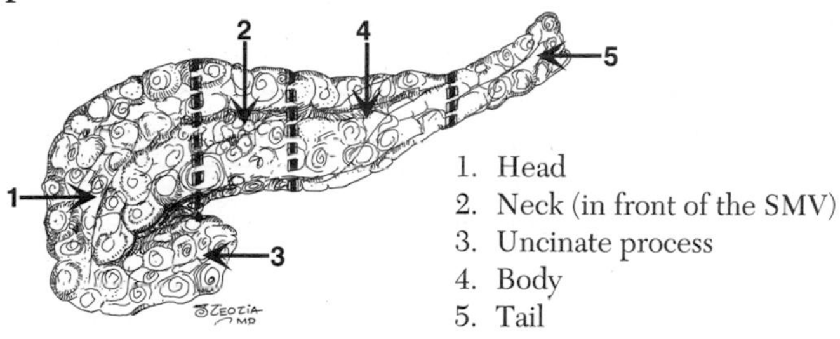

1. Head
2. Neck (in front of the SMV)
3. Uncinate process
4. Body
5. Tail

What structure is the tail of the pancreas said to "tickle"?

The spleen

Name the two pancreatic ducts.

1. Wirsung duct
2. Santorini duct

Which duct is the main duct?

The duct of Wirsung is the major duct (think: **S**antorini = **S**mall duct).

How is blood supplied to the head of the pancreas?

Celiac trunk → gastroduodenal →
- Anterior superior pancreaticoduodenal artery
- Posterior superior pancreaticoduodenal artery

Superior mesenteric artery →
- Anterior inferior pancreaticoduodenal artery
- Posterior inferior pancreaticoduodenal artery

Splenic artery →
- Dorsal pancreatic artery

Why must the duodenum be removed if the head of the pancreas is removed?

They share the same blood supply (gastroduodenal artery).

What is the endocrine function of the pancreas?

Islets of Langerhans
α-cells: glucagon
β-cells: insulin

What is the exocrine function of the pancreas?

Digestive enzymes: amylase, lipase, trypsin, chymotrypsin, carboxypeptidase

What maneuver is used to mobilize the duodenum and pancreas and evaluate the entire pancreas?

Kocher maneuver: incise the lateral attachments of the duodenum and then lift the pancreas to examine the posterior surface

PANCREATITIS

ACUTE PANCREATITIS

What is it?

Inflammation of the pancreas

What are the most common etiologies in the United States?

1. Alcohol abuse (50%)
2. Gallstones (30%)
3. Idiopathic (10%)

What acronym represents the other causes of pancreatitis?

I G.E.T. S.M.A.S.H.E.D.
I = Idiopathic

G = Gallstones
E = Ethanol
T = Trauma

S = Scorpion bite
M = Mumps (viruses)
A = Autoimmune
S = Steroids
H = Hyperlipidemia
E = ERCP
D = Drugs

What are the symptoms?

Epigastric pain (frequently radiates to another quadrant or back); nausea and vomiting

What are the signs of pancreatitis?

Epigastric tenderness
Diffuse abdominal tenderness
Decreased bowel sounds (adynamic ileus)
Fever
Dehydration/shock

What is the differential diagnosis?

Gastritis/PUD
Perforated viscus
Acute cholecystitis
SBO
Mesenteric ischemia/infarction
Ruptured AAA
Biliary colic
Inferior MI/pneumonia

What lab tests should be ordered?

CBC
LFT
Amylase/lipase
Type and cross
ABG
Ca2+
Chem 10
Coags
Serum lipids

What are the associated diagnostic findings?

Lab High amylase, high lipase, high WBC
AXR—Sentinel loop, colon cutoff, possibly gallstones (only 10% visible on x-ray)
U/S—Pseudocyst, phlegmon, abscess, cholelithiasis
CT—Pseudocyst, phlegmon, abscess, pancreatic necrosis

What is the most common sign of pancreatitis on AXR?

Sentinel loop(s)

What is the treatment?

NPO
IVF
NGT if vomiting
TPN
H_2 blocker
Analgesia (Demerol, not morphine—less sphincter of Oddi spasm)
Correction of coags/electrolytes
"Tincture of time"

What are the possible complications?

Pseudocyst
Abscess/infection
Pancreatic necrosis
Splenic/mesenteric/portal vessel rupture or thrombosis

Pancreatic ascites/pancreatic pleural effusion
Diabetes
ARDS/sepsis/MOF
Coagulopathy/DIC
Encephalopathy
Severe hypocalcemia

What is the prognosis?
Based on Ranson's criteria

What are Ranson's criteria for the following stages:

At presentation?
1. Age > 55
2. WBC > 16,000
3. Glc > 200
4. AST > 250
5. LDH > 350

During the initial 48 hours?
1. Base deficit > 4
2. BUN increase > 5 mg/dl
3. Fluid sequestration > 6 L
4. Serum Ca2+ < 8
5. Hct decrease > 10%
6. Po2 (ABG) < 60 mm Hg
   [Amylase value is NOT one of Ranson's criteria!]

What is the mortality per positive criteria:

0 to 2?
Less than 5%

3 to 4?
Approximately 15%

5 to 6?
Approximately 40%

7 to 8?
Approximately 100%

How can the admission Ranson criteria be remembered?
GA LAW ("Georgia law")
G—Glucose > 200
A—Age > 55

L—LDH > 350
A—AST > 250
W—WBC > 16,000
["Don't mess with the pancreas and don't mess with the Georgia law."]

How can Ranson's criteria at less than 48 hours be remembered?

C HOBBS ("Calvin and Hobbs")
C—Calcium < 8 mg/dl
H—Hct drop of > 10%
O—O2 < 60 (PaO2)
B—Base deficit > 4
B—Bun > 5 increase
S—Sequestration > 6 L

How can the AST versus LDH values in Ranson's criteria be remembered?

Alphabetically: A before L and 250 before 350
Therefore, AST > 250 and LDH > 350

What is the etiology of hypocalcemia with pancreatitis?

Fat saponification; fat necrosis binds to calcium

What complication is associated with splenic vein thrombosis?

Gastric varices

Can TPN with lipids be given to a patient with pancreatitis?

Yes, if the patient does not suffer from hyperlipidemia

What is the least common cause of acute pancreatitis (and possibly the most commonly asked cause on rounds!)

Scorpion bite (not the U.S. type; found on Pacific islands)

CHRONIC PANCREATITIS

What is it?

Chronic inflammation of the pancreas; causes destruction of the parenchyma, fibrosis, and calcification, resulting in loss of endocrine and exocrine tissue

What are the subtypes?

1. Chronic calcific pancreatitis
2. Chronic obstructive pancreatitis (5%)

What are the causes?

Alcohol abuse (most common; 70% of cases)
Idiopathic (15%)
Hypercalcemia (hyperparathyroidism)
Hyperlipidemia
Familial (found in families without any other risk factors)
Trauma
Iatrogenic
Gallstones

What are the symptoms?
Epigastric and/or back pain, weight loss, steatorrhea

What are the signs of pancreatic exocrine insufficiency?
Steatorrhea (fat malabsorption from lipase insufficiency—stools float in water)

What are the signs of pancreatic endocrine insufficiency?
Diabetes (glucose intolerance)

What are the common pain patterns?
Unrelenting pain
Recurrent pain

What are the associated signs?
Type 1 diabetes mellitus (up to one-third)
Steatorrhea (up to one-fourth)

What is the differential diagnosis?
PUD, biliary tract disease, AAA, pancreatic cancer, angina

What percentage of patients with chronic pancreatitis have or will develop pancreatic cancer?
Approximately 2%

What are the appropriate lab tests?
Amylase/lipase
72-hour fecal fat analysis
Glc tolerance test (IDDM)

Why may amylase/lipase be normal in a patient with chronic pancreatitis?
Because of extensive pancreatic tissue loss ("burned-out pancreas")

What radiographic tests should be performed?
CT—Has greatest sensitivity for gland enlargement/atrophy, calcifications, masses, pseudocysts
KUB—Calcification in the pancreas
ERCP—Ductal irregularities with dilation and stenosis (Chain of Lakes), pseudocysts

What is the medical treatment?
Discontinuation of alcohol use—can stop attacks, though parenchymal damage continues secondary to ductal obstruction and fibrosis
Insulin for Type 1 diabetes mellitus
Pancreatic enzyme replacement
Narcotics for pain (watch for addiction)

What is the surgical treatment?

Puestow—longitudinal pancreaticojejunostomy (pancreatic duct **must be dilated**)
Duval—distal pancreaticojejunostomy
Near-total pancreatectomy

What is the indication for surgical treatment of chronic pancreatitis?

Severe, prolonged/refractory pain

What are the possible complications of chronic pancreatitis?

Type 1 diabetes mellitus (glucose intolerance)
Steatorrhea
Malnutrition
Biliary obstruction
Splenic vein thrombosis
Gastric varices
Pancreatic pseudocyst/abscess
Narcotic addiction
Pancreatic ascites/pleural effusion
Splenic artery aneurysm

GALLSTONE PANCREATITIS

What is it?

Acute pancreatitis from a gallstone in or passing through the ampulla of Vater (the exact mechanism is unknown)

How is the diagnosis made?

Acute pancreatitis and cholelithiasis and/or choledocholithiasis and no other cause of pancreatitis (e.g., no history of alcohol abuse)

What radiologic tests should be performed?

U/S to look for gallstones
CT to look at the pancreas, if symptoms are severe

What is the treatment?

Conservative measures and early interval cholecystectomy (laparoscopic cholecystectomy or open cholecystectomy) and intraoperatic cholangiogram (IOC) 3 to 5 days (after pancreatic inflammation resolves)

Why should early interval cholecystectomy be performed on patients with gallstone pancreatitis?

Pancreatitis will recur in approximately 33% of patients within 8 weeks (so always perform early interval cholecystectomy and IOC in 3 to 5 days when pancreatitis resolves).

HEMORRHAGIC PANCREATITIS

What is it?	Bleeding into the parenchyma and retroperitoneal structures with extensive pancreatic necrosis
What are the signs?	Abdominal pain, shock/ARDS, Cullen's sign, Grey Turner's sign, Fox's sign
Define the following terms:	
Cullen's sign	**Bluish discoloration of the periumbilical area** from retroperitoneal hemorrhage tracking around to the anterior abdominal wall through fascial planes
Grey Turner's sign	**Ecchymosis or discoloration of the flank** in patients with retroperitoneal hemorrhage from dissecting blood from the retroperitoneum (think: Grey Turner = turn side to side = flank [side] hematoma)
Fox's sign	**Ecchymosis of the inguinal ligament** from blood tracking from the retroperitoneum and collecting at the inguinal ligament
What are the significant lab values?	Increased amylase/lipase Decreased Hct Decreased calcium levels
What radiologic test should be performed?	CT scan with IV contrast

PANCREATIC ABSCESS

What is it?	Infected peripancreatic purulent fluid collection
What are the signs/ symptoms?	Fever, unresolving pancreatitis, epigastric mass
What radiographic tests should be performed?	Abdominal CT with needle aspiration → send for Gram stain/culture
What are the associated lab findings?	Positive Gram stain and culture of bacteria

Which organisms are found in pancreatic abscesses?

Gram negative (most common): *Escherichia coli, Pseudomonas, Klebsiella*
Gram positive: *Staphylococcus aureus, Candida*

What is the treatment?

Antibiotics and percutaneous drain placement or operative debridement and placement of drains

PANCREATIC NECROSIS

What is it?

Dead pancreatic tissue, usually following acute pancreatitis

How is the diagnosis made?

Abdominal CT with IV contrast; dead pancreatic tissue does not take up IV contrast and is not enhanced on CT scan

What is the treatment?

Surgical debridement and drain placement IF there is infected necrosis or patient is severely ill and refractory to medical management

PANCREATIC PSEUDOCYST

What is it?

Encapsulated collection of pancreatic fluid ("pseudo" = wall formed by inflammatory fibrosis, NOT epithelial cell lining)

What is the incidence?

Approximately 1 in 10 after alcoholic pancreatitis

What are the associated risk factors?

Acute pancreatitis < chronic pancreatitis from alcohol

What is the most common cause of pancreatic pseudocyst in the United States?

Chronic alcoholic pancreatitis

What are the symptoms?

Epigastric pain
Emesis
Mild fever
Weight loss
Should be suspected when a patient with acute pancreatitis fails to resolve pain

What are the signs?
Palpable epigastric mass, tender epigastrium, ileus

What lab tests should be performed?
Amylase/lipase
Bilirubin
CBC

What are the diagnostic findings?
Lab—High amylase, leukocytosis, high bilirubin (if there is obstruction)
U/S—Fluid-filled mass
CT—Fluid-filled mass, good for showing multiple cysts
ERCP—Radiopaque contrast material fills cyst if there is a communicating pseudocyst (i.e., pancreatic duct communicates with pseudocyst)

What is the differential diagnosis of a pseudocyst?
Cystadenocarcinoma, cystadenoma

What are the possible complications of a pancreatic pseudocyst?
Infection, bleeding into the cyst, fistula, pancreatic ascites, gastric outlet obstruction

What is the treatment?
Drainage of the cyst or observation

What is the waiting period before a pseudocyst should be drained?
It takes 6 weeks for pseudocyst walls to "mature" or become firm enough to hold sutures and most will resolve in this period of time if they are going to.

What percentage of pseudocysts resolve spontaneously?
Approximately 50%

What size pseudocyst should be drained?
Controversial, but most experts say those larger than 5 cm as:
Pseudocysts larger than 5 cm have a small chance of resolving and have a higher chance of complications (e.g., bleeding, infection).
Many experts advocate close follow-up only for pancreatic pseudocysts less than 5 cm.

What are two treatment options for pancreatic pseudocyst?
Percutaneous/aspiration/drain
Operative drainage

What are the surgical options for the following conditions:

Pseudocyst adherent to the stomach?
Cystogastrostomy (drain into the stomach)

Pseudocyst adherent to the duodenum?
Cystoduodenostomy (drain into the duodenum)

Pseudocyst not adherent to the stomach or duodenum?
Roux-en-Y cystojejunostomy (drain into the Roux limb of the jejunum)

Pseudocyst in the tail of the pancreas?
Resection of the pancreatic tail with the pseudocyst

What is the other endoscopic option for drainage of a pseudocyst?
Controversial and evolving: **endoscopic** cystogastrostomy

What must be done during a surgical drainage procedure for a pancreatic pseudocyst?
Biopsy of the cyst wall to rule out a cystic carcinoma (e.g., cystadenocarcinoma)

What is the most common cause of death due to pancreatic pseudocyst?
Massive hemorrhage into the pseudocyst

PANCREATIC CARCINOMA

What is it?
Adenocarcinoma of the pancreas arising from duct cells

What are the associated risk factors?
Smoking 3× **risk,** diabetes mellitus, heavy alcohol use, chronic pancreatitis, coffee and exposure to the chemicals benzidine, β-naphthylamine may be associated

What is the male to female ratio?
3:2

What is the African-American to white ratio?
2:1

What is the average age?
Older than 60 years

What are the different types?

More than 90% are duct cell adenocarcinomas; other types include cystadenocarcinoma and acinar cell carcinoma.

What percentage arise in the pancreatic head?

Two-thirds arise in the pancreatic **head; one-third** arise in the **body and tail.**

Why are most pancreatic cancers in the tail nonresectable?

These tumors grow without symptoms until it is too late and they have already spread—head of the pancreas tumors draw attention earlier because of biliary obstruction.

What are the signs/ symptoms of tumors based on location:

Head of the pancreas?

Painless jaundice (70%) from obstruction of common bile duct; weight loss (90%); abdominal pain (75%); weakness; **pruritus** (40%) from bile salts in skin; anorexia (60%); palpable, nontender, distended gallbladder (**Courvoisier's sign**); acholic stools; dark urine

Body or tail?

Weight loss and pain (90%); migratory thrombophlebitis (10%); jaundice (< 10%); nausea and vomiting; fatigue

What percentage will have Courvoisier's sign?

33%

What is the classic presentation of pancreatic cancer in the head of the pancreas?

Painless jaundice

What are the associated lab findings?

Increased direct bilirubin and alkaline phosphatase (as a result of biliary obstruction)
Increased LFTs
Elevated pancreatic tumor markers

Which tumor markers are associated with pancreatic cancer?

CEA and CA 19–9

What diagnostic studies are performed?

Abdominal CT, U/S, cholangiography (ERCP to rule out choledocholithiasis and cell brushings), selective angiography (rarely used as CT has replaced), endoscopic U/S AJCC

What are the pancreatic cancer STAGES:

Stage I?

Tumor is limited to pancreas, with no nodes or metastases.

Stage II?

Tumor extends into bile duct, peripancreatic tissues, or duodenum; there are no nodes or metastases.

Stage III?

Same findings as stage II plus **positive nodes.**

Stage IVA?

Tumor extends to stomach, colon, spleen, or major vessels, with any nodal status and no metastases.

Stage IVB?

Distant metastases (any nodal status, any tumor size) are found.

What is the treatment based on location:

Head of the pancreas?

Whipple procedure (pancreaticoduodenectomy)

Body or tail?

Distal resection

What factors signify inoperability?

Vascular encasement (portal vein, SMV, SMA)
Liver metastasis
Peritoneal implants
Distant lymph node metastasis (periaortic/celiac nodes)
Distant metastasis

Should patients undergo preoperative biliary drainage (e.g., PTC)?

No (exceptions for symptoms/preoperative XRT, trials, etc.)

Define the Whipple procedure (pancreaticoduodenectomy).

Cholecystectomy
Truncal vagotomy
Antrectomy

Pancreaticoduodenectomy—removal of head of pancreas and duodenum
Choledochojejunostomy—anastomosis of common bile duct to jejunum
Pancreaticojejunostomy—anastomosis of distal pancreas remnant to jejunum
Gastrojejunostomy—anastomosis of stomach to jejunum

What is the complication rate after a Whipple procedure?

Approximately 25%

What mortality rate is associated with a Whipple procedure?

Approximately 3%

What is the "pylorus-preserving Whipple"?

No antrectomy; anastomose duodenum to jejunum

What are the possible post-Whipple complications?

Delayed gastric emptying (if antrectomy is performed); anastomotic leak (from the bile duct or pancreatic anastomosis), causing pancreatic/biliary fistula; wound infection; postgastrectomy syndromes; sepsis; pancreatitis

Why must the duodenum be removed if the head of the pancreas is resected?

They share the same blood supply.

What is the preoperative and/or postoperative adjuvant therapy?

Chemotherapy (5-FU) and x-ray therapy

What is the palliative treatment if the tumor is inoperable and biliary obstruction is present?

PTC or ERCP and placement of stent across obstruction

What is the prognosis at 1 year after diagnosis?

Dismal; 90% of patients die within 1 year of diagnosis

What is the survival after resection at 5 years?

Overall survival rate is 20% at 5 years after resection.

MISCELLANEOUS

What is an annular pancreas?

Pancreas encircling the duodenum; if obstruction is present, bypass, **do not resect**

What is pancreatic divisum?

Failure of the two pancreatic ducts to fuse; the normally small duct (small = **S**antorini) of Santorini acts as the main duct in pancreatic divisum (think: the two pancreatic ducts are **Di**vided = **Di**visum)

What is heterotopic pancreatic tissue?

Heterotopic pancreatic tissue usually found in the stomach, intestine, duodenum

What is a Puestow procedure?

Longitudinal filleting of the pancreas with a side-to-side anastomosis with the small bowel

What medication decreases output from a pancreatic fistula?

Somatostatin (GI-inhibitory hormone)

Which has a longer half life: amylase or lipase?

Lipase; therefore, amylase may be normal and lipase will remain elevated longer

What is the WDHA syndrome?

A pancreatic **VIP**oma (**V**asoactive **I**ntestinal **P**olypeptide tumor)

Also known as Verner-Morrison syndrome

Tumor secretes VIP, which causes:

- **W: Watery**
- **D: Diarrhea**
- **H: Hypokalemia**
- **A: Achlorhydria** (inhibits gastric acid secretion)

What is the Whipple triad of pancreatic insulinoma?

1. Hypoglycemia (Glc < 50)
2. Symptoms of hypoglycemia: mental status changes/vasomotor instability
3. Relief of symptoms with administration of glucose

What is the most common islet cell tumor?

Insulinoma

What pancreatic tumor is associated with gallstone formation?

Somatostatinoma (inhibits gallbladder contraction)

What is the triad found with pancreatic somatostatinoma tumor?

1. Gallstones
2. Diabetes
3. Steatorrhea

What are the two classic findings with pancreatic glucagonoma tumors?

1. Diabetes
2. Dermatitis/rash (necrotizing migratory erythema)

53 The Breast

ANATOMY OF THE BREAST AND AXILLA

Name the boundaries of the axilla for dissection:

Superior boundary — Axillary vein

Posterior boundary — Long thoracic nerve

Lateral boundary — Latissimus dorsi muscle

Medial boundary — Lateral to, deep to, or medial to pectoral minor muscle, depending on level of nodes taken

What four nerves must the surgeon be aware of during an axillary dissection?

1. **Long thoracic nerve**
2. **Thoracodorsal nerve**
3. Medial pectoral nerve
4. Lateral pectoral nerve

Describe the location of these nerves and the muscle each innervates.

Long thoracic nerve — Courses along lateral chest wall in midaxillary line on serratus anterior muscle; innervates serratus anterior muscle

Thoracodorsal nerve — Courses lateral to long thoracic nerve on latissimus dorsi muscle; innervates latissimus dorsi muscle

Medial pectoral nerve — Runs **lateral** to or through the pectoral minor muscle, actually lateral to the lateral pectoral nerve; innervates the pectoral minor and pectoral major muscles; also known as the medial thoracic nerve

Lateral pectoral nerve

Runs **medial** to the lateral pectoral nerve through the pectoral minor muscle (names describe orientation from the brachial plexus!); innervates the pectoral major; also known as the lateral thoracic nerve

Identify the nerves in the axilla on the illustration below.

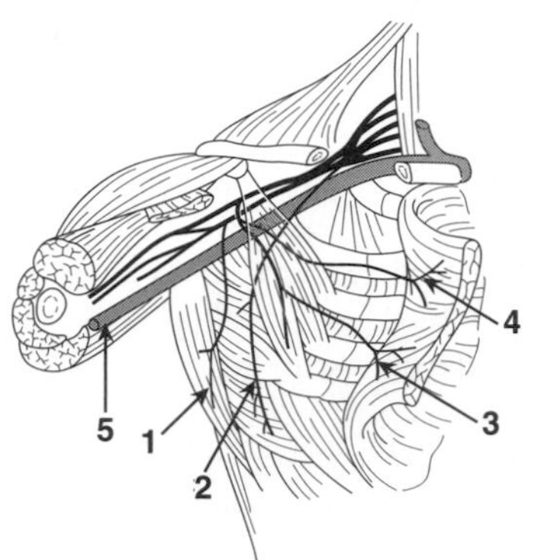

1. Thoracodorsal nerve
2. Long thoracic nerve
3. Medial pectoral nerve
4. Lateral pectoral nerve
5. Axillary vein

What is the name of the deformity if you cut the long thoracic nerve in this area?

"Winged scapula"

What is the name of the CUTANEOUS nerve that crosses the axilla in a transverse fashion? (Many surgeons try to preserve this nerve.)

Intercostobrachial nerve

What is the name of the large vein that marks the upper limit of the axilla?

Axillary vein

What is the lymphatic drainage of the breast?

Lateral: axillary lymph nodes
Medial: parasternal nodes that run with internal mammary artery

What are the levels of axillary lymph nodes?

Level I (low): lateral to pectoral minor
Level II (middle): deep to pectoral minor
Level III (high): medial to pectoral minor

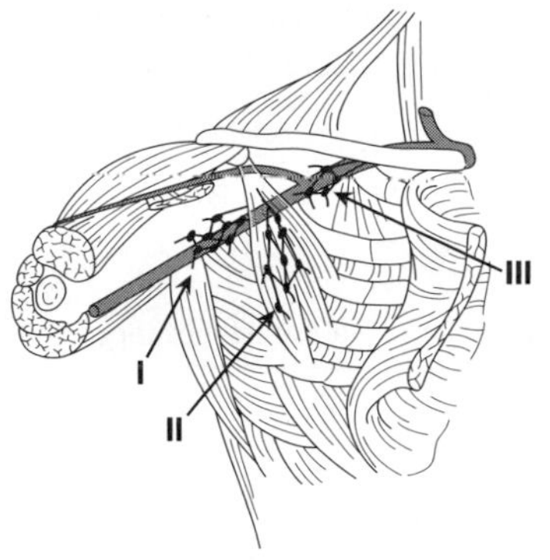

In breast cancer, a higher level of involvement has a worse prognosis, but the level of involvement is less important than the number of positive nodes. (**Think:** Levels I, II, III are in the same superior–inferior anatomic order as the LeFort facial fractures and the trauma neck zones; *I dare you to forget!*)

What are Rotter's nodes?
Nodes between the pectoralis major and minor muscles; not usually removed unless there is clinical evidence of metastasis

What are the suspensory breast ligaments called?
Cooper's ligaments

What is the mammary "milk line"?
The embryological line from shoulder to thigh where "supernumerary" breast nipples can be found

What is the "tail of Spence"?
The "tail" of breast tissue that tapers into the axilla

Which hormone is mainly responsible for breast milk production?
Prolactin

BREAST CANCER

What is the incidence of breast cancer?
12% lifetime risk

What percentage of women with breast cancer have no known risk factor?
75%!

What percentage of all breast cancers occur in women younger than 30 years?
Approximately 2%

What percentage of all breast cancers occur in women older than 70 years?

33%

What are the major breast cancer susceptibility genes?

BRCA1 and **BRCA**2 (easy **BR** = breast and **CA** = cancer)

What is the most common motivation for medicolegal cases involving the breast?

Failure to diagnose a breast carcinoma

What are the history risk factors for breast cancer?

N.A.A.C.P.
N Nulliparity
A Age at menarche (younger than 13 years)
A Age at menopause (older than 55 years)
C Cancer of the breast (in self or family)
P Pregnancy with first child (older than 30 years)

Is having a history of a breast biopsy that is benign a risk factor for breast cancer?

Yes

What are physical/anatomic risk factors for breast cancer?

CHAFED LIPS
C Cancer in the breast (3% synchronous contralateral cancer)
H Hyperplasia (moderate/florid) (2× risk)
A Atypical hyperplasia (4×)
F Female (100× male risk)
E Elderly
D DCIS

L LCIS
I Inherited genes (BRCA I and II)
P Papilloma (1.5×)
S Sclerosing adenitis (1.5×)

What is the relative risk of hormone replacement therapy?

1–1.5 controversial

Who has a higher risk of developing breast cancer over the remainder of her life: a 50-year-old woman or a 70-year old woman?

Classic trick! The 50-year-old woman, as she has on average 28 years of risk to live

Is "run of the mill" fibrocystic disease a risk factor for breast cancer?

No

What are the possible symptoms of breast cancer?

No symptoms
Mass in the breast
Pain (**most are painless**)
Nipple discharge
Local edema
Nipple retraction
Dimple
Nipple rash

Why does skin retraction occur?

Tumor involvement of Cooper's ligaments and subsequent traction on ligaments pull skin inward.

What are the signs of breast cancer?

Mass (1 cm is usually the smallest lesion that can be palpated on examination)
Dimple
Nipple rash
Edema
Axillary/supraclavicular nodes

What is the most common site of breast cancer?

Approximately one-half of cancers develop in the upper outer quadrants.

What are the major types of invasive carcinoma?

Invasive ductal carcinoma (90%)
Invasive lobular carcinoma (10%)
Inflammatory carcinoma

What is the most common type of breast cancer?

Infiltrating ductal carcinoma

What is the differential diagnosis?

Fibrocystic disease of the breast
Fibroadenoma
Intraductal papilloma
Duct ectasia
Fat necrosis
Abscess
Radial scar
Adenitis

Describe the appearance of the edema of the dermis in inflammatory carcinoma of the breast.

Peau d'orange (orange peel)

What are the screening recommendations for breast cancer:

Breast exam recommendations?

Self-exam of breasts monthly
Ages 20 to 40 years: breast exam every 2 to 3 years by a physician
Older than 40 years: Annual breast exam by physician

Mammograms?

Recommendations are controversial, but most experts say:
Baseline mammogram between 35 and 40 years
Mammogram every year or every other year for ages 40 to 50
Mammogram yearly after age 50

When is the best time for breast self exams?

One week after menstrual period

Why is mammography a more useful diagnostic tool in older than in younger women?

Breast tissue undergoes fatty replacement with age, making masses more visible. Younger women have more fibrous tissue, which makes mammograms harder to interpret.

What are the radiographic tests for breast cancer?

Mammography and breast ultrasound (MRI rarely)

Which option is best to evaluate a breast mass in a woman younger than 30 years?

Breast ultrasound

What are the methods for obtaining tissue for pathologic examination?

Fine needle aspiration (FNA), core biopsy (larger needle core sample), mammotome biopsy, and open biopsy. Open biopsy can be incisional (cutting a **piece** of the mass) or excisional (cutting out the **entire** mass).

What are the indications for biopsy?

Persistent mass after aspiration
Solid mass
Blood in cyst aspirate
Suspicious lesion by mammography
Bloody nipple discharge
Ulcer or dermatitis of nipple

Patient's concern of persistent breast abnormality

What is the process for performing a biopsy when a nonpalpable mass is seen on mammogram?

Mammotome biopsy or needle loc biopsy

What is a needle loc biopsy (NLB)?

Needle localization by radiologist, followed by biopsy. Removed breast tissue must be checked by mammogram to ensure all suspicious lesion has been excised.

What is a mammotome biopsy?

Mammogram-guided computerized stereotatic core biopsies

What is obtained first, the mammogram or the biopsy?

The mammogram is obtained first; otherwise, tissue extraction (core or open) may alter the mammographic findings. (Fine needle aspiration may be done prior to the mammogram because the fine needle will not affect the mammographic findings.)

What would be suspicious mammographic findings?

Mass, microcalcifications, stellate/spiculated mass

What is the "workup" for a breast mass?

1. Physical exam
2. Mammogram or breast ultrasound
3. Fine needle aspiration, core biopsy, or open biopsy

How do you proceed if the mass appears to be a cyst?

Aspirate it with a needle.

Is the fluid from a breast cyst sent for cytology?

Not routinely; bloody fluid should be sent for cytology

When do you proceed to open biopsy for a breast cyst?

1. In the case of a second cyst recurrence
2. Bloody fluid in the cyst
3. Palpable mass after aspiration

What is the preoperative staging workup in a patient with breast cancer?

Bilateral mammogram (cancer in one breast is a risk factor for cancer in the contralateral breast!)
CXR (to check for lung metastasis)
LFTs (to check for liver metastasis)

Serum calcium level, alkaline phosphatase. (If these tests indicate bone metastasis, proceed to bone scan.)
Other tests, depending on signs/symptoms (e.g., head CT if patient has focal neurologic deficit, to look for brain metastasis)

What hormone receptors must be checked for in the biopsy specimen?

Estrogen and progesterone receptors. This is **key for determining adjuvant treatment.** This information must be obtained on all specimens (including fine needle aspirates).

What staging system is used for breast cancer?

TMN: tumor/metastases/nodes (AJCC)

Describe the staging (simplified).

Stage I

Tumor ≤ 2 cm in diameter without metastases, **no nodes**

Stage IIA

Tumor ≤ 2 cm in diameter with mobile axillary nodes **or**
Tumor 2 to 5 cm in diameter, no nodes

Stage IIB

Tumor 2 to 5 cm in diameter with mobile axillary nodes or
Tumor larger than 5 cm **with no nodes**

Stage IIIA

Tumor larger than 5 cm with mobile axillary nodes or
Any size tumor with **fixed** axillary nodes, no metastases

Stage IIIB

Peau d'orange (skin edema) or
Chest wall invasion/fixation or
Inflammatory cancer or
Breast skin ulceration or
Breast skin satellite metastases or
Any tumor and + ipsilateral **internal mammary** lymph nodes

Stage IV

Distant metastases (including ipsilateral supraclavicular nodes)

What are the sites of metastases?

Lymph nodes (most common)
Lung/pleura
Liver
Bones
Brain

What are the major treatments of breast cancer?

Modified radical mastectomy
Lumpectomy and radiation
(Both treatments either with or without postop chemotherapy/Tamoxifen)

What breast carcinomas are candidates for lumpectomy and radiation?

Stage I and stage II (tumors < 5 cm)

What is the treatment of inflammatory carcinoma of the breast?

Chemotherapy first! Then often followed by radiation, mastectomy, or both

What is a lumpectomy and radiation?

Lumpectomy (segmental mastectomy: removal of a **part** of the breast); axillary node dissection; and course of radiation therapy **after** operation, over a period of several weeks

What is the major absolute contraindication to lumpectomy and radiation?

Pregnancy

What are other contraindications to lumpectomy and radiation?

Previous radiation to the chest
Positive margins
Collagen vascular disease
Extensive DCIS (often seen as diffuse microcalcification)
Relative contraindications:
Lesion that cannot be seen on the mammograms (i.e., early recurrence will be missed on follow-up mammograms)
Very small breast (no cosmetic advantage)

What is a modified radical mastectomy?

Breast, axillary nodes (level II, I), and nipple–areolar complex are removed.
Pectoralis major and minor muscles are **not** removed (Auchincloss modification).
Drains are placed to drain lymph fluid.

What are the potential complications after a modified radical mastectomy?	Ipsilateral arm lymphedema, infection, and injury to nerves, skin flap necrosis, hematoma/seroma, phantom breast syndrome
During an axillary dissection, should the patient be paralyzed?	NO, because the nerves (long thoracic/thoracodorsal) are stimulated with resultant muscle contraction to help identify them
How can the long thoracic and thoracodorsal nerves be identified during an axillary dissection?	The nerves can be stimulated with a forceps, which results in contraction of the latissimus dorsi (thoracodorsal nerve) or anterior serratus (long thoracic nerve).
When do you remove the drains after an axillary dissection?	When there is less than 30 cc of drainage per day, or on postop day 14 (whichever comes first)
What is a "sentinel" node biopsy?	Instead of removing all the axillary lymph nodes the **primary** draining or "sentinel" lymph node is removed.
How is the "sentinel" lymph node found?	Inject blue dye or technetium-labeled sulfur colloid
What follows a positive sentinel node biopsy?	Removal of the rest of the axillary lymph nodes
What do you do with a mammotome biopsy that returns as "atypical hyperplasia"?	Open needle loc biopsy as many will have D.C.I.S. or invasive cancer
How does tamoxifen work?	It binds estrogen receptors.
What is the treatment for local recurrence in breast after lumpectomy and radiation?	"Salvage" mastectomy (axillary dissection already completed)
Can tamoxifen prevent breast cancer?	**Yes.** In the Breast Cancer Prevention Trial of 13,000 women, tamoxifen reduced the risk of breast cancer by 50% in women who had a 1.7% 5-year risk of developing breast cancer.

What are the options for breast reconstruction?

TRAM flap, saline implant, latissimus dorsi flap

What is a TRAM flap?

Transverse **R**ectus **A**bdominis **M**yocutaneous flap

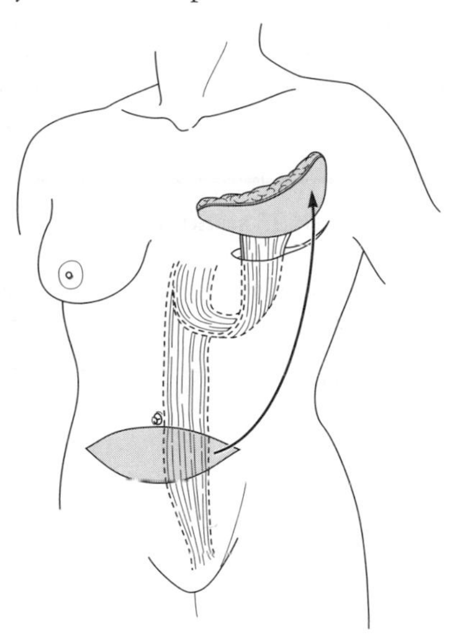

What are side effects of tamoxifen?

Endometrial cancer (2.5 relative risk), DVT, pulmonary embolus, cataracts

Give the common adjuvant therapy for the following patients with breast cancer. These are rough guidelines; check for current guidelines, as they are always changing. (ER = estrogen receptor)

Premenopausal, node +, ER −

Chemotherapy

Premenopausal, node +, ER +

Chemotherapy and tamoxifen

Premenopausal, node −, ER +

Tamoxifen

Postmenopausal, node +, ER +

Tamoxifen, +/− chemotherapy

Postmenopausal, node +, ER −	Chemotherapy (*Note:* chemotherapy is often added for high-risk tumors)
What type of chemotherapy is used for breast cancer?	CMF (cyclophosphamide, methotrexate, 5-fluorouracil) or CAM (cyclophosphamide, Adriamycin, 5-fluorouracil)

DCIS

What does DCIS stand for?	**D**uctal **C**arcinoma **I**n **S**itu
What is DCIS also known as?	Intraductal carcinoma
Describe DCIS.	Cancer cells in the duct without invasion (in situ: cells do not penetrate the basement membrane)
What are the signs/ symptoms?	Usually none; usually nonpalpable
What are the mammographic findings?	Microcalcifications
How is the diagnosis made?	Core or open biopsy
What is the most aggressive histologic type?	Comedo
What is the risk of lymph node metastasis with DCIS?	Less than 2% (usually when microinvasion is seen)
What is the major risk with DCIS?	Subsequent development of infiltrating ductal carcinoma in the **same breast**
What is the treatment for DCIS in the following cases:	
Tumor less than 1 cm (low grade)?	Remove with 1 cm margins +/− XRT
Tumor > 1 cm?	Perform lumpectomy with 1 cm margins and radiation **or** total mastectomy (**no** axillary dissection).
What is a total (simple) mastectomy?	Removal of the breast and nipple without removal of the axillary nodes (always

remove nodes with invasive cancer)

When must a simple mastectomy be performed for DCIS?

Diffuse breast involvement (e.g., diffuse microcalcifications), > 1 cm and contraindication to radiation

What is the role of axillary node dissection with DCIS?

No role in true DCIS (i.e., without microinvasion); often a "low" axillary dissection is included with a total mastectomy for a large tumor

What is chemotherapy for DCIS?

Tamoxifen (30% decrease in ipsilateral breast cancer after lumpectomy and radiation for DCIS and 50% decrease in subsequent contralateral breast cancer—NSABP B-24)

LCIS

What is LCIS?

Lobular **C**arcinoma **I**n **S**itu (carcinoma cells in the lobules of the breast without invasion)

What are the signs/symptoms?

There are none.

What are the mammographic findings?

There are none.

How is the diagnosis made?

LCIS is found **incidentally** on biopsy.

What is the major risk?

Carcinoma of **either** breast

Which breast is most at risk for developing an invasive carcinoma?

Equal risk in both breasts! (Think of LCIS as a **risk marker** for future development of cancer in either breast.)

What percentage of women with LCIS develop an invasive breast carcinoma?

About 30% in the 20 years after diagnosis of LCIS!

What type of invasive breast cancer do patients with LCIS develop?

Most commonly, **infiltrating ductal carcinoma, with equal distribution** in the contralateral and ipsilateral breasts (*Note:* counterintuitive!)

What is the treatment of LCIS?

None—close follow-up (or bilateral simple mastectomy in high-risk patients)

What is the major difference in the subsequent development of invasive breast cancer with DCIS and LCIS?	LCIS cancer develops in *either* breast; DCIS cancer develops in the ipsilateral breast.
What is the most common cause of bloody nipple discharge in a young woman?	Intraductal papilloma
What is the most common breast tumor in patients younger than 30 years?	Fibroadenoma
What is Paget's disease of the breast?	Scaling rash/dermatitis of the nipple caused by invasion of skin by cells from a ductal carcinoma
What are the common options for breast reconstruction after a mastectomy?	Saline implant TRAM flap: bring rectus muscle up and create a new breast.

MALE BREAST CANCER

What is the incidence of breast cancer in men?	< 1% of all breast cancer cases (1/150)
What is the average age at diagnosis?	65 years of age
What are the risk factors?	Increased estrogen Radiation Gynecomastia from increased estrogen Estrogen therapy Klinefelter's syndrome (XXY)
What type of breast cancer do men develop?	Nearly 100% of cases are ductal carcinoma. (Men do not usually have breast lobules.)
What are the signs/symptoms of breast cancer in men?	Breast mass (most are painless), breast skin changes (ulcers, retraction), and nipple discharge (usually blood or a blood-tinged discharge)

How is breast cancer in men diagnosed?

Biopsy and mammogram

What is the treatment?

One of the more aggressive surgical approaches (radical mastectomy or modified radical mastectomy) is used because of early involvement of the pectoralis major and the skin. **Radical mastectomy:** removal of skin, nipple, **pectoral muscles,** and axillary nodes, +/− skin graft.

BENIGN BREAST DISEASE

What is the most common cause of green, straw-colored, or brown nipple discharge?

Fibrocystic disease

What is the most common cause of breast mass after breast trauma?

Fat necrosis

What is Mondor's disease?

Thrombophlebitis of superficial breast veins

What must be ruled out with spontaneous galactorrhea (+/− amenorrhea)?

Prolactinoma (check pregnancy test and prolactin level)

CYSTOSARCOMA PHYLLODES

What is it?

It is a mesenchymal tumor arising from breast lobular tissue; most are benign. "Sarcoma" is a misnomer, as the vast majority are benign.

What is the usual age of the patient with this tumor?

Older than 30 years (she is usually older than the patient with fibroadenoma)

What are the signs/ symptoms?

Mobile, smooth breast mass that resembles a fibroadenoma on mammogram/ultrasound

How is it diagnosed?

Through core/open biopsy or excision

What is the treatment?	If benign, wide local excision; if malignant, simple total mastectomy
What is the role of axillary dissection with cystosarcoma phyllodes tumor?	Only if clinically palpable axillary nodes, as the malignant form rarely spreads to nodes (most common site of metastasis is the lung)

FIBROADENOMA

What is it?	Benign tumor of the breast consisting of collagen arranged in "swirls"
What is the clinical presentation of a fibroadenoma?	Young women younger than 30 years with a solid, mobile, **well-circumscribed** round breast mass
How is fibroadenoma diagnosed?	Negative needle aspiration looking for fluid; ultrasound; core biopsy
What is the treatment?	Surgical resection for large or growing lesions; small fibroadenomas can be observed closely
What is this disease's claim to fame?	It is the most common breast tumor in women younger than 30 years.

FIBROCYSTIC DISEASE

What is it?	A common benign breast condition consisting of fibrous (rubbery) and cystic changes in the breast
What are the signs/ symptoms?	Breast pain or tenderness that varies with the menstrual cycle; cysts; and fibrous ("nodular") fullness
How is it diagnosed?	Through breast exam, history, and aspirated cysts (usually straw-colored or green fluid)
What is the treatment for symptomatic fibrocystic disease?	**Stop caffeine** Stop tobacco Pain medications (NSAIDs) Vitamin E, evening primrose oil (danazol and OCP as last resort)

What is done if the patient has a breast cyst?

Needle drainage: if aspirate is bloody or a palpable mass remains after aspiration, an open biopsy is performed. If the aspirate is straw-colored or green, the patient is followed closely; then, if there is recurrence, a second aspiration is performed. A re-recurrence usually requires open biopsy.

MASTITIS

What is it?

Superficial infection of the breast (cellulitis)

In what circumstance does it most often occur?

Breast-feeding

What bacteria are most commonly the cause?

Staphylococcus aureus

How is mastitis treated?

Stop breast-feeding and use a breast pump instead; apply heat; administer antibiotics

Why must the patient with mastitis have close follow-up?

To make sure that she does not have inflammatory breast cancer!

BREAST ABSCESS

What are the causes?

Mammary ductal ectasia (stenosis of breast duct) and mastitis

What is the treatment of breast abscess?

Antibiotics
Needle or open drainage with cultures taken
Resection of involved ducts if recurrent
Breast pump if breast-feeding

MALE GYNECOMASTIA

What is it?

Enlargement of the male breast

What are the causes?

Medications
Illicit drugs (marijuana)
Liver failure
Increased estrogen
Decreased testosterone

What is the major differential diagnosis in the older patient?

Male breast cancer

What is the treatment?

Stop or change medications; correct underlying cause if there is a hormonal imbalance; and perform biopsy or subcutaneous mastectomy (i.e., leave nipple) if refractory to conservative measures and time.

54 Endocrine

ADRENAL GLAND

NORMAL ADRENAL PHYSIOLOGY

What is CRH?	**Corticotropin-releasing hormone:** released from anterior hypothalamus and causes release of ACTH from anterior pituitary
What is ACTH?	**AdrenoCorticoTropic Hormone:** released normally by anterior pituitary, which in turn causes adrenal gland to release cortisol
What feeds back to inhibit ACTH secretion?	Cortisol

CUSHING'S SYNDROME

What is Cushing's syndrome?	Excessive **cortisol** production
Most common cause?	Iatrogenic (i.e., prescribed prednisone)
Second most common cause?	Cushing's disease (most common noniatrogenic cause)
What is Cushing's disease?	Cushing's syndrome caused by excess production of ACTH by anterior **pituitary**
What is an ectopic ACTH source?	A tumor not found in the pituitary that secretes ACTH, which in turn causes adrenal gland to release cortisol without the normal negative feedback loop

What are the signs/ symptoms of Cushing's syndrome?	Truncal obesity, hirsutism, "moon" facies, acne, "buffalo hump," purple striae, hypertension, diabetes, weakness, depression, easy bruising, myopathy
How can cortisol levels be indirectly measured over a short duration?	By measuring urine cortisol or the breakdown product of cortisol, 17-hydroxycorticosteroid (**17-OHCS**), in the urine
What is a direct test of serum cortisol?	Serum cortisol level (highest in the morning and lowest at night in healthy patients)
Can ACTH levels be checked directly?	Yes (but many hospitals do not offer direct testing)
What initial tests should be performed in Cushing's syndrome?	Electrolytes Serum cortisol Urine-free cortisol, urine 17-OHCS Low-dose dexamethasone suppression test
What is the low-dose dexamethasone suppression test?	Dexamethasone is a synthetic cortisol that results in negative feedback on ACTH secretion and subsequent cortisol secretion in healthy patients. Patients with Cushing's syndrome do not suppress their cortisol secretion.
What test should be performed if a patient fails to suppress with the low-dose dexamethasone test?	**High**-dose dexamethasone suppression tests
What is the high-dose dexamethasone suppression test?	Dexamethasone is a **cortisol analog** that suppresses pituitary secretion of ACTH by the cortisol negative feedback. Decreased ACTH results in decreased cortisol, as measured by serum cortisol, decreased urine 17-OHCS, or both.
What is the CRH-stimulation test?	CRH is administered via IV tube, causing an increase in ACTH
Summarize the "Cushing's syndrome" lab values found in the majority of patients with the following conditions:	

Healthy patients	Normal cortisol and ACTH, suppression with low-dose or high-dose dexamethasone (< 1/2), mild increase with CRH
Cushing's disease (pituitary ACTH hypersecretion)	High cortisol and ACTH, no suppression with low-dose dexamethasone, suppression with high-dose dexamethasone, great increase in cortisol with CRH
Adrenal tumor	High cortisol, low ACTH, no suppression with low-dose or high-dose dexamethasone, no change with CRH
Ectopic ACTH-producing tumor	High cortisol and ACTH, no suppression with low-dose or high-dose dexamethasone, no change with CRH

What is the most common site of ectopic ACTH-producing tumor?

More than two-thirds are oat cell tumors of the lung.

How are the following tumors treated:

Adrenal adenoma?

Adrenalectomy (almost always **unilateral**)

Adrenal carcinoma?

Surgical excision (only one third of cases are operable)

Ectopic ACTH-producing tumor?

Surgical excision, if feasible

What medication must be given to a patient who is undergoing surgical correction of Cushing's syndrome?

Cortisol (usually hydrocortisone until PO is resumed)

What medication can be given to a patient with SEVERE cortisol excess?

Metyrapone (inhibits cortisol production by inhibiting the enzyme 11b-hydroxylase)

What is a complication of BILATERAL adrenalectomy?

Nelson's syndrome—occurs in 10% of patients after bilateral adrenalectomy

What is Nelson's syndrome?

Functional pituitary adenoma producing excessive ACTH and mass effect producing visual disturbances,

hyperpigmentation, amenorrhea, with elevated ACTH levels
Think: **N**elson = **N**uclear reaction in the pituitary

ADRENAL INCIDENTALOMA

What is an incidentaloma?
A tumor found in the adrenal gland **incidentally** on a CT scan performed for an unrelated reason

What is the incidence of incidentalomas?
1% to 4% of all CTs

What is the risk factor for carcinoma?
Solid tumor more than 6 cm in diameter

What is the treatment?
Controversial for smaller/medium-sized tumors, but almost all surgeons would agree that resection is indicated for solid incidentalomas more than 6 cm in diameter because of risk of cancer

What are the indications for removal of adrenal incidentaloma less than 6 cm?
MRI T2 signal > 2
Hormonally active = hyperfunctioning tumor
Enlarging cystic lesion
Does not look like an adenoma

What tumor must be ruled out prior to biopsy or surgery for any adrenal mass?
Pheochromocytoma

PHEOCHROMOCYTOMA

What is it?
Tumor of the adrenal **MEDULLA** and sympathetic ganglion (from chromaffin cell lines) that produces **catecholamines** (norepinephrine > epinephrine)

What is the incidence?
It is the cause of hypertension in approximately 1/500 hypertensive patients (≈10% of U.S. population has hypertension).

Which age group is most likely to be affected?
Any age (children and adults); average age is 40 to 60 years

What are the associated risk factors?	MEN-II, family history, Von Recklinghausen Disease, Von Hippel-Lindau disease
What are the signs/ symptoms?	"Classic" triad: 1. **Palpitations** 2. **Headache** 3. **Episodic diaphoresis** Also, hypertension (50%), pallor → flushing, anxiety, weight loss, tachycardia, hyperglycemia
How can the pheochromocytoma SYMPTOMS triad be remembered?	Think of the first three letters in the word **PHE**ochromocytoma: **P**alpitations **H**eadache **E**pisodic diaphoresis
What is the most common sign of pheochromocytoma?	Hypertension
What is the differential diagnosis?	Renovascular hypertension, menopause, migraine headache, carcinoid syndrome, preeclampsia, neuroblastoma, anxiety disorder with panic attacks, hyperthyroidism, insulinoma
What diagnostic tests should be performed?	Urine screen: vanillylmandelic acid **(VMA), metanephrine,** and normetanephrine (all breakdown products of the catechols) Urine/serum **epinephrine/ norepinephrine** levels
What are the other common lab findings?	Hyperglycemia (epinephrine increases glucose, norepinephrine decreases insulin) Polycythemia (resulting from intravascular volume depletion)
What is the most common site of a pheochromocytoma?	**Adrenal** > 90%
What are the other sites for pheochromocytoma?	Organ of Zuckerkandl, thorax (mediastinum), bladder, scrotum
What are the tumor localization tests?	CT, MRI, **^{131}I-MIBG,** PET scan

What does ^{131}I-MIBG stand for?

Meta**I**odo**B**enzyl**G**uanidine

How does the ^{131}I-MIBG scan work?

^{131}I-MIBG is a norepinephrine analog that collects in adrenergic vesicles and, thus, in pheochromocytomas

What is the role of PET scan?

Positron **E**mission **T**omography is helpful in localizing pheochromocytomas that do not accumulate MIBG.

What is the scan for imaging adrenal cortical pheochromocytoma?

NP-59 (a cholesterol analog)

What is the localizing option if a tumor is not seen on CT, MRI, or I-MIBG?

IVC venous sampling for catecholamines (gradient will help localize the tumor)

What is the tumor site if epinephrine is elevated?

It must be adrenal or near the adrenal gland (e.g., organs of Zuckerkandl), because nonadrenal tumors lack the capability to methylate norepinephrine to epinephrine.

What percentage of patients have malignant tumors?

Approximately 10%

Can histology be used to determine malignancy?

No; only distant metastasis or invasion can determine malignancy.

What is the classic pheochromocytoma "rule of 10's"?

10% malignant
10% bilateral
10% in children
10% multiple tumors
10% extraadrenal

What is the preoperative/medical treatment?

Increase intravascular volume with α-blockade (e.g., phenoxybenzamine or prazosin) to allow reduction in catecholamine-induced vasoconstriction and resulting volume depletion; treatment should start as soon as diagnosis is made.

What is the surgical treatment?

Tumor resection with early ligation of venous drainage (lower possibility of catecholamine release/crisis by tying off drainage) and minimal manipulation

What are the possible perioperative complications?

Anesthetic challenge: hypertensive crisis with manipulation (treat with nitroprusside), hypotension with total removal of the tumor, cardiac dysrhythmias

In the patient with pheochromocytoma, what must be ruled out?

MEN type II (almost all cases are bilateral)

What are the organs of Zuckerkandl?

Embryonic chromaffin cells around the abdominal aorta (near the inferior mesenteric artery) that normally atrophy during childhood but are a major site of extra-adrenal pheochromocytoma

CONN'S SYNDROME

What is it?

Hyper**aldosteronism** (primary)

What are the common sources?

Adrenal adenoma or adrenal hyperplasia; aldosterone is abnormally secreted by an adrenal adenoma (two-thirds) > hyperplasia > carcinoma

What is the normal physiology for aldosterone secretion?

BP in the renal afferent arteriole is low.
Low sodium and hyperkalemia cause **renin** secretion from juxtaglomerular cells.
Renin then converts angiotensinogen to angiotensin I.
Angiotensin converting enzyme in the lung then converts angiotensin I to angiotensin II.
Angiotensin II then causes the adrenal glomerulosa cells to secrete **aldosterone.**

What is the normal physiologic effect of aldosterone?

Aldosterone causes sodium retention for exchange of potassium in the kidney, resulting in fluid retention and increased BP.

What are the signs/symptoms?

Hypertension, headache, fatigue, nocturia/polydipsia

What are the two classic clues of Conn's syndrome?

1. Hypertension
2. Hypokalemia

What kind of hypertension? Diastolic hypertension

What are the renin levels with Conn's syndrome? Normal or decreased!

What are the associated lab findings? Increased serum sodium, decreased serum potassium (makes sense: aldosterone results in sodium/H_2O retention with loss of K^+), increased urinary aldosterone, **normal or low serum renin,** high urine potassium

What is secondary hyperaldosteronism? Hyperaldosteronism resulting from abnormally high renin levels (renin increases angiotensin/aldosterone)

What diagnostic tests should be performed? CT, adrenal venous sampling for aldosterone levels, iodocholesterol scanning, arteriography/venography (retrograde), Captopril test, saline infusion

What is the saline infusion test? Saline infusion will decrease aldosterone levels in normal patients but not in Conn's syndrome.

What is the Captopril test? Captopril will decrease aldosterone levels in normal patients but not in patients with Conn's syndrome.

What is the preoperative treatment? Spironolactone

What is spironolactone? An antialdosterone medication (works at the kidney tubule)

What are the causes of Conn's syndrome?
Adrenal adenoma (66%)
Bilateral idiopathic adrenal hyperplasia (30%)
Adrenal cancer (< 1%)

What is the treatment of the following conditions:

Adenoma? Unilateral adrenalectomy

Unilateral hyperplasia? Unilateral adrenalectomy

Bilateral hyperplasia? Spironolactone (or Amiloride) (no surgery)

What are the renin levels in patients with PRIMARY hyperaldosteronism?
Normal or low (key point!)

INSULINOMA

What is it?
Insulin-producing tumor arising from β cells

What is the incidence?
Number one islet cell neoplasm; half of β cell tumors of the pancreas produce insulin

What are the associated risks?
Associated with MEN-I syndrome (ppp = pituitary, pancreas, parathyroid tumors)

What are the signs/ symptoms?
Sympathetic nervous system symptoms resulting from hypoglycemia: palpitations, diaphoresis, tremulousness, irritability, weakness

What are the neurologic symptoms?
Personality changes, confusion, obtundation, seizures, coma

What is Whipple's triad?
1. Hypoglycemic symptoms produced by fasting
2. Blood glucose < 50 mg/dl during symptomatic attack
3. Relief of symptoms by administration of glucose

What is the differential diagnosis?
Reactive hypoglycemia
Functional hypoglycemia with gastrectomy
Adrenal insufficiency
Hypopituitarism
Hepatic insufficiency
Munchausen syndrome (insulin self-injections)
Nonislet cell tumor causing hypoglycemia (hemangiopericytoma, fibrosarcoma, leiomyosarcoma, hepatoma, adrenocortical carcinoma)
Surreptitious administration of insulin by others

What lab tests should be performed?
Glucose and insulin levels during fast; proinsulin levels (if self-injection of

	insulin is a concern, as insulin injections have **no** proinsulin)
What diagnostic tests should be performed?	Fasting hypoglycemia with inappropriately high levels of insulin **72-hour fast,** then check glucose and insulin levels every 6 hours (monitor very closely because patient can develop hypoglycemic crisis)
What localizing tests should be performed?	CT, A-gram, endoscopic US, venous catheterization (to sample blood along portal and splenic veins to measure insulin and localize tumor), intraoperative US
What is the medical treatment?	Diazoxide, to suppress insulin release
What is the surgical treatment?	Surgical resection
What is the prognosis?	Approximately 80% of patients have a benign solitary adenoma that is cured by surgical resection.

GLUCAGONOMA

What is it?	Glucagon-producing tumor
Where is it located?	Pancreas (usually in the tail)
What are the symptoms?	**Necrotizing migratory erythema** (usually below the waist), glossitis, stomatitis, diabetes
What are the skin findings?	Necrotizing migratory erythema is a red often psoriatic-appearing rash with serpiginous borders over the trunk and limbs.
What are the associated lab findings?	Hyperglycemia, low amino acid levels, high glucagon levels
What stimulation test is used for glucagonoma?	Tolbutamide stimulation test: IV tolbutamide results in elevated glucagon levels
What test is used for localization?	CT

What is the medical treatment of necrotizing migratory erythema?	Somatostatin, IV amino acids
What is the treatment?	Surgical resection

ZOLLINGER-ELLISON SYNDROME

What is it?	**Gastrinoma:** Non-β islet cell tumor of the pancreas (or other locale) that produces gastrin, causing gastric hypersecretion of HCl acid, resulting in GI **ulcers**
What is the incidence?	1/1000 in patients with peptic ulcer disease, but nearly 2% in patients with **recurrent ulcers**
What is the associated syndrome?	MEN-I syndrome
What percentage of patients with ZE have MEN-I syndrome?	Approximately 25% (75% of cases of ZE are "sporadic")
What percentage of patients with MEN-I will have ZE syndrome?	Approximately 50%
What are the signs/symptoms?	Peptic ulcers, diarrhea, weight loss, abdominal pain
What causes the diarrhea?	Massive acid hypersecretion and destruction of digestive enzymes
What are the signs?	**PUD:** epigastric pain, hematemesis, melena, hematochezia, GERD, diarrhea, **recurrent ulcers,** ulcers in unusual locations (e.g., proximal jejunum)
What are the possible complications?	GI hemorrhage/perforation, gastric outlet obstruction/stricture, metastatic disease
What is the differential diagnosis of increased gastrin?	Postvagotomy Gastric outlet obstruction Antral G-cell hyperplasia/hyperfunction Pernicious anemia Atrophic gastritis Short gut syndrome

Renal failure
H_2 blocker, omeprazole (remember: a gastric pH < 2 inhibits gastrin in normal patients)

Which patients should have a gastrin level checked?

Those with recurrent ulcer; ulcer in unusual position (e.g., jejunum) or refractory to medical management; before any operation for ulcer

What lab tests should be performed?

Fasting gastrin level
Postsecretin challenge gastrin level
Calcium (screen for MEN-I)
Chem 7

What are the associated gastrin levels?

NL fasting = 100 pg/ml
ZES fasting = 200–1000 pg/ml
Basal acid secretion; (ZES > 15 mEq/hr, nl < 10mEq/hr)

What is the secretin stimulation test?

IV secretin is administered and the gastrin level is determined. Patients with ZE have a paradoxic increase in gastrin.

Lab results with secretin challenge:
NL—Decreased gastrin
ZE—Increased gastrin (increased by > 200 pg/ml)

What tests are used to evaluate ulcers?

EGD, UGI, or both

What tests are used to localize the tumor?

Abdominal CT, MRE **octreotide scan,** selective angiography, selective venous sampling for gastrin

What is the most common site?

Pancreas

What is the most common NONpancreatic site?

Duodenum

What are some other sites?

Stomach, lymph nodes, liver, kidney, ovary

Define the "gastrinoma triangle."

A triangle drawn from the following points:
1. Cystic duct

2. Junction of the second and third portions of the duodenum
3. Neck of the pancreas (90% of gastrinomas are in this triangle)

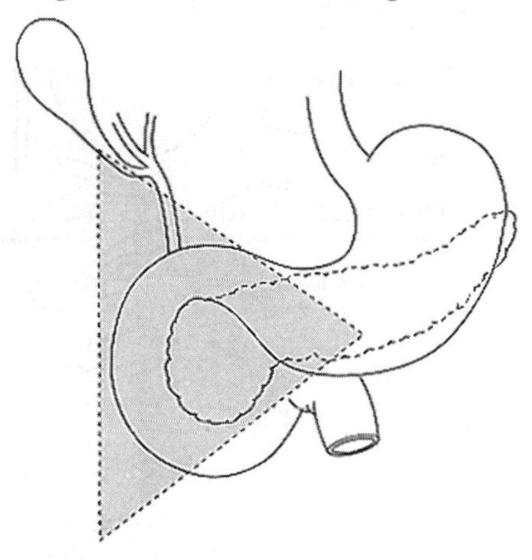

What is the next step if the tumor cannot be localized?

Exploratory surgery (if tumor is not in pancreas, open duodenum and look), proximal gastric vagotomy if not found

What is the medical treatment?

H_2 blockers, omeprazole, somatostatin

What is the surgical treatment?

If tumor is in head of pancreas, remove (enucleation); if tumor is in body/tail of pancreas, perform distal pancreatic resection; if tumor is in duodenum, remove locally.

What percentage have malignant tumors?

Two thirds

What is the most common site of metastasis?

Liver

What is the treatment of patients with liver metastasis?

Excision, if technically feasible

What is the surgical option if gastrinoma is in duodenum/ head of pancreas and is too large or has too many lymph node metastases for local resection?

Whipple procedure

What is the treatment of widely metastatic or incurable gastrinoma?	Debulking surgery Chemotherapy: 5-FU, streptozotocin, doxorubicin
What is the prognosis with the following procedures:	
Complete excision?	90% 10-year survival
Incomplete excision?	25% 10-year survival

MULTIPLE ENDOCRINE NEOPLASIA

What is it also known as?	MEN syndrome
What is it?	Inherited condition of propensity to develop multiple endocrine tumors
How is it inherited?	Autosomal dominant (but with a significant degree of variation in penetrance)
Which patients should be screened for MEN?	All family members of patients diagnosed with MEN

MEN TYPE I

What is the common eponym?	Wermer's syndrome (think: Wermer = Winner = # 1 = type **1**)
What are the most common tumors and their incidences?	**PPP:** **P**arathyroid hyperplasia (≈ 90%) **P**ancreatic islet cell tumors (≈ 66%) Gastrinoma: ZE syndrome (50%) Insulinoma (20%) **P**ituitary tumors (≈ 50%)
How can tumors for MEN-I be remembered?	Think: type 1 = primary, primary, primary = **PPP** = parathyroid, pancreas, pituitary
How can the P's associated with MEN-I be remembered?	All the P's are followed by a vowel: PA, PA, PI
What percentage of patients with MEN-I have parathyroid hyperplasia?	Approximately 90%
What percentage of patients with MEN-I have a gastrinoma?	Approximately 50%

What other tumors (in addition to PPP) are associated with MEN- I?	Adrenal (30%) and thyroid (15%) adenomas

MEN TYPE IIA

What is the common eponym?	Sipple's syndrome (think: Sipple = Second = # 2 = type **2**)
What are the most common tumors and their incidences?	**MPH:** **M**edullary thyroid carcinoma (100%) Calcitonin secreted **P**heochromocytoma (> 33%) Catecholamine excess **H**yperparathyroidism (about 50%) Hypercalcemia
How can the tumors involved with MEN-II be remembered?	Think: type 2 = 2 **MPH** or 2 **M**iles **P**er **H**our = **MPH** = **M**edullary, **P**heochromocytoma, **H**yperparathyroid
How can the P of MPH be remembered?	Followed by the consonant "H" PHEOCHROMOCYTOMA (remember, the P's of MEN-I are followed by vowels)
What percentage of patients with MEN-IIA have medullary carcinoma of the thyroid?	100%

MEN TYPE IIB

What are the most common abnormalities, their incidences, and symptoms?	**MMMP:** **M**ucosal neuromas (100%)—in the nasopharynx, oropharynx, larynx, and conjunctiva **M**edullary thyroid carcinoma (≈ 85%)—more aggressive than in MEN-IIa **M**arfanoid body habitus (long/lanky) **P**heochromocytoma (≈ 50%) and found bilaterally**
How can the features of MEN-IIB be remembered?	MMMP (think: **3M P**lastics)
What is the anatomic distribution of medullary thyroid carcinoma in MEN- II?	**Almost always bilateral;** sporadic cases are almost always **unilateral!**

What are the physical findings/signs of MEN-IIB?	Mucosal neuromas (e.g., mouth, eyes) Marfanoid body habitus Pes cavus/planum (large arch of foot/flatfooted) Constipation
What is the most common GI complaint of patients with MEN-IIB?	**Constipation** resulting from ganglioneuromatosis of GI tract
What percentage of pheochromocytomas in MEN-IIA/B are bilateral?	Approximately 70% (but found bilaterally in only 10% of all patients diagnosed with pheochromocytoma)
What is the major difference between MEN-IIA and MEN-IIB?	MEN-IIa = parathyroid hyperplasia MEN-IIb = **no** parathyroid hyperplasia (and neuromas, marfanoid habitus, pes cavus [extensive arch of foot], etc.)
What type of parathyroid disease is associated with MEN-I and MEN-IIA?	**Hyperplasia** (treat with removal of all parathyroid tissue with autotransplant of some of the parathyroid tissue to the forearm)
What percentage of patients with ZE have MEN-I?	Approximately 25%

55 Thyroid Gland

THYROID DISEASE

ANATOMY

Identify the following structures:

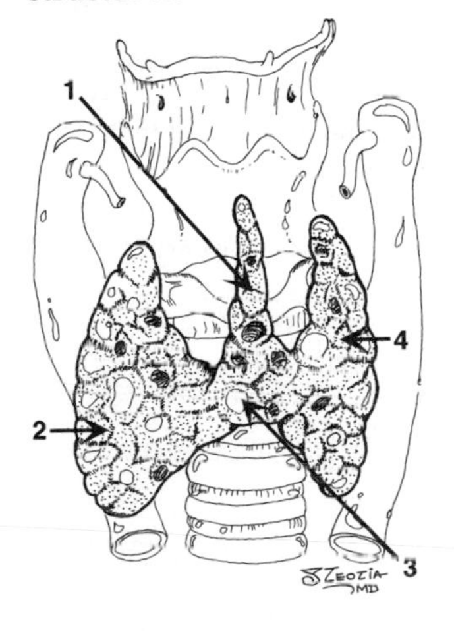

1. Pyramidal lobe
2. Right lobe
3. Isthmus
4. Left lobe

Define the arterial blood supply to the thyroid.

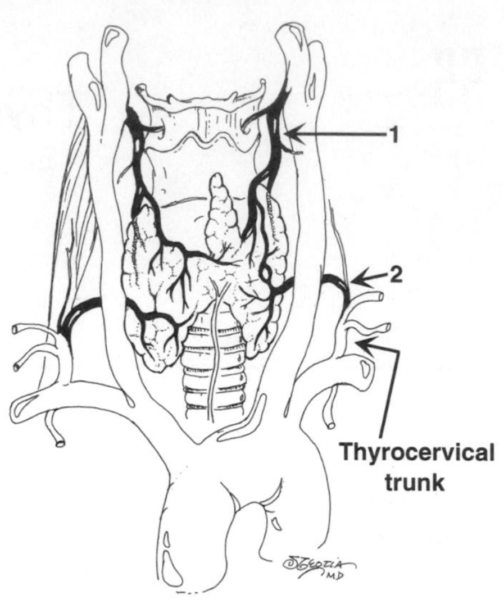

Two arteries:

1. Superior thyroid artery (first branch of the external carotid artery)
2. Inferior thyroid artery (branch of the thyrocervical trunk) (IMA artery rare)

What is the venous drainage of the thyroid?

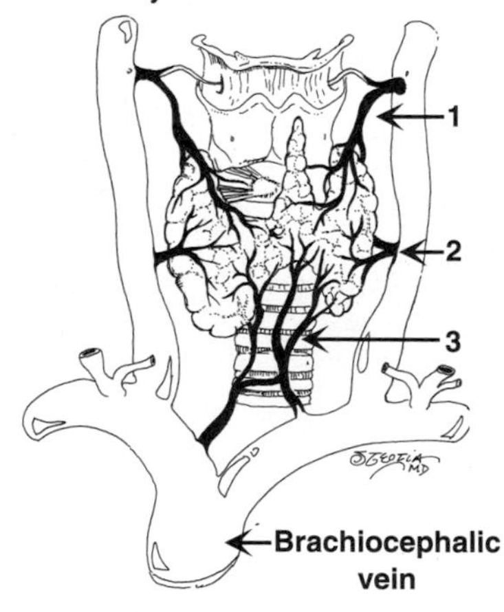

Three veins:

1. Superior thyroid vein
2. **Middle** thyroid vein
3. Inferior thyroid vein

Name the thyroid lobe appendage coursing toward the hyoid bone from around the thyroid isthmus?

Pyramidal lobe

What percentage of patients have a pyramidal lobe?

Approximately 50%

Name the lymph node group around the pyramidal thyroid lobe?	Delphian lymph node group
What is the thyroid isthmus?	Midline tissue border between the left and right thyroid lobes
Which ligament connects the thyroid to the trachea?	Ligament of Berry
What is the IMA (not I.M.A.) artery?	A small inferior artery to the thyroid from the aorta or innominate artery
What percentage of patients have an IMA artery?	Approximately 3%
Name the most posterior extension of the lateral thyroid lobes.	Tubercle of Zuckerkandl
Which paired nerves must be carefully identified during a thyroidectomy?	The **recurrent laryngeal nerves,** which are found in the tracheoesophageal grooves and dive behind the cricothyroid muscle; damage to these nerves paralyzes laryngeal abductors and causes hoarseness if unilateral and airway obstruction is bilateral.
What other nerve is at risk during a thyroidectomy and what are the symptoms?	**Superior laryngeal nerve;** if damaged, patient will have a deeper and quieter voice (unable to hit high pitches)
What is the name of the famous opera singer whose superior laryngeal nerve was injured during thyroidectomy?	**Urban legend** has it that it was Amelita Galli-Curci, but no objective data support such a claim (ANN SURG 233:588. April 2001).

PHYSIOLOGY

What is TRH?	**T**hyrotropin-**R**eleasing **H**ormone released from the hypothalamus; causes release of TSH
What is TSH?	**T**hyroid-**S**timulating **H**ormone released by the anterior pituitary; causes release of thyroid hormone from the thyroid

What are the thyroid hormones?
T3 and T4

What is the most active form of thyroid hormone?
T3

What is a negative feedback loop?
T3 and T4 feed back negatively on the anterior pituitary (causing decreased release of TSH in response to TRH).

What is the most common site of conversion of T4 to T3?
Peripheral (e.g., liver)

What is Synthroid (levothyroxine): T3 or T4?
T4

What is the half-life of Synthroid (levothyroxine)?
7 days

What do parafollicular cells secrete?
Calcitonin

THYROID NODULE

What percentage of people have a thyroid nodule?
About 5% (but only about 10–15% of excised nodules are malignant)

What is the differential diagnosis of a thyroid nodule?
Multinodular goiter
Adenoma
Hyperfunctioning adenoma
Cyst
Thyroiditis
Carcinoma/lymphoma
Parathyroid carcinoma

Name three types of nonthyroidal neck masses.
1. Inflammatory lesions (e.g., abscess, lymphadenitis)
2. Congenital lesions (i.e., thyroglossal duct [midline], branchial cleft cyst [lateral])
3. Malignant lesions: lymphoma, metastases, squamous cell carcinoma

What studies can be used to evaluate a thyroid nodule?
US—solid or cystic nodule
Fine needle aspirate (FNA) → cytology
Radioiodide

	^{123}I or ^{99m}Tc scan—hot or cold nodule Thyroid antibody TSH Serum calcium
What is meant by a hot versus a cold nodule?	Nodule uptake of IV ^{131}I or ^{99}mT **Hot**—Increased ^{123}I or ^{99}mT uptake = functioning/hyperfunctioning nodule **Cold**—Decreased ^{123}I or ^{99}mT uptake = nonfunctioning nodule
What is the DIAGNOSTIC test of choice for thyroid nodule?	FNA
What is the percentage of false negative results on FNA for thyroid nodule?	Approximately 5%
What is the role of thyroid suppression of a thyroid nodule?	Diagnostic and therapeutic; administration of thyroid hormone suppresses TSH secretion, and up to half of the benign thyroid nodule will disappear!
In evaluating thyroid nodules, what history, labs, symptoms, and signs suggest carcinoma?	History of radiation therapy to the neck History of rapid development Vocal cord paralysis (recurrent laryngeal nerve paralysis) Cervical adenopathy Invasion outside the thyroid Hard fixed mass in the thyroid Elevated serum calcitonin
What is the most common cause of thyroid enlargement?	Multinodular goiter
What are indications for surgery with multinodular goiter?	Cosmetic deformity, compressive symptoms, cannot rule out cancer
What is Plummer's disease?	Toxic multinodular goiter

MALIGNANT THYROID NODULES

What percentage of cold thyroid nodules are malignant?	Approximately 25% in adults

What are the risk factors for a malignant nodule?

History of neck irradiation, young > old, cold nodule, solitary nodule > multiple nodules

What percentage of multinodular masses are malignant?

Approximately 1%

What are the pros and cons of FNA?

Pros—Safe, cost-effective diagnosis of papillary, medullary, and anaplastic carcinomas
Cons—false negative results; FNA cannot accurately distinguish between benign and malignant follicular or Hürthle cell tumors

What is the treatment of a patient with a history of radiation exposure, thyroid nodule, and negative FNA?

Most experts would remove the nodule surgically (because of the high risk of radiation).

What should be done with thyroid cyst aspirate?

Send to cytopathology

THYROID CARCINOMA

Name the FIVE main types of thyroid carcinoma and their relative percentages.

1. Papillary carcinoma: 80% (**P**opular = **P**apillary)
2. Follicular carcinoma: 10%
3. Medullary carcinoma: 5%
4. Hürthle cell carcinoma: 4%
5. Anaplastic/undifferentiated carcinoma: 1% to 2%

What are the signs/symptoms?

Mass/nodule, lymphadenopathy; most are **euthyroid** (rarely hyperfunctioning)

What comprises the work-up?

Thyroid US, **FNA,** TSH, calcium level, CXR, +/− radioisotope scan

What oncogenes are associated with thyroid cancers?

Ras gene family and RET proto-oncogene

PAPILLARY ADENOCARCINOMA

With what condition is it associated?

Gardner's syndrome and neck irradiation

What are the associated histologic findings?

Psammoma bodies (remember, **P** = **P**sammoma = **P**apillary, which constitute

80% of thyroid tumors; therefore, **P**apillary = **P**opular)

Describe the route and rate of spread.

Most spread via lymphatics (cervical adenopathy); spread occurs slowly.

^{131}I uptake?

Good uptake

What is the 10-year survival rate?

Approximately 95%

What is the treatment for:

< 1.5 CM and no history of neck radiation exposure?

Options:
1. Thyroid lobectomy and isthmectomy
2. Near-total thyroidectomy
3. Total thyroidectomy

> 1.5 cm, bilateral, + cervical node mets OR history of radiation exposure?

Total thyroidectomy

What is the treatment for palpable cervical lymph nodes?

Modified neck dissection (ipsilateral)

Do positive cervical nodes affect the prognosis?

NO!

What postoperative medication should be administered?

Thyroid hormone replacement, to suppress TSH

What is a postoperative treatment option for papillary carcinoma?

Postoperative ^{131}I scan can locate residual tumor and distant metastasis that can be treated with ablative doses of ^{131}I.

What are the "P's" of papillary thyroid cancer?

Papillary cancer:
Popular (most common type)
Psammoma bodies
Palpable lymph nodes (spreads most commonly by lymphatics, seen in up to one-third of patients)
Positive ^{131}I uptake
Positive prognosis
Postoperative ^{131}I scan to diagnose/treat metastases

FOLLICULAR ADENOCARCINOMA

What percentage of thyroid cancers does it comprise?
Approximately 10%

Describe the nodule consistency.
Rubbery, encapsulated

What is the route of spread?
Hematogenous, more aggressive than papillary adenocarcinoma

What is the male:female ratio?
1:3

^{131}I uptake?
Good uptake

What is the overall 10-year survival rate?
Approximately 85%

Can the diagnosis be made by FNA?
No; tissue structure is needed for a diagnosis of cancer.

What histologic findings define malignancy in follicular cancer?
Capsular or blood vessel invasion

What is the most common site of distant metastasis?
Bone

What is the treatment:

< 2cm?
Near total thyroidectomy or lobectomy/isthmectomy vs. total thyroidectomy

> 2cm?
Total thyroidectomy

What is the postoperative treatment option if malignant?
Postoperative ^{131}I scan for diagnosis/treatment

What are the "F's" of follicular cancer?
Follicular cancer:
Far-away metastasis (spreads hematogenously)
Female (3 to 1 ratio)
FNA . . . NOT (FNA CANNOT diagnose cancer)
Favorable prognosis

HÜRTHLE CELL THYROID CANCER

What is it?	Thyroid cancer of Hürthle cells
What percentage of thyroid cancers does it comprise?	Approximately 4%
What is the cell of origin?	Follicular cells
^{131}I uptake?	No uptake
How is the diagnosis made?	FNA can identify cells, but malignancy can be determined only by tissue histology (like follicular cancer).
What is the route of metastasis?	Lymphatic > hematogenous
What is the treatment?	Same guidelines as for follicular cancer

MEDULLARY CARCINOMA

What percentage of all thyroid cancers does it comprise?	Approximately 5%
With what other conditions is it associated?	MEN type II; autosomal-dominant genetic transmission
Histology?	Amyloid (a**M**yloid = **M**edullary)
What does it secrete?	Calcitonin
What is the appropriate stimulation test?	Pentagastrin
Describe the route and rate of spread.	Lymphatic and hematogenous distant metastasis
How is the diagnosis made?	FNA
^{131}I uptake?	Poor uptake
What is the prognosis?	Ten-year survival rate is 50%; cure rate is 95% when occult tumors are found in MEN family members being screened for elevated calcitonin. If detected when clinically palpable, cure rate is < 20%.

What is the treatment?	Total thyroidectomy and **median lymph node dissection** Modified neck dissection, if lateral cervical nodes are positive
What are the "M's" of medullary carcinoma?	**M**edullary cancer: **MEN II** a**M**yloid **M**edian lymph node dissection **M**odified neck dissection if lateral nodes are positive

ANAPLASTIC CARCINOMA

What is it also known as?	Undifferentiated carcinoma
What is it?	An undifferentiated cancer arising in approximately 75% of previously differentiated thyroid cancers (most commonly, follicular carcinoma)
What percentage of all thyroid cancers does it comprise?	Approximately 1% to 2%
What is the gender preference?	Women > men
What are the associated histologic findings?	Giant cells, spindle cells
^{131}I uptake?	Very poor uptake
How is the diagnosis made?	FNA (large tumor)
What is the major differential diagnosis?	Thyroid lymphoma (much better prognosis!)
What is the treatment of the following disorders:	
Small tumors?	Total thyroidectomy ± external beam x-ray therapy
Airway compromise?	Debulking surgery and tracheostomy
What is the prognosis?	Dismal, because most patients are at stage IV at presentation (distant metastasis); survival past 2 years is rare

MISC

What laboratory value must be followed postoperatively after a thyroidectomy?

Calcium decreased secondary to parathyroid damage; during lobectomy, the parathyroids must be spared and their blood supply protected; if blood supply is compromised intraoperatively, they can be autografted into the sternocleidomastoid muscle or forearm

What is the differential diagnosis of postoperative dyspnea after a thyroidectomy?

Neck hematoma (remove sutures and clot at the **bedside**)
Bilateral recurrent laryngeal nerve damage

What is a "lateral aberrant rest" of the thyroid?

A misnomer; it is **papillary** cancer of a lymph node from metastasis.

BENIGN THYROID DISEASE

What is the most common cause of hyperthyroidism?

Graves' disease

What is Graves' disease?

Diffuse goiter with hyperthyroidism, exophthalmos, and pretibial myxedema

What is the etiology?

Caused by circulating **antibodies** that stimulate TSH receptors on follicular cells of the thyroid and cause deregulated production of thyroid hormones (i.e., hyperthyroidism)

What is the female:male ratio?

6:1

What specific physical finding is associated with Graves'?

Exophthalmos

How is the diagnosis made?

Increased T3, T4, and anti-TSH receptor antibodies, decreased TSH, global uptake of ^{131}I radionuclide

Name treatment option modalities for Graves' disease.

1. **Medical blockade:** iodide, propranolol, propylthiouracil (PTU), methimazole, Lugol's solution (potassium iodide)
2. **Radioiodide ablation:** most popular therapy
3. **Surgical resection:** (bilateral subtotal thyroidectomy)

What are the possible indications for surgical resection?	Suspicious nodule; if patient is non-compliant or refractory to medicines, pregnant, a child, or if patient refuses radioiodide therapy
What is the major complication of radioiodide or surgery for Graves' disease?	Hypothyroidism
What does PTU stand for?	**P**ropyl**T**hio**U**racil
How does PTU work?	1. Inhibits incorporation of iodine into T4/T3 (by blocking peroxidase oxidation of iodide to iodine) 2. Inhibits peripheral conversion of T4 to T3
How does methimazole work?	Inhibits incorporation of iodine into T4/T3 **only** (by blocking peroxidase oxidation of iodide to iodine)

TOXIC MULTINODULAR GOITER

What is it A.K.A.?	Plummer's disease
What is it?	**Multiple** thyroid nodules with one or more nodules producing thyroid hormone, resulting in hyperfunctioning thyroid (hyperthyroidism or a "toxic" thyroid state)
How is the hyperfunctioning nodule(s) localized?	I^{131} radionuclide scan
What is the treatment?	Surgically remove hyperfunctioning nodule(s) with lobectomy or near total thyroidectomy

THYROIDITIS

What are the features of acute thyroiditis?	Painful, swollen thyroid; fever; overlying skin erythema; dysphagia
What is the cause of ACUTE thyroiditis?	Bacteria (usually *Streptococcus* or *Staphylococcus*), usually caused by a thyroglossal fistula or anatomic variant
What is the treatment of ACUTE thyroiditis?	Antibiotics, drainage of abscess, needle aspiration for culture; most patients need

definitive surgery later to remove the fistula

What are the features of subacute thyroiditis?

Glandular swelling, tenderness, often follows URI, elevated ESR

What is the cause of subacute thyroiditis?

Viral infection

What is the treatment of subacute thyroiditis?

Supportive: NSAIDS, ± steroids

What is De Quervain's thyroiditis?

Just another name for subacute thyroiditis caused by a virus (think: De Quer**V**AIN: **V**IRUS)

How can the differences between etiologies of ACUTE and SUBACUTE thyroiditis be remembered?

Alphabetically: **A** before **S, B** before **V** (i.e., **A**cute before **S**ubacute and **B**acterial before **V**iral and thus: **A**cute = **B**acterial and **S**ubacute = **V**iral)

What are the common causative bacteria in acute suppurative thyroiditis?

Streptococcus or *Staphylococcus*

What are the two types of chronic thyroiditis?

1. Hashimoto's thyroiditis
2. Riedel's thyroiditis

What are the features of Hashimoto's (chronic) thyroiditis?

Firm and rubbery gland, 95% in women, lymphocyte invasion

What is the claim to fame of Hashimoto's disease?

Most common cause of hypothyroidism in the United States

What is the etiology of Hashimoto's disease?

Autoimmune (think: HashimOTO = AUTO; thus, Hashimoto = autoimmune)

What lab tests should be performed to diagnose Hashimoto's disease?

Antithyroglobulin and microsomal antibodies

What is Riedel's thyroiditis?

Benign inflammatory thyroid enlargement **with fibrosis** of thyroid
Patients present with painless, large thyroid.
Fibrosis may involve surrounding tissues.

56 Parathyroid

ANATOMY

How many parathyroids are there?	Usually **four** (two superior and two inferior)
What percentage of patients have five parathyroid glands?	Approximately 5% (think 5 = 5)
What % of patients have three parathyroid glands?	Approximately 10%
What is the usual position of the inferior parathyroid glands?	Posterior and lateral behind the thyroid and below the inferior thyroid artery
What is the most common site of an "extra" gland?	Thymus gland
What percentage of patients have a parathyroid gland in the mediastinum?	Approximately 1%
If only three parathyroid glands are found at surgery, where can the fourth one be hiding?	Thyroid gland Thymus/mediastinum Carotid sheath Tracheoesophageal groove Behind the esophagus
What is the embryologic origin of the following structures:	
Superior parathyroid glands?	Fourth pharyngeal pouch
Inferior parathyroid glands?	Third pharyngeal pouch (counterintuitive)

What supplies blood to the parathyroid glands?

Inferior thyroid artery

What percentage of patients have all four parathyroid glands supplied by the inferior thyroid arteries exclusively?

Approximately 80%

What is DiGeorge's syndrome?

Congenital absence of the parathyroid glands and the thymus

PHYSIOLOGY

What cell type produces PTH?

Chief cells

What are the major actions of parathyroid hormone (PTH)?

Increases blood **calcium** levels (takes from bone breakdown, GI absorption, increased resorption from kidney, excretion of phosphate by kidney)

How does vitamin D work?

Increases intestinal absorption of calcium and phosphate

Where is calcium absorbed?

Duodenum and proximal jejunum

HYPERPARATHYROIDISM (HPTH)

Define primary HPTH.

Increased secretion of PTH by parathyroid gland(s); marked by elevated calcium, low phosphorus

Define secondary HPTH.

Increased serum PTH resulting from calcium wasting caused by **renal failure or decreased GI calcium absorption;** calcium levels are normal or **low**

Define tertiary HPTH

Persistent HPTH after correction of secondary hyperparathyroidism; results from autonomous PTH secretion not responsive to the normal negative feedback due to elevated Ca^{++} levels

What are the methods of imaging the parathyroids?

Surgical operation
Ultrasound

	Sestamibi scan ^{201}TI(technetium)—thallium subtraction scan CT/MRI A-gram (rare) Venous sampling for PTH (rare)
What are the indications for a localizing preoperative study?	**Reoperation** for recurrent hyperparathyroidism

PRIMARY HYPERPARATHYROIDISM (HPTH)

What is the most common cause of primary HPTH?	Adenoma (> 85%)
What are the etiologies of primary HPTH and percentages?	**Adenoma** (~ 85%) Hyperplasia (~ 10%) Carcinoma (~ 1%)
What is the incidence of primary HPTH in the United States?	Approximately 1/1000–4000
What are the risk factors for primary HPTH?	Family history, MEN I and IIa, irradiation
What are the signs/symptoms of primary HPTH hypercalcemia?	"**Stones, bones, groans, and psychiatric overtones**": **Stones:** Kidney stones **Bones:** Bone pain, pathologic fractures, subperiosteal resorption **Groans:** Muscle pain and weakness, pancreatitis, gout, constipation **Psychiatric overtones:** Depression, anorexia, anxiety **Other symptoms:** Polydipsia, weight loss, HTN (10%), polyuria, lethargy
What is the "33 to 1" rule?	Patients with primary HPTH have a ratio of serum [Cl^-] to phosphate $\geq$ 33.
What plain x-ray findings are associated with HPTH?	Subperiosteal bone resorption (usually in hand digits; said to be "pathognomonic" for HPTH!)
How is primary HPTH diagnosed?	Labs—elevated PTH (hypercalcemia, ↑ phosphorus, ↑ chloride); urine calcium

should be checked for familial hypocalciuric hypercalcemia

What is familial hypocalciuric hypercalcemia?

Familial (autosomal-dominant) inheritance of a condition of **asymptomatic** hypercalcemia and low urine calcium, with or without elevated PTH; in contrast, hypercalcemia from HPTH results in high levels of urine calcium

Surgery to remove parathyroid glands is not indicated for this diagnosis.

How many of the glands are USUALLY affected by the following conditions:

Hyperplasia?

Four

Adenoma?

One

Carcinoma?

One

What percentage of adenomas are not single but are found in more than one gland?

Approximately 5%

What is the differential diagnosis of hypercalcemia?

"CHIMPANZEES":
Calcium overdose
Hyperparathyroidism (1°/2°/3°)
Hyperthyroidism, **H**ypocalciuric **H**ypercalcemia (familial)
Immobility/iatrogenic (thiazide diuretics)
Metastasis/milk alkali syndrome (rare)
Paget's disease (bone)
Addison's disease/acromegaly
Neoplasm (colon, lung, breast, prostate, multiple myeloma)
Zollinger Ellison syndrome
Excessive vitamin D
Excessive vitamin A
Sarcoid

What is the initial medical treatment of hypercalcemia (1° HPTH)?

Medical—IV fluids, furosemide—**NOT** thiazide diuretics

What is the definitive treatment of HPTH in the following cases:

Primary HPTH resulting from HYPERPLASIA?
Neck exploration removing all parathyroid glands and leaving at least 30 mg of parathyroid tissue placed in the forearm muscles (nondominant arm, of course!)

Primary HPTH resulting from parathyroid ADENOMA?
Surgically remove adenoma (send for frozen section) and biopsy all abnormally enlarged parathyroid glands (some experts biopsy all glands).

Primary HPTH resulting from parathyroid CARCINOMA?
Remove carcinoma, ipsilateral thyroid lobe, and all enlarged lymph nodes.

Secondary HPTH?
Correct calcium and phosphate; perform renal transplantation (no role for parathyroid surgery).

Tertiary HPTH?
Correct calcium and phosphate; perform surgical operation to remove all parathyroid glands and reimplant 30 to 40 mg in the forearm if **REFRACTORY** to medical management.

Why place 30 to 40 mg of sliced parathyroid gland in the forearm?
To retain parathyroid function. If HPTH recurs, remove some of the parathyroid gland from the easily accessible forearm.

What must be ruled out in the patient with HPTH from hyperplasia?
MEN type I and MEN type IIa

What carcinomas are commonly associated with hypercalcemia?
Breast cancer metastases, prostate cancer, kidney cancer, lung cancer, pancreatic cancer, multiple myeloma

What is the most likely diagnosis if a patient has a PALPABLE neck mass, hypercalcemia, and elevated PTH?
Parathyroid carcinoma (vast majority of other causes of primary HPTH have nonpalpable parathyroids)

PARATHYROID CARCINOMA

What is it?
Primary carcinoma of the parathyroid gland

What is the number of glands usually affected?	One
What are the signs/ symptoms?	Hypercalcemia, elevated PTH, **PALPABLE** parathyroid gland (50%), pain in neck, recurrent laryngeal nerve paralysis (change in voice), hypercalcemic crisis (usually associated with calcium levels > 13)
What is the common tumor marker?	Human chorionic gonadotrophin
What is the treatment?	Surgical resection of parathyroid mass with ipsilateral thyroid lobectomy, ipsilateral lymph node resection
What percentage of all cases of primary HPTH are caused by parathyroid carcinoma?	1%

POSTOPERATIVE COMPLICATIONS OF PARATHYROIDECTOMY

What are the possible postoperative complications after a parathyroidectomy?	Recurrent nerve injury (unilateral: voice change; bilateral: airway obstruction), neck hematoma (open at bedside if breathing is compromised), hypocalcemia, superior laryngeal nerve injury
What is "hungry bone syndrome"?	Severe hypocalcemia seen after surgical correction of HPTH as chronically calcium-deprived bone aggressively absorbs calcium
What are the signs/ symptoms of postoperative hypocalcemia?	Perioral tingling, paresthesia, positive Chvostek's sign, positive Trousseau's sign, positive tetany
What is the treatment of hypoparathyroidism?	Acute: IV calcium Chronic: PO calcium, and vitamin D

57 Spleen and Splenectomy

Which arteries supply the spleen?	The splenic artery, a branch of the celiac trunk, and the short gastric arteries that arise from the gastroepiploic arteries
What is the venous drainage of the spleen?	The **portal** vein, via the splenic vein and the left gastroepiploic vein
What is said to "tickle" the spleen?	The tail of the pancreas
What percentage of people have an accessory spleen?	Approximately 20%
What percentage of the total body platelets are stored in the spleen?	33%
What are the functions of the human spleen?	Filters abnormal RBCs (does NOT store RBCs like canine spleen!), stores platelets, produces tuftsin and properdin (opsins), produces antibodies (especially IGM), is site of phagocytosis
What is the spleen's claim to fame?	The **spleen** is the **most common** intra-abdominal organ injured in **blunt trauma.**
What is "delayed splenic rupture"?	A subcapsular hematoma may rupture some time after blunt trauma, causing "delayed splenic rupture." Rupture classically occurs about 2 weeks after the injury and presents with shock/abdominal pain.
What are the signs/ symptoms of ruptured/ injured spleen?	Hemoperitoneum and Kehr's sign, LUQ abdominal pain, Ballance's sign

What is Kehr's sign?

Left shoulder pain seen with splenic rupture

What is Balance's sign?

LUQ dullness to percussion

What is Seagesser's sign?

Phrenic nerve manual compression causing neck tenderness in splenic rupture

How is a spleen injury diagnosed?

Abdominal CT, **if the patient is stable;** DPL or FAST exam if the patient is unstable

What is the treatment?

1. Nonoperative in a stable patient with an isolated splenic injury without hilar involvement/complete rupture, or if the patient can be stabilized
2. If patient is unstable, DPL/FAST laparotomy with splenorrhaphy or splenectomy

What is a splenorrhaphy?

Splenic salvage operation: wrapping vicral mesh, aid of topical hemostatic agents or partial splenectomy (VAST majority of pediatric patients undergo nonoperative treatment for blunt spleen injury)

What are the other indications for splenectomy:

Malignant diseases?

Hodgkin's staging not conclusive by CT (rare)
Splenic tumors (primary/metastatic/locally invasive)
Hypersplenism caused by other leukemias/nonHodgkin's lymphomas

Anemias?

Medullary fibrosis with myeloid metaplasia
Hereditary elliptocytosis
Sickle-cell anemia (rare, most autosplenectomize)
Pyruvate kinase deficiency
Autoimmune hemolytic anemia
Hereditary spherocytosis
Thalassemias (e.g., β-thalassemia major A.K.A. Cooley's)

Thrombocytopenia?	ITP (idiopathic thrombocytopenic purpura) TTP (thrombotic thrombocytopenic purpura)
Miscellaneous indications?	Variceal bleeding with splenic vein thrombosis, Gaucher's disease, splenic abscess, refractory splenic cysts, hypersplenism, Felty's syndrome
Is G6PD deficiency an indication for splenectomy?	NO
What are the possible post-splenectomy complications?	Thrombocytosis, subphrenic abscess, atelectasis, pancreatitis gastric dilation, and **overwhelming postsplenectomy sepsis (OPSS)**
What causes OPSS?	Increased susceptibility to fulminant bacteremia, meningitis, or pneumonia because of loss of splenic function
What is the incidence of OPSS in adults?	$< 1\%$
What is the incidence and overall mortality of OPSS in children?	1% to 2% with 50% mortality rate
What is the typical presentation of OPSS?	Fever, lethargy, common cold, sore throat, URI followed by confusion, shock, and coma with death ensuing within 24 hours in up to 50% of patients
What are the common organisms associated with OPSS?	**Encapsulated:** *Streptococcus pneumoniae, Neisseria meningitides, H. influenzae*
What is the most common bacteria in OPSS?	*Streptococcus*
What is the preventive treatment of OPSS?	**Vaccinations** for **pneumococcus,** *H. influenza,* and meningococcus Prophylactic penicillin for all minor infections/illnesses and immediate medical care if febrile illness develops
What is the best time to give immunizations to splenectomy patients?	**Preoperatively,** if at all possible

Why is an NG tube necessary after splenectomy?

To prevent gastric distention, which can blow out suture ties used to control the short gastric vessels resulting in postoperative bleeding

What lab tests are abnormal after splenectomy?

WBC count increases by 50% over the baseline; marked **thrombocytosis** occurs; RBC smear is abnormal.

What are the findings on postsplenectomy RBC smear?

Peripheral smear will show Pappenheimer bodies, Howell-Jolly bodies, and Heinz bodies.

When and how should thrombocytopenia be treated?

When platelet count is > 1 million, most surgeons will treat with **aspirin.**

What is the most common cause of splenic vein thrombosis?

Pancreatitis

What opsonins does the spleen produce?

Properdin, tuftsin (think: "PROfessionally TUF spleen")

What is the most common cause of ISOLATED GASTRIC varices?

Splenic vein thrombosis (usually from pancreatitis)

What is the treatment of gastric varices caused by splenic vein thrombosis?

Splenectomy

Which patients develop hyposplenism?

Patients with ulcerative colitis

What vaccinations should every patient with a splenectomy receive?

Pneumococcus
Meningococcus
Haemophilus influenzae type B

Define hypersplenism.

Hyperfunctioning spleen
Documented loss of blood elements (WBC, Hct, platelets)
Large spleen (splenomegaly)
Hyperactive bone marrow (trying to keep up with loss of blood elements)

Define splenomegaly.

Enlarged spleen

What is ITP?

Autoimmune (antiplatelet antibodies IgG in > 90% of patients) platelet destruction leading to troublesome bleeding and purpura

What is the most common cause of failure to correct thrombocytopenia after splenectomy for ITP?

Missed accessory spleen

What are the "I's" of ITP?

Immune etiology (**I**gG antiplatelets ABs)
Immunosuppressive treatment (initially treated with steroids)
Immune globulin
Improvement with splenectomy (75% of patients have improved platelet counts after splenectomy)

What is the treatment of choice for TTP?

Plasmapheresis (splenectomy reserved as a last resort)

What is the most common physical finding of portal hypertension?

Splenomegaly

58

Surgically Correctable HTN

What is it?

Hypertension caused by conditions that are amenable to surgical correction

What percentage of patients with HTN have a surgically correctable cause?

Approximately 7%

What are diseases that cause HTN that are surgically correctable?

Renal artery stenosis
Pheochromocytoma
Unilateral renal parenchymal disease
Cushing's syndrome
Conn's syndrome (primary hyperaldosteronism)
Hyperparathyroidism/hyperthyroidism
Coarctation of the aorta
Cancer
Neuroblastoma
Increased intracranial pressure

What is the formula for pressure?

Pressure = flow × resistance or P = F × R (think: **P**ower **F**o**R**ward); thus, an increase in flow, resistance, or both results in an increase in pressure

59 Soft Tissue Sarcomas and Lymphomas

SOFT TISSUE SARCOMAS

What are they?
Soft tissue tumors, derived from mesoderm

Sarcoma means what in GREEK?
Fish flesh

Sarcomas are more common in upper or lower extremities?
50% of sarcomas are in the extremities and are 3.5 times **more** common in the **lower** extremity (thigh).

How common are they?
They comprise 1% of malignant tumors.

What are the risk factors?
R.A.L.E.S.:
R = **R**adiation
A = **A**IDS(Immunosuppression)
L = **L**ymphedema
E = **E**xposure to chemicals
S = **S**yndromes (Gardner's/Le-Fraumeni)

Name the following types of malignant sarcoma:

Fat
Liposarcoma

Smooth muscle
Leiomyosarcoma

Myofibroblast
Malignant fibrous histiocytoma

Striated muscle
Rhabdomyosarcoma

Vascular endothelium
Angiosarcoma

Fibroblast
Fibrosarcoma

Lymph vessel
Lymphangiosarcoma

Peripheral nerve	Malignant neurilemmoma or schwannoma
AIDS	Kaposi's sarcoma
Lymphedema	Lymphangiosarcoma
What are the signs/ symptoms?	Soft tissue mass; pain from compression of adjacent structures, often noticed after minor trauma to area of mass
How do most sarcomas metastasize?	Hematogenously (i.e., via blood)
What is the most common location and route of metastasis?	**Lungs** via hematogenous route
What tests should be done in the preoperative work-up?	CXR, ± chest CT, LFTs
What are the three most common malignant sarcomas in adults?	Fibrous histiocytoma (25%), liposarcoma (20%), leiomyosarcoma (15%)
What are the two most common in children?	Rhabdomyosarcoma (about 50%), fibrosarcoma (20%)
What is the most common type to metastasize to the lymph nodes?	Malignant fibrous histiocytoma
What is the most common sarcoma of the retro-peritoneum?	Liposarcoma
How do sarcomas locally invade?	Usually along anatomic planes such as fascia, vessels, etc.
How is the diagnosis made?	Imaging work-up—MRI is superior to CT at distinguishing the tumor from adjacent structures Mass less than 3 cm: excisional biopsy **Mass more than 3 cm:** incisional biopsy or **core biopsy**

Define excisional biopsy.
Biopsy by removing the **entire** mass

Define incisional biopsy.
Biopsy by removing a **piece** of the mass

What is the orientation of incision for incisional biopsy of a suspected extremity sarcoma?
Longitudinal, not transverse, so that the incision can be incorporated in a future resection if biopsy for sarcoma is positive

Define core biopsy.
A large-bore needle that takes a core of tissue (like an earth core sample)

American Joint Committee for Cancer Staging (AJCC) Sarcoma Stages:

Stage I?
Well differentiated (**grade**), any size, no nodes, no metastases

Stage II?
Moderately differentiated (**grade**), any size, no nodes, no metastases

Stage III?
Poorly differentiated or undifferentiated (**grade**), any size tumor, no nodes, no metastases

Stage IV?
Positive nodes or distant metastases

What is a pseudocapsule and what is its importance?
It is the outer layer of a sarcoma that represents compressed malignant cells. Microscopic extensions of tumor cells invade through the pseudocapsule into adjacent structures. Thus, definitive therapy must include a wide margin of resection to account for this phenomenon and not just be "shelled-out" like a benign growth.

What is the most important factor in the prognosis?
Histologic grade of the primary lesion

What is the treatment?
Surgical resection and radiation (postoperative, ± preoperative)

What is the treatment of pulmonary metastasis?
Surgical resection for isolated lesions

What tests should be done in the follow-up?
Physical examination, CXR, repeat CT/MRI of the area of resection to look for recurrence

What syndrome of lymphangiosarcoma arises in chronic lymphedema after axillary dissection for breast cancer?

Stewart-Treves syndrome

What syndrome is associated with breast cancer and soft tissue sarcoma?

Le-Fraumeni syndrome (p53 tumor suppressor gene mutation)

LYMPHOMA

How is the diagnosis made?

Cervical or axillary node excisional biopsy

What cell type is associated with the histology of Hodgkin's disease?

Reed-Sternberg cells

What are the four histopathologic types of Hodgkin's disease?

1. Nodular sclerosing (most common; about 50% of cases)
2. Mixed cellularity
3. Lymphocyte predominant (best prognosis)
4. Lymphocyte depleted

What are the indications for a "staging laparotomy" in Hodgkin's disease?

Controversial; usually performed for the low stages because they are treated differently than advanced stages

Some experts rely on CT scans and do not perform laparotomy.

What is a staging laparotomy for Hodgkin's lymphoma?

A laparotomy to distinguish between advanced and low-stage disease to define proper therapy. It includes:

1. **Splenectomy**
2. Iliac crest bone aspiration
3. Biopsies of splenic hilar, celiac, mesenteric, porta hepatis, para-aortic, and iliac **lymph nodes**
4. **Liver biopsy**
5. **Oophoropexy:** if the patient is a woman of childbearing years, the ovaries are marked with metallic clips and then tacked behind the uterus for protection from the radiation field.

Define the stages (Ann Arbor) of Hodgkin's disease:	
Stage I	Single lymph node region (think stage 1 = 1 region)
Stage II	Two or more lymph node regions on **the same side of the diaphragm** (think stage 2 = > 2 regions)
Stage III	Involvement on **both** sides of the diaphragm
Stage IV	Diffuse and/or disseminated involvement
What is stage A Hodgkin's?	Asymptomatic (think: **A**symptomatic = stage **A**)
What is stage B Hodgkin's?	Symptomatic: weight loss, fever, night sweats, etc. Think, stage **B** = **B**ad
What is the "E" on the staging?	Extralymphatic site involvement (E = **E**xtralymphatic)
What treatments are used for low versus advanced stage Hodgkin's lymphoma?	Low stage: radiotherapy Advanced stage: chemotherapy
What percentage of patients with Hodgkin's disease can be cured?	Approximately 80%

GI LYMPHOMA

What is it?	Non-Hodgkin's lymphoma arising in the GI tract
What are the signs/ symptoms?	Abdominal pain, obstruction, GI hemorrhage, GI tract perforation, fatigue
What is the treatment for gastric lymphoma?	Controversial: chemoradiation vs. surgical resection
What is the treatment of intestinal lymphoma?	Resection with removal of draining lymph nodes and chemotherapy ± radiation
What is the most common site of primary GI tract lymphoma?	The stomach (66%)

60 Skin Lesions

What are the most common skin cancers?

1. Basal cell carcinoma (75%)
2. Squamous cell carcinoma (20%)
3. Melanoma (4%)

What is the most common skin cancer that causes death?

Melanoma

What is malignant melanoma?

A redundancy! All melanomas are considered malignant.

SQUAMOUS CELL CARCINOMA

What is it?

Carcinoma arising from epidermal cells

What are the most common sites?

Head, neck, and hands

What are the risk factors?

Sun exposure, pale skin, chronic inflammatory process, immunosuppression, xeroderma pigmentosum, arsenic

What is a precursor skin lesion?

Actinic keratosis

What are the signs/ symptoms?

Raised, slightly pigmented skin lesion; ulceration/exudate; chronic scab; itching

How is the diagnosis made?

Small lesion—excisional biopsy
Large lesions—needle or incisional biopsy

What is the treatment?

Small lesion (< 1 cm): excise with 0.5 cm margin
Large lesion > 1 cm: resect with 1 to 2 cm margins of normal tissue (large lesions may require skin graft/flap)

What is the dreaded sign of metastasis?	Palpable lymph nodes (remove involved lymph nodes)
What is Marjolin's ulcer?	Squamous cell carcinoma that arises in an area of chronic inflammation (e.g., chronic fistula, burn wound, osteomyelitis)
What is the prognosis?	Excellent if totally excised (95% cure rate); most patients with positive lymph-node metastasis eventually die from metastatic disease
What is the treatment for solitary metastasis?	Surgical resection

BASAL CELL CARCINOMA

What is it?	Carcinoma arising in the germinating basal cell layer of epithelial cells
What are the risk factors?	Sun exposure, fair skin, radiation, chronic dermatitis, xeroderma pigmentosum
What are the most common sites?	Head, neck, and hands
What are the signs/ symptoms?	Slow-growing skin mass (chronic, scaly); scab; ulceration, with or without pigmentation
How is the diagnosis made?	Excisional or incisional biopsy
What is the treatment?	Resection with 5-mm margins (2-mm margin in cosmetically sensitive areas)
What is the risk of metastasis?	Very low (recur locally)

MISCELLANEOUS SKIN LESIONS

What is an epidermal inclusion cyst?	EIC = A benign subcutaneous cyst filled with epidermal cells (should be removed surgically) filled with waxy material; no clinical difference from a sebaceous cyst
What is a sebaceous cyst?	A benign subcutaneous cyst filled with sebum (waxy, paste-like substance) from a

blocked sweat gland (should be removed with a small area of skin that includes the blocked sweat gland); may become infected; much less common than EIC

What is actinic keratosis?

A premalignant skin lesion from sun exposure; seen as a scaly skin lesion (surgical removal eliminates the 20% risk of cancer transformation)

What is seborrheic keratosis?

Benign pigmented lesion in the elderly; observe or treat by excision (especially if there is any question of melanoma), curettage, or topical agents

How to remember actinic keratosis vs. seborrheic keratosis malignant potential?

Actinic keratosis = AK = asset kicker = premalignant
Seborrheic keratosis = SK = soft kicker = benign

What is Bowen's disease of the skin?

Squamous carcinoma in situ (should be removed surgically, thereby removing the problem)

What is "MOHS" surgery?

MOHS technique or surgery: repeats thin excision until margins are clear by microscopic review (named after Dr. MOHS)—used to minimize collateral skin excision (e.g., on the face)

61

Melanoma

What is it?

Neoplastic disorder produced by malignant transformation of the melanocyte; melanocytes are derived from neural crest cells

Which patients are at greatest risk?

White patients with blonde/red hair, fair skin, freckling, a history of blistering sunburns, blue/green eyes, actinic keratosis
Male > female

What are the most common sites?

#1: Skin
#2: Eyes
#3: Anus
Think: **SEA** = **S**kin, **E**yes, **A**nus

What is the most common site in African Americans?

Palms of the hands, soles of the feet (acral lentiginous melanoma)

What characteristics are suggestive of melanoma?

Usually a pigmented lesion with an irregular border, irregular surface, or irregular coloration
Other clues: darkening of a pigmented lesion, development of pigmented satellite lesions, irregular margins or surface elevations, notching, recent or rapid enlargement, erosion or ulceration of surface, pruritus

What are the "A, B, C, D's" of melanoma?

A: Asymmetry
B: Border irregularity
C: Color variation
D: Diameter > 6 mm and dark lesion

What are the associated risk factors?

Severe sunburn before age 18, giant congenital nevi, family history, race (white), ultraviolet radiation (sun), multiple dysplastic nevi

How does location differ in men and women?
Men get more lesions on the trunk; women get more on the extremities.

Which locations are unusual?
Noncutaneous regions, such as mucous membranes of the vulva/vagina, anorectum, esophagus, and choroidal layer of the eye

What is the most common site of melanoma in men?
Back (one-third)

What is the most common site of melanoma in women?
Legs (one-third)

What are the four major histologic types?
1. Superficial spreading
2. Lentigo maligna
3. Acral lentiginous
4. Nodular

Define the following terms:

Superficial spreading melanoma
Occurs in both sun-exposed and nonexposed areas
Superficial spread is the most common type (75% of melanomas).

Lentigo maligna melanoma
Malignant cells that are superficial, found usually in elderly patients on the head or neck
Called "Hutchinson's freckle" if noninvasive
Least aggressive type; very good prognosis
Accounts for $< 10\%$ of melanomas

Acral lentiginous melanoma
Occurs on the palms, soles, subungual areas, and mucous membranes
Accounts for $\approx 5\%$ of melanomas (most common melanoma in African-American patients $\approx 50\%$)

Nodular melanoma
Vertical growth predominates
Lesions are usually dark
Most aggressive type; worst prognosis
Accounts for $\approx 15\%$ of melanomas

Amelanotic melanoma
Melanoma from melanocytes but with obvious lack of pigment

What is the most common type of melanoma?

Superficial spreading (> 70%) (think **super**ficial = **super**ior)

What type of melanoma arises in Hutchinson's freckle?

Lentigo maligna melanoma

What is Hutchinson's freckle?

Lentigo melanoma in the radial growth phase without vertical extension (noninvasive); usually occurs on the faces of elderly women

STAGING

What is Clark's classification (microstaging of tumor)

I?

Tumor confined to the epidermis; recurrence rate of 0% to 5%

II?

Tumor invading the papillary dermis; 5-year recurrence rate of 5%

III?

Tumor cells up to the junction of the papillary and reticular dermis; 5-year recurrence rate of 33%

IV?

Invasion into the reticular dermis; 5-year recurrence rate of approximately 66%

V?

Invasion into subcutaneous fat; 5-year recurrence rate of approximately 75%

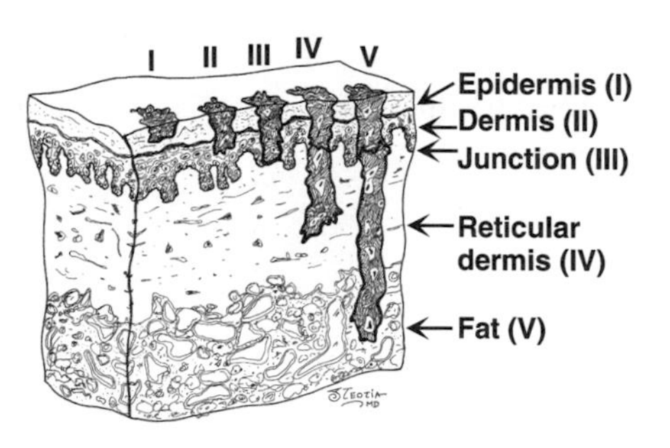

How can Clark's stages be remembered?

Think: **E**pidermis (I), **P**apillary dermis (II), **J**unction of papillary/reticular dermis (III), **R**eticular dermis (IV), and **F**at (V) = **E**very **P**igmented **J**unction **R**equires **F**ormalin

What is the Breslow classification (microstaging of tumor)?

Staging by actually measuring the depth of the lesion:
Less than 0.76 mm thickness has more than 90% cure with excision.
More than 4.0 mm has at least an 80% risk of local recurrence or metastasis in 5 years.

How can Breslow versus Clarke's classifications be remembered?

Think: Bres**low** = **low** = depth by measurement

Which tumor staging is more accurate in predicting survival?

The Breslow classification (a more consistent measure of tumor thickness)

What are the American Joint Committee on Cancer (AJCC) stages simplified:

I?

Less than 1.5 mm depth

II?

More than 1.5 mm depth

III?

Positive nodes (regional nodal basin)

IV?

Metastases (including NONregional nodal basin)

What are the common sites of metastasis?

Nodes local
Distant skin recurrence, lung, liver, bone, heart, and brain
Melanoma has a specific attraction for small bowel mucosa and distant cutaneous sites.
Brain metastases are a common cause of death.

What are the metastatic routes?

Both lymphatic and hematogenous

How is the diagnosis made?

Excisional biopsy (complete removal leaving only normal tissue) or incisioned biopsy for very large lesions
(Early diagnosis is crucial.)

What is the role of shave biopsy?

No role

What is the "sentinel node" biopsy?	Inject Lymphazurin blue dye, colloid with a radiolabel, or both around the melanoma; the first LN in the draining chain is identified as the "sentinel lymph node" and reflects the metastatic status of the group of lymph nodes.
When is elective lymph node dissection recommended?	Controversial—possible advantage in melanomas 1 to 2 mm in depth but jury still out. Sentinel node biopsy if >1 mm is getting very common. Remember, lymph node dissection is fraught with morbidity (e.g., lymphedema).
What is the recommended size of the surgical margin for depth of invasion:	
Melanoma in situ?	0.5 cm margin
1 mm thick?	1 cm margin
> 1 mm thick	2 cm margin
What is the treatment for digital melanoma?	Amputation
What is the treatment of palpable lymph node metastasis?	Lymphadenectomy
What factors determine the prognosis?	Depth of invasion and metastasis are the most important factors. (Superficial spreading and lentigo maligna have a better prognosis because they have a longer horizontal phase of growth and are thus diagnosed at an earlier stage. Nodular has the worst prognosis because it grows predominantly vertically and metastasizes earlier.)
What is the workup to survey for metastasis in the patient with melanoma?	Physical exam, LFTs, CXR (bone scan/ CT/MRI reserved for symptoms)
What is the treatment of intestinal metastasis?	Surgical resection to prevent bleeding/obstruction

Which malignancy is most likely to metastasize to the bowel?
Melanoma

What is the surgical treatment of nodal metastasis?
Lymphadenectomy

What is FDA-approved adjuvant therapy?
Interferon-alfa (in patients with thick tumors T4 and nodal metastases)

What is the treatment of unresectable brain metastasis?
Radiation

What is the treatment of isolated adrenal metastasis?
Surgical resection

What is the treatment of isolated lung metastasis?
Surgical resection

What is the most common symptom of anal melanoma?
Bleeding

What is the treatment of anal melanoma?
APR or wide excision (no survival benefit from APR, but better local control)

What other experimental therapy is available for metastatic disease?
1. IL-2
2. Monoclonal antibodies
3. Chemotherapy (e.g., dacarbazine)
4. Vaccinations

62 Surgical Intensive Care

INTENSIVE CARE UNIT (ICU) BASICS

How is an ICU note written?
The note is by **systems:**
- Neurologic (e.g., GCS, MAE, pain control)
- Pulmonary (e.g., vent settings)
- CVS (e.g., pressors, Swan numbers)
- Heme (CBC)
- FEN (e.g., Chem 10, nutrition)
- Renal (e.g., urine output, bun, cr)
- ID (e.g., Tmax, WBC, antibiotics)
- Assessment
- Plan
- (**FEN** = **F**luids, **E**lectrolytes, **N**utrition); physical exam included in each section

What are the possible causes of fever in the ICU?
Central line infection
UTI, urosepsis
Pneumonia/atelectasis
Intra-abdominal abscess
Sinusitis
DVT
Thrombophlebitis
Drug fever
Fungal infection, meningitis, wound infection
Endocarditis

What is the most common bacteria in ICU pneumonia?
Gram-negative rods

INTENSIVE CARE UNIT FORMULAS AND TERMS YOU SHOULD KNOW

What is CO?
Cardiac **O**utput: HR (heart rate) × SV (stroke volume)

What is the normal CO? Between 4 and 8 L/min

What factors increase CO? Increased contractility, heart rate, and preload; decreased afterload

What is CI? **C**ardiac **I**ndex: CO/BSA (body surface area)

What is the normal CI? Between 2.5 and 3.5 L/min/M_2

What is SV? **S**troke **V**olume: the amount of blood pumped out of the ventricle each beat; simply, end diastolic volume minus the end systolic volume **or** CO/HR

What is the normal SV? Between 60 and 100 cc

What is CVP? **C**entral **V**enous **P**ressure: indirect measurement of intravascular volume status

What is the normal CVP? Between 4 and 11

What is PCWP? **P**ulmonary **C**apillary **W**edge **P**ressure: indirectly measures left atrial pressure, which is an estimate of intravascular volume (LV filling pressure)

What is the normal PCWP? Between 5 and 15

What is anion gap? $Na^+ - (Cl^- + HCO^-_3)$

What is the normal anion gap? Between 10 and 14

What are the causes of increased anion gap acidosis in surgical patients? ACRONYM : **S.A.L.U.D.:**
S: Starvation
A: Alcohol (ethanol/methanol)
L: Lactic acidosis
U: Uremia
D: DKA

Define MODS. **M**ultiple **O**rgan **D**ysfunction **S**yndrome

What is SVR? **S**ystemic **V**ascular **R**esistance: MAP − CVP / CO × 80 (remember, P = F × R, **P**ower **F**o**R**ward; and calculating resistance: **R** = **P/F**)

What is SVRI?	**S**ystemic **V**ascular **R**esistance **I**ndex: SVR/BSA
What is the normal SVRI?	Between 1500 and 2400
What is MAP?	**M**ean **A**rterial **P**ressure: diastolic blood pressure + **1/3 (systolic–diastolic pressure)** *Note:* Not the mean between diastolic and systolic blood pressure because diastole lasts longer than systole
What is PVR?	**P**ulmonary **V**ascular **R**esistance: $PA_{(MEAN)} - PCWP / CO \times 80$ (PA is pulmonary artery pressure and LA is left atrial or PCWP pressure)
What is the normal PVR value?	100 ± 50
What is the formula for arterial oxygen content?	Hemoglobin $\times$ O_2 saturation (SaO_2)
What is the formula for oxygen delivery?	CO $\times$ (hemoglobin $\times$ SaO_2)
What factors can increase oxygen delivery?	Increased CO by increasing SV, HR, or both; increased O_2 content by increasing the hemoglobin content, SaO_2, or both
What is mixed venous oxygen saturation?	SvO_2; simply, the O_2 saturation of the blood in the right ventricle or pulmonary artery; an indirect measure of peripheral oxygen supply and demand
Which lab values help assess adequate oxygen delivery?	SvO_2 (low with inadequate delivery), lactic acid (elevated with inadequate delivery), pH (acidosis with inadequate delivery)
What is FENA?	Fractional excretion of sodium: $(U_{Na^+} \times P_{cr} / P_{Na}{}^+ \times U_{cr}) \times 100$
What is the memory aid for calculating FENA?	**Think: "You need pee" = You (Urine) need (Na^+) pee (plasma);** therefore, $\mathbf{U_{Na}{}^+ \times P_{Cr}}$; and for the denominator switch everything, or $P_{Na}{}^+ \times U_{Cr}$
What is the prerenal FENA value?	< 1.0; renal failure from decreased renal blood flow (e.g., cardiogenic, hypovolemia, arterial obstruction, etc.)

How long does Lasix effect last?

6 hours = **LASIX** = **LA**sts **SIX** hours

What is the formula for flow/pressure/resistance?

Remember **P**ower **F**o**R**ward:
Pressure = **F**low × **R**esistance

What is the "10 for 0.08 rule" of acid-base?

For every increase of $PaCO_2$ by 10 mm Hg, the pH falls by 0.08.

What is the "40, 50, 60 for 70, 80, 90 rule" for O_2 sats?

A PaO_2 of **40, 50, 60** corresponds roughly to an O_2 sat of **70, 80, 90,** respectively.

One liter of O_2 via nasal cannula raises FiO_2 by how much?

Approximately 3% to 4%

What is pure respiratory acidosis?

Low pH (acidosis), increased $PaCO_2$, normal bicarbonate (or high with compensation)

What is pure respiratory alkalosis?

High pH (alkalosis), decreased $PaCO_2$, normal bicarbonate (or low with compensation)

What is pure metabolic acidosis?

Low pH, low bicarbonate, normal (or low with compensation) $PaCO_2$

What is pure metabolic alkalosis?

High pH, high bicarbonate, normal (or high with compensation) $PaCO_2$

What does MOF stand for?

Multiple **O**rgan **F**ailure

What does SIRS stand for?

Systemic **I**nflammatory **R**esponse **S**yndrome

SICU DRUGS

DOPAMINE

What is the site of action and effect at the following levels: Low dose (1–3 μg/kg/min)?

++ dopa agonist; **renal vasodilation** (A.K.A. "renal dose dopamine")

Intermediate dose (4–10 μg/kg/min)?

+ $alpha_1$, ++ $beta_1$; positive inotropy and some vasoconstriction

High dose (> 10 μg/kg/min)? +++ $alpha_1$ agonist; marked afterload increase from arteriolar vasoconstriction

DOBUTAMINE

What is the site of action? +++ $beta_1$ agonist, ++ $beta_2$

What is the effect? ↑ inotropy; ↑ chronotropy, **decrease in systemic vascular resistance**

ISOPROTERENOL

What is the site of action? +++ $beta_1$ and $beta_2$ agonist

What is the effect? ↑ inotropy; ↑ chronotropy; (+ vasodilation of skeletal and mesenteric vascular beds)

EPINEPHRINE (EPI)

What is the site of action? $Alpha_1$, $alpha_2$, $beta_1$, and $beta_2$ agonist

What is the effect? ↑ inotropy; ↑ chronotropy

What is the effect at high doses? Vasoconstriction

NOREPINEPHRINE (NE)

What is the site of action? $Alpha_1$, $alpha_2$, and $beta_1$ agonist

What is the effect? ↑ inotropy; ↑ chronotropy; ++ increase in blood pressure

What is the effect at high doses? Severe vasoconstriction

NITROGLYCERINE (NTG)

What is the site of action? +++ venodilation; + arteriolar dilation

What is the effect? Increased venous capacitance, decreased preload, coronary arteriole vasodilation

SODIUM NITROPRUSSIDE (SNP)

What is the site of action? +++ venodilation; +++ arteriolar dilation

What is the effect?	Decreased preload and afterload (allowing blood pressure titration)
What is the major toxicity of SNP?	**Cyanide** toxicity

INTENSIVE CARE PHYSIOLOGY

Define the following terms:	
Preload	Load on the heart muscle that stretches it to end-diastolic volume (end-diastolic pressure) = intravascular volume
Afterload	Load or resistance the heart must pump against = vascular tone = SVR
Contractility	Force of heart muscle contraction
Compliance	Distensibility of heart by the preload
What is the Frank-Starling curve?	Cardiac output increases with increasing preload up to a point.
What is the clinical significance of the steep slope of the Starling curve relating end-diastolic volume to cardiac output?	It demonstrates the importance of preload in determining cardiac output.
What factors influence the oxygen content of whole blood?	Oxygen content is composed largely of that oxygen bound to hemoglobin, and is thus determined by the hemoglobin concentration and the arterial oxygen saturation; the partial pressure of oxygen dissolved in plasma plays a minor role.
What determines the oxygen delivery to the tissues?	The oxygen content of whole blood and the cardiac output
What factors influence mixed venous oxygen saturation?	Oxygen delivery (hemoglobin concentration, arterial oxygen saturation, cardiac output) and oxygen extraction by the peripheral tissues
What lab test for tissue ischemia is based on the shift from aerobic to anaerobic metabolism?	Serum lactic acid levels

Define the following terms:

Dead space

That part of the inspired air that will not participate in gas exchange (e.g., the gas in the large airways/ET tube not in contact with capillaries)
Think: space = air

Shunt fraction

That fraction of pulmonary venous blood that did not participate in gas exchange
Think: shunt = blood

What causes increased dead space?

Overventilation (emphysema, excessive PEEP) or underperfusion (pulmonary embolus, low cardiac output, pulmonary artery vasoconstriction)

At high shunt fractions, what is the effect of increasing FiO_2 on arterial PO_2?

At high shunt fractions (> 50%), changes in FiO_2 have almost no effect on arterial PO_2 because the blood that does "see" the O_2 is already at maximal O_2 absorption and, thus, increasing the FiO_2 has no effect (FiO_2 can be minimized to prevent oxygen toxicity).

Define ARDS.

Acute **R**espiratory **D**istress **S**yndrome (previously known as **A**dult **R**espiratory **S**yndrome) = noncardiac pulmonary edema

What is the ARDS diagnostic triad?

C.X.R.:
C: Capillary wedge pressure < 18
X: X-ray of chest with bilateral infiltrates
R: Ratio of PaO_2 To FiO_2 < 200

At what concentration does O_2 toxicity occur?

FiO_2 of > 60% × 48 hours; thus, try to keep FiO_2 below 50% at all times

What are the main causes of carbon dioxide retention?

Hypoventilation, increased dead space ventilation, and increased carbon dioxide production (as in hypermetabolic states)

Why are carbohydrates minimized in the diet/TPN of patients having difficulty with hypercapnia?

The respiratory quotient (RQ) is the ratio of CO_2 production to O_2 consumption and is highest for carbohydrates (1.0) and lowest for fats (0.7). By minimizing carbohydrate consumption, the CO_2 production at any metabolic rate is minimized.

HEMODYNAMIC MONITORING

Why are indwelling arterial lines used for blood pressure monitoring in critically ill patients?

Because of the need for frequent measurements, the inaccuracy of frequently repeated cuff measurements, the inaccuracy of cuff measurements in hypotension, and the need for frequent arterial blood sampling/labs

Which pressures/values are obtained from a Swan-Ganz catheter?

CVP, PA pressures, PCWP, CO, PVR, SVR, mixed venous o_2 saturation

Identify the Swan-Ganz waveforms.

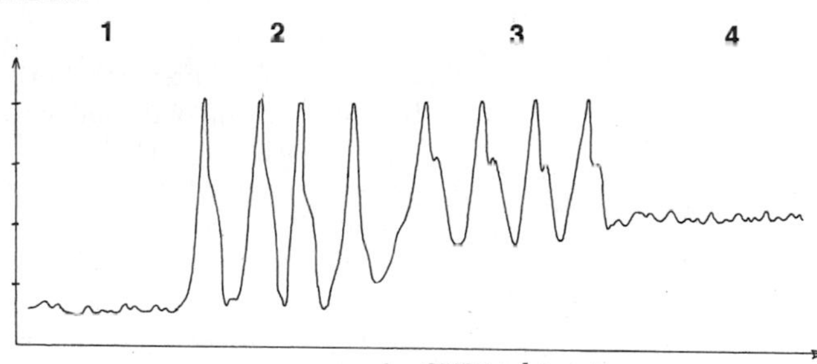

1. CVP/right atrium
2. Right ventricle
3. Pulmonary artery
4. Wedge

What does the abbreviation PCWP stand for?

Pulmonary **C**apillary **W**edge **P**ressure

Give other names for PCWP.

Wedge or wedge pressure

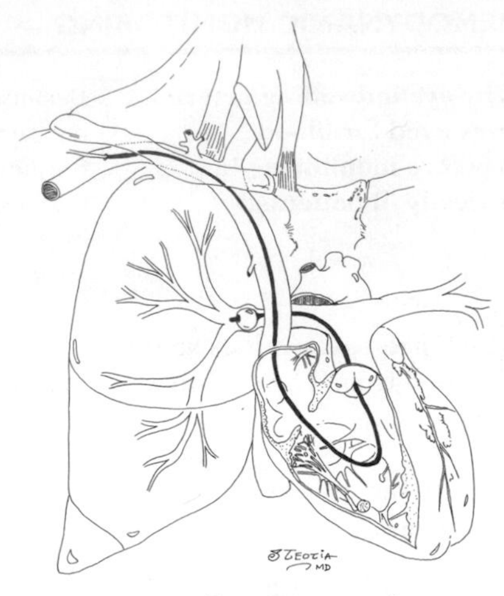

What is it?

Pulmonary capillary pressure after balloon occlusion of the pulmonary artery, which is equal to left atrial pressure because there are no valves in the pulmonary system.

Left atrial pressure is essentially equal to left ventricular end diastolic pressure (LVEDP): left heart preload, and, thus, intravascular volume status

What is the primary use of the PCWP?

As an indirect measure of preload = intravascular volume

At what point in the respiratory cycle is PCWP most accurate?

Ventilated patient—at end expiration

Nonventilated patient—at peak inspiration

Think: "Peaks and valleys"

Peaks—**P**atient breathing on his own = **P**eak of inspiration

Valleys—**V**entilated patient = **V**alley of expiration

In which clinical situations is PCWP not an accurate estimate of preload?

Pulmonary disease, such as ARDS; pulmonary hypertension; valvular heart disease; ischemic heart disease with a noncompliant ventricle; high levels of PEEP; tamponade; PTX

How does thermodilution determine the cardiac output (CO)?

The temperature of a proximal saline injection or heater probe is determined at a point distal (pulmonary artery) to its origin. The temperature difference determines amount of blood flow and, thus, CO.

MECHANICAL VENTILATION

Define ventilation.

Air through the lungs; monitored by PCO_2

Define oxygenation.

Oxygen delivery to the alveoli; monitored by O_2 sats and PO_2

What can increase ventilation to decrease PCO_2?

Increased respiratory rate (RR), increased tidal volume (minute ventilation)

What is minute ventilation?

Volume of gas ventilated through the lungs (RR × tidal volume)

Define tidal volume.

Volume delivered with each breath; should be 7 to 10 cc/kg on the ventilator

Are ventilation and oxygenation related?

Basically no; you can have an O_2 sat of 100% and a PCO_2 of 150. O_2 sats do not tell you anything about the PCO_2 (key point!).

What can increase PO_2 (oxygenation) in the ventilated patient?

Increased FIO_2
Increased PEEP

What can decrease PCO_2 in the ventilated patient?

Increased RR
Increased tidal volume (i.e., increase minute ventilation)

Modes defined

IMV?

Intermittent mandatory ventilation: mode with intermittent mandatory ventilations at a predetermined rate; patients can also breathe on their own above the mandatory rate **without** help from the ventilator

SIMV?

Synchronous IMV: mode of IMV that delivers the mandatory breath synchronously with patient's initiated effort; if no breath is initiated, the ventilator delivers the predetermined mandatory breath

A-C?

Assist-control ventilation: mode in which the ventilator delivers a breath when the patient initiates a breath, or the ventilator "assists" the patient to breathe; if the patient does not initiate a breath, the ventilator takes "control" and delivers a breath at a predetermined rate

In contrast to IMV, all breaths are by the ventilator.

CPAP? — **C**ontinuous **P**ositive **A**irway **P**ressure: positive pressure delivered **continuously** (during expiration and inspiration) by ventilator, but no volume breaths (patient breathes on own)

Pressure support? — Pressure is delivered only **with an initiated breath**. Pressure support decreases the work of breathing by overcoming the resistance in the ventilator circuit.

What are the effects of positive pressure ventilation in a patient with hypovolemia or low lung compliance? — Venous return and cardiac output are decreased.

Define PEEP. — **P**ositive **E**nd **E**xpiration **P**ressure: positive pressure maintained at the end of a breath; keeps alveoli open

What is "physiologic PEEP"? — PEEP of 5 cm H_2O; thought to approximate normal pressure in normal nonintubated people caused by the closed glottis

What are the side effects of increasing levels of PEEP? — Barotrauma (injury to airway = pneumothorax), decreased CO from decreased preload

What are the typical initial ventilator settings:

Mode? — Intermittent mandatory ventilation

Tidal volume? — 7 to 10 ml/kg

Ventilator rate? — 10 breaths/min

FiO_2? — 100% and wean down

PEEP? — 5 cm H_2O
From these parameters, change according to blood-gas analysis

What clinical situations cause increased airway resistance? — Airway or endotracheal tube obstruction, bronchospasm, ARDS, mucus plug, CHF (pulmonary edema)

What are the presumed advantages of PEEP?

Prevention of alveolar collapse and atelectasis, improved gas exchange, increased pulmonary compliance, decreased shunt fraction

What are the possible disadvantages of PEEP?

Decreased cardiac output, especially in the setting of hypovolemia; decreased gas exchange; ↓ compliance with high levels of PEEP, fluid retention, increased intracranial pressure, barotraumas

What parameters must be evaluated in deciding if a patient is ready to be extubated?

Patient alert and able to protect airway, gas exchange ($Pao_2 > 70$, $Paco_2 < 50$), tidal volume (> 5 cc/kg), minute ventilation (< 10 L/min), negative inspiratory pressure (< −20 cm H_20 or more negative), $Fio_2 \subseteq 40\%$, PEEP 5, pH > 7.25

What is a possible source of fever in a patient with an NG or nasal endotracheal tube?

Sinusitis (diagnosed by sinus films/CT)

What is the 35–45 rule of blood gas values?

Normal values:
pII = 7.**35**–7.**45**
PCO = **35–45**

Which medications can be delivered via an endotracheal tube?

N.A.V.E.L.:
Narcan
Atropine
Vasopressin
Epinephrine
Lidocaine

63 Vascular Surgery

What is atherosclerosis?	A diffuse disease process in arteries; atheromas containing cholesterol and lipid form within the intima and inner media, often accompanied by ulcerations and smooth muscle hyperplasia
What is the common theory of how atherosclerosis is initiated?	Endothelial injury → platelets adhere → growth factors released → smooth muscle hyperplasia/plaque deposition
What are the risk factors for atherosclerosis?	Hypertension, **smoking,** diabetes mellitus, family history, hypercholesterolemia, high LDL, obesity, and sedentary lifestyle
What are the common sites of plaque formation in arteries?	Branch points (carotid bifurcation), tethered sites (superficial femoral artery [SFA] in Hunter's canal in the leg)
What must be present for a successful arterial bypass operation?	1. Inflow (e.g., patent aorta) 2. Outflow (e.g., open distal popliteal artery) 3. Run off (e.g., patent trifurcation vessels down to the foot)
What is the major principle of safe vascular surgery?	Get **proximal** and **distal** control of the vessel to be worked on!
What does it mean to "POTTS" a vessel?	Place a vessel loop twice around a vessel so that if you put tension on the vessel loop, it will occlude the vessel.
What is the suture needle orientation through graft versus diseased artery in a graft to artery anastomosis?	Needle "in to out" of the lumen in diseased artery to help **tack down the plaque** and the needle "out-to-in" on the graft

What are the layers of an artery?

1. Intima
2. Media
3. Adventitia

Which arteries supply the blood vessel itself?

Vasovasorum

What is a true aneurysm?

Dilation (> 2× nl diameter) of all three layers of a vessel

What is a false (pseudo)aneurysm?

Dilation of artery not involving all three layers (e.g., hematoma with fibrous covering)
Often connects with vessel lumen and blood swirls inside the false aneurysm

PERIPHERAL VASCULAR DISEASE

Define the arterial anatomy.

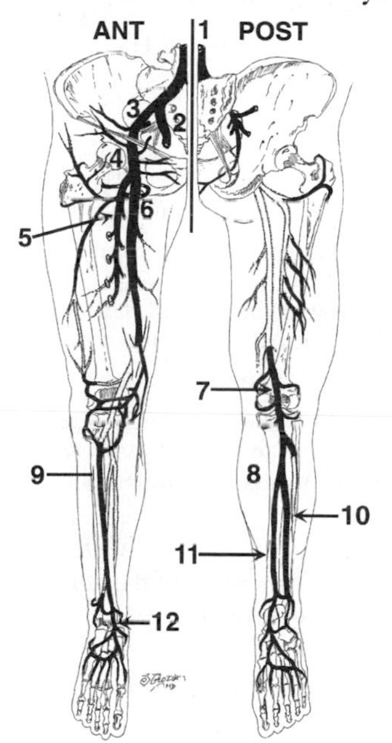

1. Aorta
2. Internal iliac (hypogastric)
3. External iliac
4. Common femoral artery
5. Profundi femoral artery
6. Superficial femoral artery (SFA)
7. Popliteal artery
8. Trifurcation
9. Anterior tibial
10. Peroneal artery
11. Posterior tibial artery
12. Dorsalis pedis artery

How can you remember the orientation of the lower exterior arteries below the knee on A-Gram?

Use the acronym **L.A.M.P.**:
Lateral **A**nterior tibial
Medial **P**osterior tibial

What is peripheral vascular disease (PVD)?	Occlusive atherosclerotic disease in the lower extremities
What is the most common site of arterial atherosclerotic occlusion in the lower extremities?	Occlusion of the SFA in Hunter's canal
What are the symptoms of PVD?	Intermittent claudication, rest pain, erectile dysfunction, sensorimotor impairment, tissue loss
What is intermittent claudication?	Pain, cramping, or both of the lower extremity, usually the calf muscle, after walking a specific distance; then the pain/cramping resolves after stopping for a specific amount of time while standing; this pattern is reproducible
What is rest pain?	Pain in the foot, usually over the distal metatarsals; this pain arises at rest (classically at night, awakening the patient)
What classically resolves rest pain?	Hanging the foot over the side of the bed or standing; gravity affords some extra flow to the ischemic areas
How can vascular causes of claudication be differentiated from nonvascular causes, such as neurogenic claudication or arthritis?	History (in the vast majority of patients) and noninvasive tests; remember, vascular claudication appears after a specific distance and resolves after a specific time of rest while standing (not so with most other forms of claudication)
What is the differential diagnosis of lower extremity claudication?	Neurogenic (e.g., nerve entrapment/discs), arthritis, coarctation of the aorta, popliteal artery syndrome, chronic compartment syndrome, neuromas, anemia, diabetic neuropathy pain
What are the signs of PVD?	Absent pulses, bruits, muscular atrophy, decreased hair growth, thick toenails, tissue necrosis/ulcers/infection
What is the site of a PVD ulcer vs. a venous stasis ulcer?	PVD arterial insufficiency ulcer—usually on the toes/foot Venous stasis ulcer—medial malleolus (ankle)

What is the ABI?

The **A**nkle to **B**rachial **I**ndex (**ABI**); simply, the ratio of the systolic blood pressure at the ankle to the systolic blood pressure at the arm (brachial artery) A:B; ankle pressure taken with Doppler; the ABI is noninvasive

What ABIs are associated with normals, claudicators, and rest pain?

Normal ABI— ≥ 1.0
Claudicator ABI— < 0.6
Rest pain ABI— < 0.4

Who gets false ABI readings?

Patients with calcified arteries, especially those with diabetes

What are PVRs?

Pulse **V**olume **R**ecordings; pulse wave forms are recorded from lower extremities representing volume of blood per heart beat at sequential sites down leg
A large wave form means good collateral blood flow.
(Noninvasive using pressure cuffs)

Prior to surgery for chronic PVD, what diagnostic test will every patient receive?

A-gram (arteriogram: dye in vessel and x-rays) maps disease and allows for best treatment option (i.e., angioplasty vs. surgical bypass vs. endarterectomy)
Gold standard for diagnosing PVD

What is the bedside management of a patient with PVD?

1. Sheep skin (easy on the heels)
2. Foot cradle (keeps sheets/blankets off the feet)
3. Skin lotion to avoid further cracks in the skin that can go on to form a fissure and then an ulcer

What are the indications for surgical treatment in PVD?

1. Rest pain
2. Tissue necrosis
3. Infection
4. Severe claudication refractory to conservative treatment that affects quality of life/livelihood (e.g., can't work because of the claudication)

What is the treatment of claudication?

For the vast majority, conservative treatment, including exercise, smoking cessation, treatment of HTN, diet, aspirin, with or without Trental (pentoxifylline)

How can you remember the medical conservative treatment for claudication?

The acronym P.A.C.E.:
P = **P**entoxifylline
A = **A**spirin
C = **C**essation of smoking
E = **E**xercise

How does aspirin work?

Inhibits platelets (inhibits cyclo-oxygenase)

How does Trental (pentoxifylline) work?

Results in increased RBC deformity and flexibility (think: pento**X**ifylline = RBC fle**X**ibility)

What is the risk of limb loss with claudication?

Five percent limb loss at 5 years (think: 5 in 5)

What is the risk of limb loss with rest pain?

More than 50% of patients will have amputation of the limb at some point.

In the patient with PVD, what is the main postoperative concern?

Cardiac status, because most patients with PVD have coronary artery disease; about 20% have an AAA
MI is the most common cause of postoperative death after a PVD operation.

What is Leriche's syndrome?

Impotence, buttock claudication, and gluteus muscle atrophy from occlusive disease of the iliacs/distal aorta
Think **C.I.A.:**
C: Claudication
I: Impotence
A: Atrophy
(think the CIA spy Leriche)

What are the treatment options for severe PVD?

1. Surgical graft bypass
2. Angioplasty—balloon dilation
3. Endarterectomy—remove diseased intima and media
4. Surgical patch angioplasty (place patch over stenosis)

What is a FEM-POP bypass?

Bypass SFA occlusion with a graft from the femoral artery to the popliteal artery

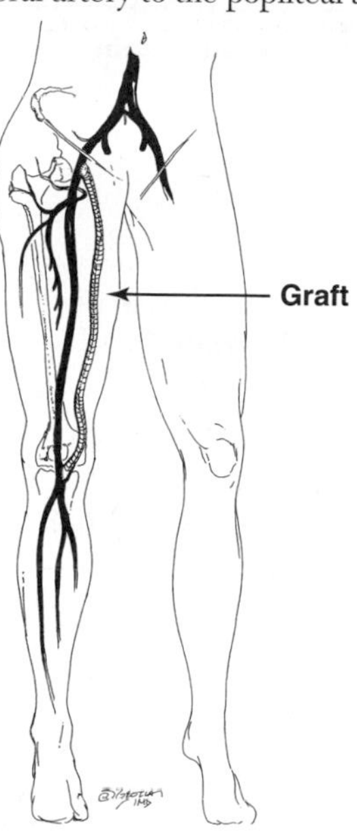

What is a FEM DISTAL bypass?

Bypass from the femoral artery to a distal artery (peroneal artery, anterior tibial artery, or posterior tibial artery)

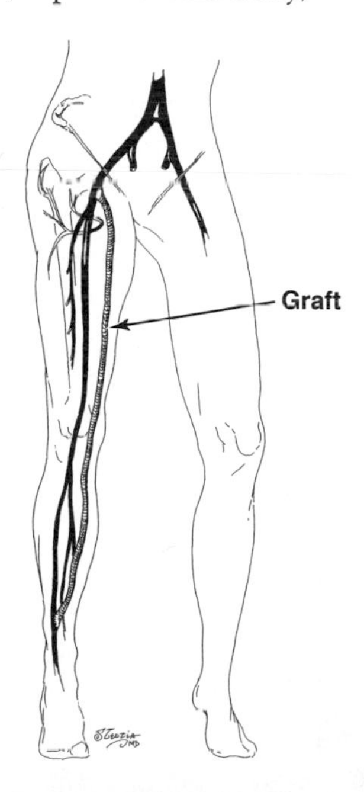

What graft material has the longest patency rate?
Autologous vein graft

What is an "in situ" vein graft?
Saphenous vein is more or less left in place, all branches are ligated, and the vein valves are broken with a small hook or cut out. A vein can also be used if reversed so that the valves do not cause a problem.

What type of graft is used for above-the-knee FEM POP bypass?
Either vein or Gortex® graft; vein still has better patency

What type of graft is used for below the knee FEM POP or FEM distal bypass?
Must use vein graft; prosthetic grafts have a prohibitive thrombosis rate

What is DRY gangrene?
Dry necrosis of tissue without signs of infection ("mummified tissue")

What is WET gangrene?
Moist necrotic tissue with signs of infection

LOWER EXTREMITY AMPUTATIONS

What are the indications?
Irreversible tissue ischemia (no hope for revascularization bypass) and necrotic tissue, severe infection, severe pain with no bypassable vessels, or if patient is not interested in a bypass procedure

Identify the level of the following amputations:

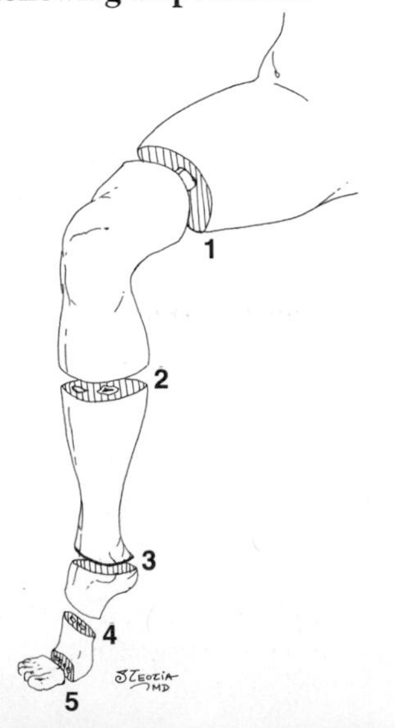

1. Above-the-knee amputation (AKA)
2. Below-the-knee amputation (BKA)
3. Symes amputation
4. Transmetatarsal amputation
5. Toe amputation

What is a Ray amputation?
Removal of toe and head of metatarsal

ACUTE ARTERIAL OCCLUSION

What is it?
Acute occlusion of an artery, usually by embolization; other causes include acute thrombosis of an atheromatous lesion, vascular trauma

What are the classic signs/ symptoms of acute arterial occlusion?
The "six P's": pain, paralysis, pallor, paresthesia, polar (some say poikilothermia—you pick), pulselessness (you **must** know these!)

What is the classic timing of pain with acute arterial occlusion from an embolus?
Acute onset; the patient can classically tell you exactly when and where it happened

What is the immediate preoperative management?
1. Anticoagulate with IV heparin (bolus followed by constant infusion)
2. A-gram

What are the sources of emboli?
1. Heart—85% (e.g., clot from AFib, clot forming on dead muscle after MI, endocarditis, myxoma)
2. Aneurysms
3. Atheromatous plaque (atheroembolism)

What is the most common cause of embolus from the heart?
AFib

What is the most common site of arterial occlusion by an embolus?
Common femoral artery (SFA is the most common site of arterial occlusion from atherosclerosis)

What diagnostic studies are in order?
1. A-gram
2. EKG (looking for MI, AFib)
3. Echocardiogram (±) looking for clot, MI, valve vegetation

What is the treatment?
Surgical embolectomy via cutdown and Fogarty balloon (bypass is reserved for embolectomy failure)

What is a Fogarty?
Fogarty balloon catheter—catheter with a balloon tip that can be inflated with saline; used for embolectomy/

thrombectomy by insinuating the catheter with the balloon deflated past the embolus and then inflating the balloon and pulling the catheter out; the balloon brings the embolus with it

How many mm in diameter is a 12 French Fogarty catheter?

Simple; to get mm from French measurements, divide the French number by pi or 3.14; thus, a 12 French catheter is 12/3 = 4 mm in diameter

What must you look for postoperatively after reperfusion of a limb?

Compartment syndrome, hyperkalemia, renal failure from myoglobinuria, MI

What is compartment syndrome?

The leg (calf) is separated into compartments by very unyielding fascia; **tissue swelling** from reperfusion can increase the intracompartmental pressure, resulting in decreased capillary flow, ischemia, and myonecrosis; myonecrosis may occur after the intra-compartment pressure reaches only 30 mm Hg.

What are the signs/ symptoms of compartment syndrome?

Classic signs include pain, especially after passive flexing/extension of the foot, paralysis, paresthesias, and pallor; **pulses are present** in most cases because systolic pressure is much higher than the minimal 30 mm Hg needed for the syndrome!

Can a patient have a pulse and compartment syndrome?

YES!

How is the diagnosis made?

History/suspicion, compartment pressure measurement

What is the treatment of compartment syndrome?

Treatment includes opening compartments via bilateral calf-incision fasciotomies of all four compartments in the calf.

ABDOMINAL AORTIC ANEURYSMS

What is it also known as?

AAA, or "triple A"

25% have aortoiliac or femoral popliteal occlusive Disease
20% chance 1st degree relative will have Aneurysm

What is it?
woman-3.5cm

An abnormal dilation of the abdominal aorta (> 1.5–2× normal), forming a true aneurysm

Type A-prox. to subclav

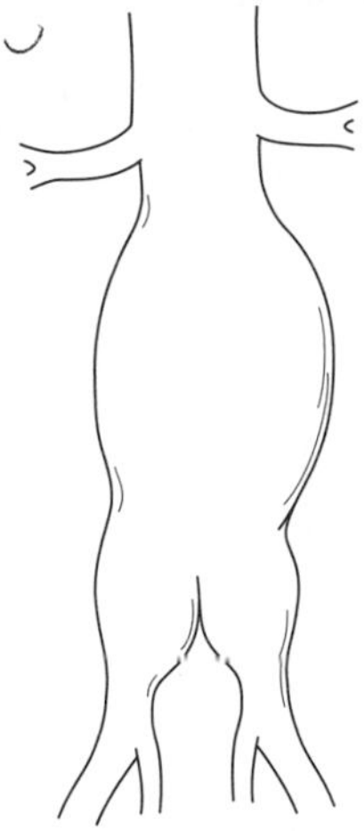

What is the male to female ratio?

M:F = approximately 4:1

thorac Aneur. more common in women

What is the common etiology?

Believed to be a**therosclerotic** in 95% of cases; 5% inflammatory

Also moyamoya, Ehlers Danlos, collagenase def.

What is the most common site?

Infrarenal (95%) -vasovasorum missing in infrarenal- relative ischemia of wall

What is the incidence?

Five percent of all adults older than 60 years of age; approximately 4% of white men (highest risk group)

About 1 in 5 patients with PVD will have an AAA; thus, rule out AAA in all your patients with PVD!

What percentage of patients with AAA have a peripheral arterial aneurysm?

20%

What are the risk factors?

Atherosclerosis, hypertension, smoking, male gender, advanced age

What are the symptoms?
compression surrounding structures

Most AAAs are **asymptomatic** and discovered during routine abdominal exam by primary care physicians; in the remainder, symptoms range from vague epigastric discomfort to back and abdominal pain.

What are the risk factors for rupture?

Increasing aneurysm diameter, COPD, HTN

What are the signs of rupture?

Classic triad of ruptured AAA:

1. **Abdominal pain**
2. **Pulsatile abdominal mass**
3. **Hypotension**

Pulsatile mass is usually left of the midline and above the umbilicus. Severe back or flank pain and signs of blood loss suggest ruptured/leaking AAA; if a patient has the classic triad, take him straight to the OR.

What are the risk factors for rupture?

Recent rapid expansion, large diameter, hypertension, COPD, symptomatic

By how much each year do AAAs grow?

Approximately 2 to 4 mm/year on average (larger AAAs grow faster than smaller AAAs)

Why do larger AAAs rupture more often and grow faster than smaller AAAs?

Probably because of Laplace's law (wall tension = pressure × diameter)

What is the risk of rupture per year based on AAA diameter size?

Less than 5 cm = 4%
Between 5 and 7 cm = 7%
More than 7 cm = 20%

Where does the aorta bifurcate?

At the level of the **umbilicus;** therefore, when palpating for an AAA, palpate above the umbilicus and below the xiphoid process

What is the differential diagnosis?

Acute pancreatitis, aortic dissection, mesenteric ischemia, MI, perforated ulcer, diverticulosis, renal colic, etc.

What are the diagnostic tests?

Use U/S to follow AAA clinically; other tests involve contrast CT and A-gram; A-gram will assess lumen patency and iliac/renal involvement.

What is the limitation of A-gram?

AAAs often have large mural thrombi, which result in a falsely reduced diameter because only the patent lumen is visualized.

What are the signs of AAA on AXR?

Calcification in the aneurysm wall, best seen on lateral projection (A.K.A. egg-shell calcifications)

What are the indications for surgical repair of AAA?

AAA more than 5 cm in diameter, if the patient is not an overwhelming high risk for surgery; also, rupture of the AAA, rapid growth, symptoms

What is the treatment?

Prosthetic graft placement, with rewrapping of the native aneurysm adventitia around the prosthetic graft after the thrombus is removed; when rupture is strongly suspected, **proceed to immediate laparotomy; there is no time for diagnostic tests!**

Why wrap the graft in the native aorta?

To reduce the incidence of enterograft fistula formation

What type of repair should be performed with AAA and iliacs severely occluded or iliac aneurysm(s)?

Aortobi-iliac or aortobifemoral graft replacement (bifurcated graft)

What is the treatment if the patient has abdominal pain, pulsatile abdominal mass, and hypotension?

Take the patient to the **O.R.** for emergent AAA repair

What is the treatment if the patient has known AAA and new onset of abdominal pain or back pain?

Take the patient straight to the O.R. for surgical repair

What is the mortality rate associated with the following types of AAA treatment:

Elective?
Good; less than 4% operative mortality

Ruptured?
More than 50% operative mortality

What is the leading cause of postoperative death in a patient undergoing elective AAA treatment?
Myocardial infarction (MI)

What are the other etiologies of AAA?
Inflammatory (connective tissue diseases), mycotic (a misnomer because most result from bacteria, not fungi)

What is the mean normal abdominal aortic diameter?
2 cm

What are the possible operative complications?
Atheroembolism, declamping hypotension, acute renal failure (especially if aneurysm involves the renal arteries), ureteral injury, hemorrhage

Why is colonic ischemia a concern in the repair of AAAs?
Often the IMA is sacrificed during surgery; if the collaterals are not adequate, the patient will have colonic ischemia.

What are the signs of colonic ischemia?
Heme-positive stool, or bright red blood per rectum (BRBPR), diarrhea, abdominal pain

What is the study of choice to diagnose colonic ischemia?
Colonoscopy

When is colonic ischemia seen postoperatively?
Usually in the first week

What is the treatment of necrotic sigmoid colon from colonic ischemia?
1. Resection of necrotic colon
2. Hartmann's pouch or mucus fistula
3. End colostomy

What is the possible long-term complication that often presents with both upper/lower GI bleeding?
Aortoenteric fistula (fistula between aorta and duodenum)

What are the other possible postoperative complications?
Erectile dysfunction (sympathetic plexus injury), retrograde ejaculation, aortovenous fistula (to IVC), graft infection, **anterior spinal syndrome**

What is the anterior spinal syndrome?

Classically:
1. Paraplegia
2. Loss of bladder/bowel control
3. Loss of pain/temperature sensation below level of involvement
4. **Sparing of proprioception**

Which artery is involved in anterior spinal cord syndrome?

Artery of **Adamkiewicz**—supplies the anterior spinal cord

What are the most common bacteria involved in aortic graft infections?

1. *Staphylococcus aureus*
2. *Staphylococcus epidermidis* (usually late)

How is a graft infection and an aortoenteric fistula treated?

Perform an **extra-anatomic bypass** with resection of the graft

What is an extra-anatomic bypass graft?

Axillofemoral bypass graft— **graft not in a normal vascular path;** usually, the graft goes from the axillary artery to the femoral artery and then from one femoral artery to the other (fem-fem bypass)

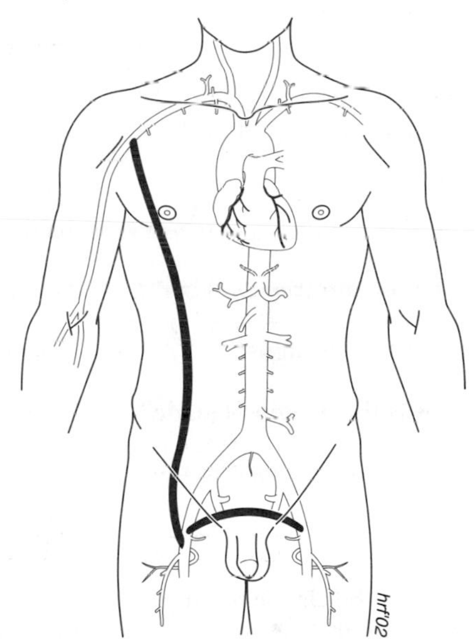

What is an endovascular repair?

Placement of a stent proximal and distal to an AAA through a distant percutaneous access (usually through the groin); less invasive; long-term results pending

CLASSIC INTRAOP QUESTIONS DURING AAA REPAIR

Which vein crosses the neck of the AAA proximally?
The renal vein

What part of the small bowel crosses in front of the AAA?
The duodenum

Which large vein runs to the left of the AAA?
IMV

Which artery comes off the middle of the AAA and runs to the left?
IMA

Which vein runs behind the RIGHT common iliac artery?
The **LEFT** common iliac vein

MESENTERIC ISCHEMIA

CHRONIC MESENTERIC ISCHEMIA

What is it?
Chronic intestinal ischemia from long-term occlusion of the intestinal arteries; most commonly results from athero-sclerosis; usually in two or more arteries because of the extensive collaterals

What are the symptoms?
Weight loss, postprandial abdominal pain, anxiety/fear of food because of postprandial pain, ± heme occult, ± diarrhea/vomiting

What is "intestinal angina"?
Postprandial pain from gut ischemia

What are the signs?
Abdominal bruit is commonly heard.

How is the diagnosis made?
A-gram

What supplies blood to the gut?
1. SMA
2. IMA
3. Celiac axis vessels

What is the classic finding on A-gram?
Two of the three mesenteric arteries are occluded, and there is atherosclerotic narrowing of the third patent artery.

What are the treatment options?
Bypass, endarterectomy

ACUTE MESENTERIC ISCHEMIA

What is it?
Acute onset of intestinal ischemia

What are the causes?
1. **Emboli** to a mesenteric vessel from the heart
2. **Acute thrombosis** of long-standing atherosclerosis of mesenteric artery

What are the causes of emboli from the heart?
AFib, MI, cardiomyopathy, valve disease/endocarditis, mechanical heart valve

What drug has been associated with acute intestinal ischemia?
Digitalis

To which intestinal artery do emboli preferentially go?
Superior mesenteric artery (SMA)

What are the signs/symptoms of acute mesenteric ischemia?
Severe pain—classically **"pain out of proportion to physical exam,"** no peritoneal signs until necrosis, vomiting/diarrhea/hyperdefecation, ± heme stools

What is the classic triad of acute mesenteric ischemia?
1. Acute onset of pain
2. Vomiting, diarrhea, or both
3. History of AFib or heart disease

How is the diagnosis made?
History/physical exam → A-gram (waste no time!)

What is the treatment of a mesenteric embolus?
Perform Fogarty catheter embolectomy, resect obviously necrotic intestine, and leave marginal looking bowel until a second look laparotomy is performed 24 to 72 hours postoperatively.

What is the treatment of acute thrombosis?
Papaverine vasodilator via A-gram catheter until **patient is in the O.R.;** then, most surgeons would perform a supraceliac aorta graft to the involved intestinal artery or endarterectomy; intestinal resection/second look as needed

MEDIAN ARCUATE LIGAMENT SYNDROME

What is it?
Mesenteric ischemia resulting from narrowing of the celiac axis vessels by

extrinsic compression by the median arcuate ligament

What are the symptoms? Postprandial pain, weight loss

What are the signs? Abdominal bruit in almost all patients

How is the diagnosis made? A-gram

What is the treatment? Release arcuate ligament surgically

CAROTID VASCULAR DISEASE

ANATOMY

Identify the following structures:

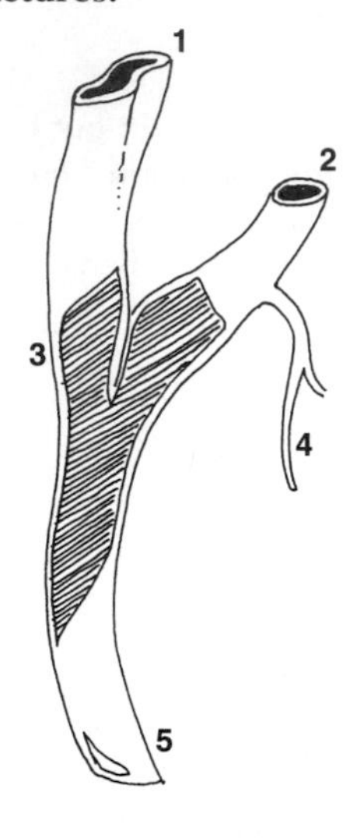

1. Internal carotid artery
2. External carotid artery
3. Carotid "bulb"
4. Superior thyroid artery
5. Common carotid artery

Shaded area: common site of plaque formation

What are the signs/symptoms? Amaurosis fugax, TIA, RIND, CVA

Define the following terms:

Amaurosis fugax Temporary monocular blindness ("curtain coming down"): seen with microemboli to retina; example of TIA

TIA **T**ransient **I**schemic **A**ttack: focal neurologic deficit with resolution of all symptoms within 24 hours

RIND **R**eversible **I**schemic **N**eurologic **D**eficit: transient neurologic impairment (without any lasting sequelae) lasting 24 to 72 hours

CVA

Cerebro**V**ascular **A**ccident (stroke): neurologic deficit with permanent brain damage

What is the risk of a CVA in patients with TIA?

About 10% a year

What is the noninvasive method of evaluating carotid disease?

Carotid ultrasound/Doppler: gives general location and degree of stenosis

What is the gold standard invasive method of evaluating carotid disease?

A-gram

What is the surgical treatment of carotid stenosis?

Carotid endarterectomy (CEA): the removal of the diseased intima and media of the carotid artery, often performed with a shunt in place

What are the indications for CEA in the ASYMPTOMATIC patient?

Carotid artery stenosis > 60%

What are the indications for CEA in the SYMPTOMATIC (CVA, TIA, RIND) patient?

Carotid stenosis > 50%

Before performing a CEA in the symptomatic patient, what study other than the A-gram should be performed?

Head CT

In bilateral high-grade carotid stenosis, on which side should the CEA be performed in the asymptomatic, right-handed patient?

Left CEA first, to protect the dominant hemisphere and speech center

What is the dreaded complication after a CEA?

Stroke

What are the possible postoperative complications after a CEA?

CVA, MI, hematoma, wound infection, hemorrhage, hypotension/hypertension, thrombosis, vagus nerve injury (change in voice), hypoglossal nerve injury (tongue deviation toward side of injury—"wheelbarrow" effect), intracranial hemorrhage

What is the mortality rate after CEA?
About 1%

What is the stroke rate after CEA?
Between 1% and 5% (higher in the symptomatic patient)

What is the risk of ipsilateral stroke after a CEA in the asymptomatic patient?
0.5%/year (1/200)

What is the risk of ipsilateral stroke after a CEA in the symptomatic patient?
About 2%

What is the postoperative medication?
Aspirin (inhibits platelets by inhibiting cyclo-oxygenase)

What is the most common cause of death during the early postoperative period after a CEA?
MI

CLASSIC CEA INTRAOP QUESTIONS

What thin muscle is cut right under the skin in the neck?
Platysma muscle

What are the extracranial branches of the internal carotid artery?
None

Which vein crosses the carotid bifurcation?
The facial vein

What is the first branch of the external carotid?
The superior thyroidal artery

Which muscle crosses the common carotid proximally?
Omohyoid muscle

Which muscle crosses the carotid artery distally?
Digastric muscle (think: **D**igastric = **D**istal)

Which nerve crosses approximately 1 cm distal to the carotid bifurcation?

Hypoglossal nerve; cut it and you get a tongue deviating toward the side of the injury (the "wheelbarrow effect")

Which nerve crosses the internal carotid near the ear?

Facial nerve (marginal branch)

What is in the carotid sheath?

1. Carotid artery
2. Internal jugular vein
3. **Vagus** nerve (lies posteriorly in 98% of patients and anterior in 2%)
4. Deep cervical lymph nodes

SUBCLAVIAN STEAL SYNDROME

What is it?

Arm fatigue and vertebrobasilar insufficiency from obstruction of the left subclavian artery or innominate proximal to the vertebral artery branch point; ipsilateral arm movement causes increased blood flow demand, which is met by retrograde flow from the vertebral artery, thereby "stealing" from the vertebrobasilar arteries

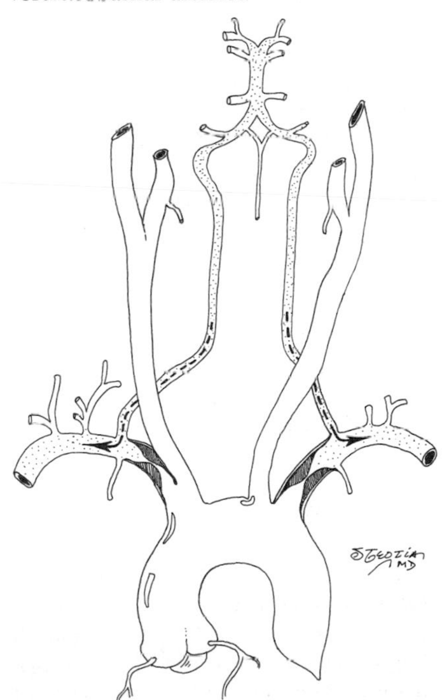

Which artery is most commonly occluded?
Left subclavian

What are the signs/symptoms?
Upper extremity claudication and signs of vertebrobasilar insufficiency: syncopal attacks, vertigo, confusion, dysarthria, blindness, or ataxia

What are the signs?
Upper extremity blood pressure discrepancy, bruit (above the clavicle)

What is the treatment?
Surgical bypass

RENAL ARTERY STENOSIS

What is it?
Stenosis of renal artery, resulting in decreased perfusion of the juxtaglomerular apparatus and subsequent activation of the renin-angiotensin-aldosterone system (i.e., hypertension from renal artery stenosis)

What is the incidence?
~ 10% to 15% of the U.S. population has HTN; of these, approximately 4% have potentially correctable renovascular HTN
Also note that 30% of malignant HTN has a renovascular etiology

What is the etiology of the stenosis?
~ two-thirds result from atherosclerosis (men > women), ~ one-third result from fibromuscular dysplasia (women > men, average age 40 years, and 50% with bilateral disease)
Note: another rare cause is hypoplasia of the renal artery

What is the classic profile of a patient with renal artery stenosis from fibromuscular dysplasia?
A young woman with hypertension

What are the associated risks/clues?
Family history, early onset of HTN, HTN refractory to medical treatment

What are the signs/symptoms?
Most patients are asymptomatic but may have headache, **diastolic** HTN, flank bruits (present in 50%), and decreased renal function.

What are the diagnostic tests?

A-gram: Maps artery and extent of stenosis; gold standard

IVP: 80% of patients have delayed nephrogram phase (i.e., delayed filling of contrast)

Renal vein renin ratio (RVRR): If sampling of renal vein renin levels shows ratio between the two kidneys ≥ 1.5, then diagnostic for a unilateral stenosis

Captopril provocation test: Will show a drop in BP

Are renin levels in serum ALWAYS elevated?

No; systemic renin levels may also be measured but are only increased in malignant HTN, as the increased intravascular volume dilutes the elevated renin level in most patients.

What is the invasive nonsurgical treatment?

Percutaneous renal transluminal angioplasty (PRTA)
Much better results with fibromuscular dysplasia but also good for isolated short-segment atherosclerotic lesions away from the ostium of the renal artery
With FM dysplasia: 85% to 100% success rate using PRTA and 5% restenosis rate
With atherosclerosis: 40% to 90% success using PRTA and about one-fourth restenosis

What is the surgical treatment?

Resection, bypass, vein/graft interposition, or endarterectomy

What antihypertensive medication is CONTRAINDICATED in patients with hypertension from renovascular stenosis?

ACE inhibitors (result in renal insufficiency)

SPLENIC ARTERY ANEURYSM

What is it?

Aneurysm of the splenic artery

What are the causes?

Women—medial dysplasia
Men—atherosclerosis

How is the diagnosis made? Usually by abdominal pain → U/S, in the OR after rupture, or incidentally **by egg-shell calcifications seen on AXR**

What is the risk factor for rupture? Pregnancy

POPLITEAL ARTERY ANEURYSM

What is it? Aneurysm of the popliteal artery caused by atherosclerosis and, rarely, bacterial infection

How is the diagnosis made? Usually by physical exam → A-gram, U/S

Why examine the contra-lateral popliteal artery? Half of all patients with a popliteal artery aneurysm have a popliteal artery aneurysm in the contralateral popliteal artery

Why examine the rest of the arterial tree (especially the abdominal aorta)? **Three-fourths of all patients with popliteal aneurysms have additional aneurysms elsewhere;** more than half of these are located in the abdominal aorta/iliacs.

MISCELLANEOUS

Define the following terms:

"Milk leg" A.K.A. phlegmasia alba dolens (alba = white): often seen in pregnant women with occlusion of iliac vein resulting from extrinsic compression by the uterus (thus, the leg is "white" because of subcutaneous edema)

Phlegmasia cerulea dolens In comparison, phlegmasia cerulea dolens is secondary to severe venous outflow obstruction and results in a cyanotic leg. The extensive venous thrombosis results in arterial inflow impairment.

Raynaud's phenomenon Vasospasm of digital arteries with color changes of the digits; usually initiated by cold/emotion

White (spasm), then blue (cyanosis), then red (hyperemia)

Takayasu's arteritis	Arteritis of the aorta and aortic branches, resulting in stenosis/occlusion/aneurysms Seen mostly in women
Buerger's disease	A.K.A. thromboangiitis obliterans: occlusion of the small vessels of the hands and feet; seen in **young men who smoke;** often results in digital gangrene → amputations
What is the treatment for Buerger's disease?	Smoking **cessation,** +/− sympathectomy
What is blue toe syndrome?	Microembolization from proximal atherosclerotic disease of the aorta resulting in blue, painful, ischemic toes
What is a "paradoxical embolus"?	Venous embolus gains access to the left heart after going through a intracardiac defect, most commonly a patent foramen ovale, and then lodges in a peripheral artery.

Section III

Subspecialty Surgery

64 Pediatric Surgery

What is the motto of pediatric surgery?
"Children are NOT little adults!"

What is a simple way to distract a pediatric patient when examining the abdomen for tenderness?
Listen to the abdomen with the stethoscope and then push down on the abdomen with the stethoscope to check for tenderness.

PEDIATRIC IV FLUIDS AND NUTRITION

What is the estimated blood volume of infants and children?
About 8% of body weight (more than adults), or approximately 80 cc/kg

What is the maintenance IV fluid for children?
D5 1/4 NS + 20 mEq KCl

Why ¼ NS?
Children (especially those younger than 4 years of age) cannot concentrate their urine—clear the sodium.

How are maintenance fluid rates calculated in children?
4, 2, 1 per hour:
- **4 cc/kg for the first 10 kg of body weight**
- **2 cc/kg for the second 10 kg of body weight**
- **1 cc/kg for every kilogram over the first 20** (e.g., the rate for a child weighing 25 kg is 4 × 10 = 40 plus 2 × 10 = 20 plus 1 × 5 = 5, for an IVF rate of 65 cc/hr)

What is the minimal urine output for children?
From 1 to 2 ml/kg/hr

What is the best way to present urine output measurements on rounds?
Urine output total per shift THEN cc/kg/hr

What is the major difference between adult and pediatric nutritional needs?

Premature infants/infants/children need more calories and protein/kg/day.

What are the caloric requirements by age for the following patients:

Premature infants?

80 Kcal/kg/day and then go up

Children younger than 1 year?

Approximately 100 Kcal/kg/day (90–120)

Children aged 1 to 7?

Approximately 85 Kcal/kg/day (75–90)

Children aged 7 to 12?

Approximately 70 Kcal/kg/day (60–75)

Youths aged 12 to 18

Approximately 40 Kcal/kg/day (30–60)

What are the protein requirements by age for the following patients:

Children younger than 1 year?

3 g/kg/day (2–3.5)

Children aged 1 to 7?

2 g/kg/day (2–2.5)

Children aged 7 to 12?

2 g/kg/day

Youths aged 12 to 18?

1.5 grams/kg/day

How many calories are in breast milk?

20 Kcal/30 cc (same as most formulas)

FETAL CIRCULATION

What is the number of umbilical veins?

1 (usually)

What is the number of umbilical arteries?

2

Which umbilical vessel carries oxygenated blood?

Umbilical vein

The oxygenated blood travels through the liver to the IVC through which structure?

Ductus venosus

Oxygenated blood passes from the right atrium to the left atrium through which structure?

Foramen ovale

Unsaturated blood goes from the right ventricle to the descending aorta through which structure?

Ductus arteriosus

What are the ADULT structures of the following fetal structures:

Ductus venosus?

Ligamentum venosus

Umbilical vein?

Ligamentum teres

Umbilical artery?

Medial umbilical ligament

Ductus arteriosus

Ligamentum arteriosus

Urachus?

Median umbilical ligament

Tongue remnant of thyroid's descent?

Foramen cecum

Persistent remnant of vitelline duct?

Meckel's diverticulum

ECMO

What is ECMO?

Extra**C**orporeal **M**embrane **O**xygenation chronic cardiopulmonary bypass—for complete respiratory support

What are the types of ECMO?

Venovenous: Blood from vein → oxygenated → back to vein
Venoarterial: Blood from vein (IJ) → oxygenated → back to artery (carotid)

What are the indications?

Severe hypoxia, usually from congenital diaphragmatic hernia, meconium aspiration, persistent pulmonary hypertension, sepsis

What are the contra-indications?

Weight < 2 kg, IVH (intraventricular hemorrhage in brain contraindicated because of heparin in line)

NECK

What is the major differential diagnosis of a pediatric neck mass?

Thyroglossal duct cyst (midline), branchial cleft cyst (lateral), lymphadenopathy, abscess, cystic hygroma, hemangioma, teratoma/dermoid cyst, thyroid nodule, lymphoma/leukemia (also parathyroid tumors, neuroblastoma, histiocytosis X, rhabdomyosarcoma, salivary gland tumors, neurofibroma)

THYROGLOSSAL DUCT CYST

What is it?

Remnant of the diverticulum formed by migration of thyroid tissue; normal development involves migration of thyroid tissue from the foramen cecum at the base of the tongue through the hyoid bone to its final position around the tracheal cartilage

What is the average age at diagnosis?

Usually presents around 5 years of age

How is the diagnosis made?

Ultrasound

What are the complications?

Enlargement, infection, and fistula formation between oropharynx or salivary gland; aberrant thyroid tissue may masquerade as thyroglossal duct cyst, and if it is not cystic, deserves a thyroid scan

What is the anatomic location?

Almost always in the **midline**

What is the treatment?

Antibiotics if infection is present, then excision, which must include the midportion of the hyoid bone and entire tract to foramen cecum (Sistrunk procedure)

BRANCHIAL CLEFT ANOMALIES

What is it?

Remnant of the primitive branchial clefts in which epithelium forms a sinus tract between the pharynx (second cleft), or the external auditory canal (first cleft), and the skin of the anterior neck; if the sinus ends blindly, a cyst may form

What is the common presentation?
Infection because of communication between pharynx and external ear canal

What is the anatomic position?
Second cleft anomaly—**lateral to the midline** along anterior border of the sternocleidomastoid, anywhere from angle of jaw to clavicle
First cleft anomaly—less common than second cleft anomalies; tend to be located higher under the mandible

What is the most common cleft remnant?
Second; thus, these are found most often laterally versus thyroglossal cysts, which are found centrally (key point)

What is the treatment?
Antibiotics if infection is present, then surgical excision of cyst and tract once inflammation is resolved

What is the major anatomic difference between thyroglossal cyst and branchial cleft cyst?
Thyroglossal cyst = **midline**
Branchial cleft cyst = **lateral**

STRIDOR

What is stridor?
A harsh, high-pitched sound heard on breathing caused by obstruction of the trachea or larynx

What are the signs/symptoms?
Dyspnea, cyanosis, difficulty with feedings

What is the differential diagnosis?
Laryngomalacia—leading cause of stridor in infants; results from inadequate development of supporting laryngeal structures; usually self-limited and treatment is expectant unless respiratory compromise is present
Tracheobronchomalacia—similar to laryngomalacia, but involves the entire trachea
Vascular rings and slings—abnormal development or placement of thoracic

large vessels resulting in obstruction of trachea/bronchus

What are the symptoms of vascular rings?

Stridor, dyspnea on exertion, or dysphagia

How is the diagnosis of vascular rings made?

Barium swallow revealing typical configuration of esophageal compression
Echo/arteriogram

What is the treatment of vascular rings?

Surgical division of the ring, if the patient is symptomatic

CYSTIC HYGROMA

What is it?

Congenital abnormality of lymph sac resulting in lymphangioma

What is the anatomic location?

Occurs in sites of primitive lymphatic lakes and can occur virtually anywhere in the body, most commonly in the floor of mouth, under the jaw, or in the neck, axilla, or thorax

What is the treatment?

Early total surgical removal because they tend to enlarge; sclerosis may be needed if the lesion is unresectable

What are the possible complications?

Enlargement in critical regions, such as the floor of the mouth or paratracheal region, may cause airway obstruction; also, they tend to insinuate onto major structures (although not malignant), making excision difficult and hazardous

ASPIRATED FOREIGN BODY (FB)

Which bronchus do FBs go into more commonly (left or right)?

Younger than age 4—50/50
Age 4 and older—most go into right bronchus because it develops into a straight shot (less of an angle)

What is the most commonly aspirated object?

Peanut

What is the associated risk with peanut aspiration?

Lipoid pneumonia

How can an FB result in "air trapping and hyperinflation"?

By forming a "ball valve" (i.e., air in, no air out) as seen on CXR as a hyperinflated lung on expiratory film

How can you tell on A-P CXR if a coin is in the esophagus or the trachea?

Coin in **esophagus** results in the coin lying "en face" with face of the coin viewed as a **round object** because of compression by anterior and posterior structures

If coin is in the **trachea,** it is viewed as a **side projection** due to the U-shaped cartilage with membrane posteriorly

What is the treatment of tracheal or esophageal FB?

Remove FB with **rigid** bronchoscope or **rigid** esophagoscope

CHEST

What is the differential diagnosis of a lung mass?

Bronchial adenoma (carcinoid is most common), pulmonary sequestration, pulmonary blastoma, rhabdomyosarcoma, chondroma, hamartoma, leiomyoma, mucus gland adenoma, metastasis

What is the differential diagnosis of mediastinal tumor/mass?

1. Neurogenic tumor (ganglioneuromas, neurofibromas)
2. Teratoma
3. Lymphoma
4. Thymoma

(T's: teratoma, terrible lymphoma, thymoma, thyroid tumor)

Rare: pheochromocytoma, hemangioma, rhabdomyosarcoma, osteochondroma

PECTUS DEFORMITY

What heart abnormality is associated with pectus abnormality?

Mitral valve prolapse (many patients receive preoperative echocardiogram)

PECTUS EXCAVATUM

What is it?

Chest wall deformity with sternum caving inward (think: ex**CAV**atum = **CAVE**)

What is the cause?

Abnormal, unequal overgrowth of rib cartilage

What are the signs/ symptoms?	Often asymptomatic; mental distress, dyspnea on exertion, chest pain
What is the treatment?	Open perichondrium, remove abnormal cartilage, place substernal strut; new cartilage grows back in the perichondrium in normal position; remove strut 6 months later
What is the NUSS procedure?	Placement of metal strut to elevate sternum **without** removing cartilage

PECTUS CARINATUM

What is it?	Chest wall deformity with sternum outward (pectus = chest, carinatum = pigeon); much less common than pectus excavatum
What is the cause?	Abnormal, unequal overgrowth of rib cartilage
What is the treatment?	Open perichondrium and remove abnormal cartilage. Place substernal strut. New cartilage grows into normal position. Remove strut 6 months later.

ESOPHAGEAL ATRESIA WITHOUT TRACHEOESOPHAGEAL (TE) FISTULA

What is it?	Blind-ending esophagus from atresia
What are the signs?	Excessive oral secretions and inability to keep food down
How is the diagnosis made?	Inability to pass NG tube; plain x-ray shows tube coiled in upper esophagus and no gas in abdomen
What is the primary treatment?	Suction blind pouch, IVFs, (gastrostomy to drain stomach if prolonged preoperative esophageal stretching is planned)
What is the definitive treatment?	Surgical with 1° anastomosis, often with preoperative stretching of blind pouch (other options include colonic or jejunal

interposition graft or gastric tube formation if esophageal gap is long)

ESOPHAGEAL ATRESIA WITH TRACHEOESOPHAGEAL (TE) FISTULA

What is it?

Esophageal atresia occurring with a fistula to the trachea; occurs in more than 90% of cases of esophageal atresia

What is the incidence?

One in 1500 to 3000 births

Define the following types of fistulas/atresias:

Type A

Esophageal atresia without TE fistula (8%)

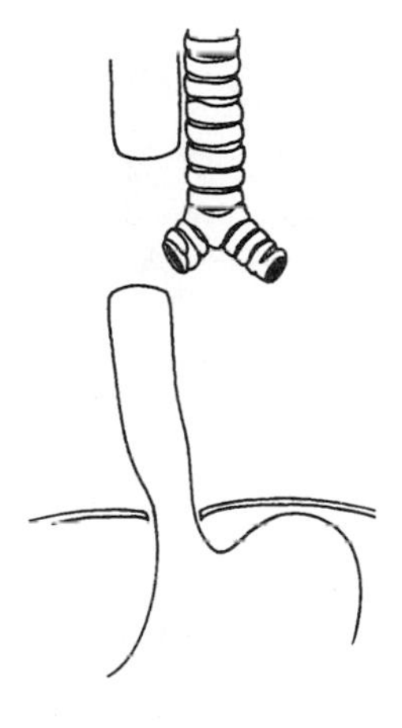

Type B

Proximal esophageal atresia with proximal TE fistula (1%)

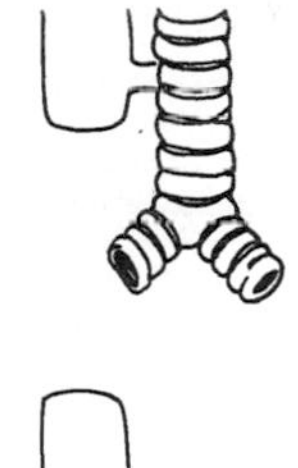

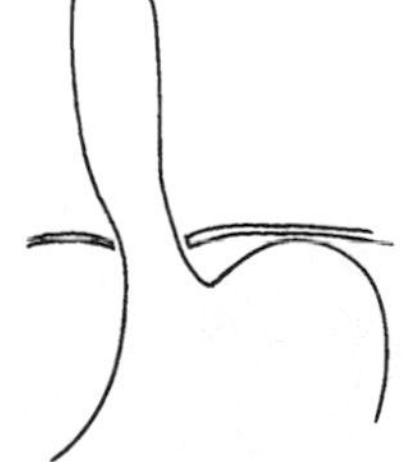

Type C Proximal esophageal atresia with distal TE fistula (85%); most common type

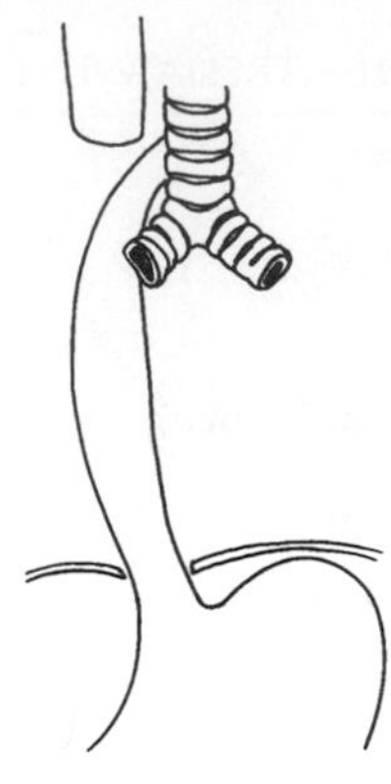

Type D Proximal esophageal atresia with both proximal and distal TE fistulas (2%) (think D = double connection to trachea)

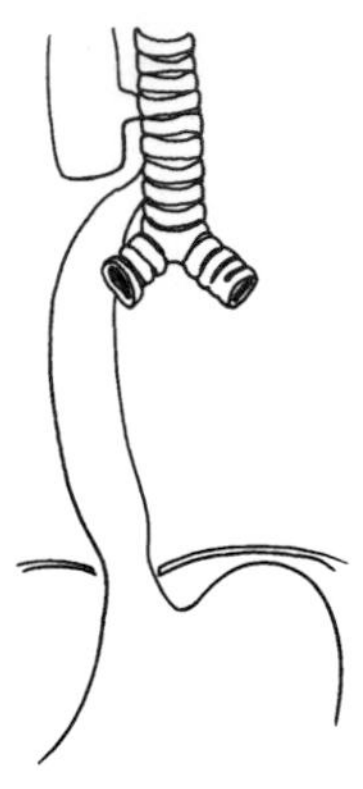

Type E "H-type" TE fistula without esophageal atresia (4%)

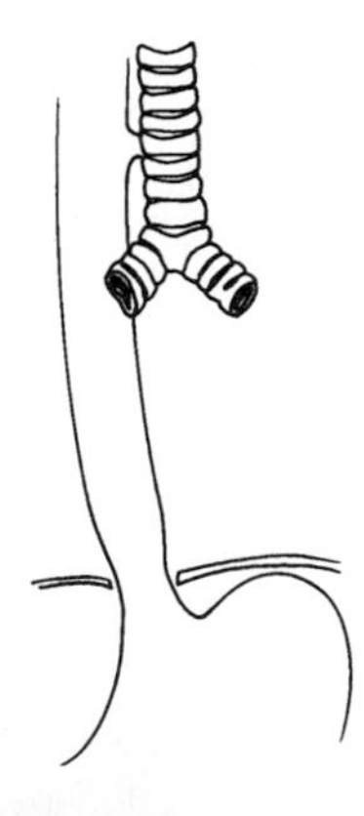

How do you remember which type is most common?
Simple: the most Common type is type C.

What are the symptoms?
Excessive secretions caused by an accumulation of saliva (may not occur with type E)

What are the signs?
Obvious respiratory compromise, aspiration pneumonia, postprandial regurgitation, gastric distention as air enters the stomach directly from the trachea

How is the diagnosis made?
Failure to pass an NG tube (although this will not be seen with type E); plain film demonstrates tube coiled in the upper esophagus, "pouchogram" (contrast in esophageal pouch); gas on AXR (tracheo-esophageal fistula)

What is the initial treatment?
Directed toward minimizing complications from aspiration:
1. Suction blind pouch (NPO/TPN)
2. Upright position of child
3. Prophylactic antibiotics (Amp/gent)

What is the definitive treatment?
Surgical correction via a thoracotomy, usually through the right chest with division of fistula and end-to-end esophageal anastomosis, if possible

What can be done to lengthen the proximal esophageal pouch?
Delayed repair: with or without G-tube and daily **stretching** of proximal pouch

Which type should be fixed via a right neck incision?
"H-Type" (type E) is high in the thorax and can most often be approached via a right neck incision.

What is the work up of a patient with a T-E fistula?
To evaluate the T-E fistula and **associated anomalies:** CXR, AXR, US of kidneys, cardiac echo (rest of work-up directed by physical exam)

What are the associated anomalies?
VACTERL cluster (present in about 10% of cases):
Vertebral or **v**ascular, **A**norectal, **C**ardiac, **TE** fistula, **E**sophageal atresia

Radial limb and **r**enal abnormalities, **L**umbar and limb
Previously known as **VATER:** **V**ertebral, **A**nus, **TE** fistula, **R**adial

What is the significance of a "gasless" abdomen on AXR?
No air to the stomach and, thus, no tracheoesophageal fistula

CONGENITAL DIAPHRAGMATIC HERNIA

What is it?
Failure of complete formation of the diaphragm, leading to a defect through which abdominal organs are herniated

What is the incidence?
One in 2100 live births; males are more commonly affected

What are the types of hernias?
Bochdalek and Morgagni

What are the associated positions?
Bochdalek—posterolateral with L > R (think: "Bochdalek = back to the left")
Morgagni—anterior parasternal hernia, relatively uncommon

What are the signs?
Respiratory distress as the bowel in the thorax impedes lung development with lung hypoplasia in both lungs and pulmonary hypertension; dyspnea, tachypnea, retractions, and cyanosis; at birth, swallowed air further distends the intestine, compressing the lung and causing a mediastinal shift, impeding venous return to thorax, and ventilation of contralateral lung; may also auscultate bowel sounds in the chest

What is the treatment?
NG tube, ET tube, stabilization, and if patient is stable, surgical repair; if patient is unstable, to the ECMO then to the OR, when deemed feasible

PULMONARY SEQUESTRATION

What is it?
Abnormal benign lung tissue with separate blood supply that **DOES NOT** communicate with the normal tracheobronchial airway

Define the following terms:

Interlobar — Sequestration in the normal lung tissue covered by normal visceral pleura

Extralobar — Sequestration not in the normal lung covered by its own pleura

What are the signs/symptoms? — Asymptomatic, recurrent pneumonia

How is the diagnosis made? — CXR, chest CT, A-gram, U/S with Doppler flow to ascertain blood supply

What is the treatment of each type:

Extralobar? — Surgical resection

Intralobar? — Lobectomy

What is the major risk during operation for sequestration? — Anomalous blood supply from below the diaphragm (can be cut and retracted into the abdomen and result in exsanguination!); always document blood supply by A-gram or U/S with Doppler flow

ABDOMEN

What is the differential diagnosis of pediatric upper GI bleeding? — Gastritis, esophagitis, gastric ulcer, duodenal ulcer, esophageal varices, foreign body, epistaxis, coagulopathy, vascular malformation, duplication cyst

What is the differential diagnosis of pediatric lower GI bleeding? — Upper GI bleeding, anal fissures, NEC (premature infants), midgut volvulus (usually children younger than 1 year), strangulated hernia, intussusception, Meckel's diverticulum, infectious diarrhea, polyps, IBD, hemolytic uremic syndrome, Henoch-Schönlein purpura, vascular malformation, coagulopathy

What is the differential diagnosis of neonatal bowel obstruction? — Malrotation with volvulus, intestinal atresia, duodenal web, annular pancreas, imperforate anus, Hirschsprung's disease, NEC, intussusception (rare), Meckel's diverticulum, incarcerated hernia, meconium ileus, meconium plug, maternal narcotic abuse (ileus), maternal hypermagnesemia (ileus), sepsis ileus

What is the differential diagnosis of infant constipation?

Hirschsprung's disease, CF, anteriorly displaced anus, polyps

INGUINAL HERNIA

What is the most commonly performed procedure by U.S. pediatric surgeons?

Indirect inguinal hernia repair

What is the most common inguinal hernia in children?

Indirect

What is an indirect inguinal hernia?

Hernia lateral to Hesselbach's triangle into the internal inguinal ring and down the inguinal canal (think: through the abdominal wall indirectly into the internal ring and out through the external inguinal ring)

What is Hesselbach's triangle?

A triangle formed by:

1. Epigastric vessels
2. Inguinal ligament
3. Lateral border of the rectus sheath

What type of hernia goes through Hesselbach's triangle?

A direct hernia from a weak abdominal floor; rare in children (0.5% of all inguinal hernias)

What is the incidence of indirect inguinal hernia in all children?

Approximately 3%

What is the incidence in premature infants?

Up to 30%

What is the male to female ratio?

6:1

What are the risk factors for an indirect inguinal hernia?

Male gender, ascites, V-P shunt, prematurity, family history, meconium ileus, abdominal wall defect elsewhere, hypo/epispadias, connective tissue disease, bladder exstrophy, undescended testicle, CF

Which side is affected more commonly?

Right (about 60%:40%)

What percentage are bilateral?	Approximately 15%
What percentage have a family history of indirect hernias?	Approximately 10%
What are the signs/ symptoms?	Groin bulge, scrotal mass, thickened cord, silk glove sign
What is the silk glove sign?	The hernia sac rolls under the finger like the finger of a silk glove.
Why should it be repaired?	Risk of incarcerated/strangulated bowel or ovary; will not go away on its own
How is a pediatric inguinal hernia repaired?	High ligation of hernia sac (no repair of the abdominal wall floor, which is a big difference between the procedure in children and adults; high refers to high position on the sac neck next to the peritoneal cavity)
Which infants need over-night apnea monitoring/ observation?	Premature infants; infants younger than 3 months of age
What is the risk of recur-rence after high ligation of an indirect pediatric hernia?	Approximately 1%
Describe the steps in the repair of an indirect inguinal hernia from skin to skin.	Cut skin, then fat, then Scarpa's fascia, then external oblique fascia through the external inguinal ring; find hernia sac anteriomedially and bluntly separate from the other cord structures; ligate sac high at the neck at the internal inguinal ring; resect sac and allow sac stump to retract into the peritoneal cavity; close external oblique; close Scarpa's fascia; close skin.
Define the following terms:	
Cryptorchidism	Failure of the testicle to descend into the scrotum
Hydrocele	Fluid-filled sac (i.e., fluid in a patent processus vaginalis or in the tunica vaginalis around the testicle)

Communicating hydrocele — Hydrocele that communicates with the peritoneal cavity and thus fills and drains peritoneal fluid or gets bigger, then smaller

Noncommunicating hydrocele — Hydrocele that does not communicate with the peritoneal cavity; stays about the same size

Can a hernia be ruled out if an inguinal mass transilluminates? — NO; baby bowel is very thin and will often transilluminate.

CLASSIC INTRAOPERATIVE QUESTIONS DURING REPAIR OF AN INDIRECT INGUINAL HERNIA

From what abdominal muscle layer is the cremaster muscle derived? — Internal oblique muscle

From what abdominal muscle layer is the inguinal ligament (A.K.A. Poupart's ligament) derived? — External oblique muscle

What nerve travels with the spermatic cord? — Ilioinguinal nerve

What is in the spermatic cord (5 structures)?

1. Cremasteric muscle fibers
2. Vas deferens
3. Testicular artery
4. Testicular pampiniform venous plexus
5. With or without hernia sac

What is the hernia sac made of? — Basically peritoneum or a patent processus vaginalis

What is the name of the fossa between the testicle and epididymis? — Fossa of Gerald

What attaches the testicle to the scrotum? — The gubernaculum

How can the opposite side be assessed for a hernia intraoperatively? — Many surgeons operatively explore the opposite side when they repair the affected side.

A laparoscope is placed into the abdomen

via the hernia sac and the opposite side internal inguinal ring is examined.

Name the remnant of the processus vaginalis around the testicle.

Tunica vaginalis

What is a Littre's inguinal hernia?

Hernia with a Meckel's diverticulum in the hernia sac

What may a yellow/orange tissue that is not fat be on the spermatic cord/testicle?

Adrenal rest

What is the most common organ in an inguinal hernia sac in boys?

Small intestine

What is the most common organ in an inguinal hernia sac in girls?

Ovary/fallopian tube

What lies in the inguinal canal in girls instead of the vas?

Round ligament

Where in the inguinal canal does the hernia sac lie in relation to the other structures?

Anteriomedially

What is a "cord lipoma"?

Preperitoneal fat on the cord structures (pushed in by the hernia sac); not a real lipoma
Should be removed surgically, if feasible

Within the spermatic cord, do the vessels or the vas lie medially?

The vas is medial to the testicular vessels.

What is a small outpouching of testicular tissue off of the testicle?

Testicular appendage (A.K.A. the appendix testes); should be removed with electrocautery

What is a "blue dot sign"?

A blue dot on the scrotal skin from a twisted testicular appendage

How is a transected vas treated?

Repair with primary anastomosis

How do you treat a transected ilioinguinal nerve?
Should not be repaired; many surgeons place a metallic clip on it to inhibit neuroma formation

What happens if you cut the ilioinguinal nerve?
Loss of sensation to the medial aspect of the inner thigh and scrotum/labia; loss of cremasteric reflex

MISCELLANEOUS

Define the following terms:

Phimosis
Fibrous attachment of the foreskin to the underlying penile glans; the foreskin will not retract

Paraphimosis
Inability to place the foreskin over the glans of the penis (foreskin stays retracted) (Think: Para = around)

Posthitis
Foreskin infection

What is the disadvantage of a foreskin?
Associated with: phimosis, paraphimosis, posthitis, hygiene, UTIs, penile cancer (very small, but real, risk)

TESTICULAR TORSION

What is it?
Torsion (twist) of the spermatic cord resulting in venous outflow obstruction and subsequent arterial occlusion → infarction of the testicle

What is the classic history?
Acute onset of scrotal pain after vigorous activity or minor trauma

What is a "Bell clapper" deformity?
Bilateral nonattachment of the testicles by the gubernaculum to the scrotum (like the clappers of a bell)

What are the symptoms?
Pain in the scrotum, suprapubic pain

What are the signs?
Very tender, swollen, elevated testicle; nonillumination

What is the differential diagnosis?
Testicular trauma, inguinal hernia, epididymitis, appendage torsion

How is the diagnosis made?
Surgical exploration, U/S (solid mass) and Doppler flow study, cold Tc-99m scan

What is the treatment?
Surgical detorsion and bilateral orchiopexy to scrotum

Within how much time from the onset of symptoms must the testicle be detorsed?
Less than 6 hours will yield the best results.

GERD

What is it?
Gastro **E**sophageal **R**eflux **D**isease

What are the causes?
LES malfunction/malposition, hiatal hernia, gastric outlet obstruction, partial bowel obstruction, common in cerebral palsy

What are the signs/ symptoms?
Spitting up, emesis, URTI, pneumonia, laryngospasm from aspiration of gastric contents into the tracheobronchial tree, failure to thrive

How is the diagnosis made?
24 hour Ph probe, bronchoscopy, UGI (manometry, EGD, US)

What cytologic aspirate finding on bronchoscopy can diagnose aspiration of gastric contents?
Lipid-laden macrophages (from phagocytosis of fat)

What is the medical/ conservative treatment?
H_2 blockers
Small meals
Elevation of head

What is the surgical treatment?
Nissen 360° fundoplication, with or without G tube

CONGENITAL PYLORIC STENOSIS

What is it?
Hypertrophy of smooth muscle of pylorus, resulting in obstruction of outflow

What are the associated risks?
Family history, firstborn males are affected most commonly, decreased incidence in African-American population

What is the incidence?
One in 750 births, male to female ratio = 4:1

What is the average age at onset?
Usually from 2 weeks after birth to about 2 months (2 to 2)

What are the symptoms?
Increasing frequency of regurgitation, leading to eventual nonbilious projectile vomiting

What are the signs?
Abdominal mass or "olive" in epigastric region (85%), hypokalemic hypochloremic metabolic alkalosis, icterus (10%), visible gastric peristalsis, paradoxic aciduria, hematemesis (< 10%)

What is the differential diagnosis?
Pylorospasm, milk allergy, increased ICP, hiatal hernia, GERD, adrenal insufficiency, uremia, malrotation, duodenal atresia, annular pancreas, duodenal web

How is the diagnosis made?
Usually by history and physical exam alone
U/S—demonstrates elongated (> 15 mm) pyloric channel and thickened muscle wall (> 3.5 mm)
If U/S is nondiagnostic, then barium swallow—shows "string sign" or "double railroad track sign"

What is the initial treatment?
Hydration and correction of alkalosis with D10 NS plus 20 mEq of KCl; *Note:* the infant's liver glycogen stores are very small; therefore, use D10; Cl^- and hydration will correct the alkalosis.

What is the definitive treatment?
Surgical, via Fredet-Ramstedt pyloromyotomy (division of circular muscle fibers without entering the lumen/mucosa)

What are the postoperative complications?
Unrecognized incision through the duodenal mucosa, bleeding, wound infection, aspiration pneumonia

What is the appropriate postoperative feeding?
Between 6 and 12 hours postoperative feeding with Pedialyte, advanced to full-strength formula over 24 hours

Which vein crosses the pylorus?
Vein of Mayo

DUODENAL ATRESIA

What is it?
Complete obstruction or stenosis of duodenum caused by an ischemic insult during development or failure of recanalization

What is the anatomic location?
85% are distal to the ampulla of Vater, 15% are proximal to the ampulla of Vater (these present with nonbilious vomiting).

What are the signs?
Bilious vomiting (if distal to the ampulla), epigastric distention

What is the differential diagnosis?
Malrotation with Ladd's bands, annular pancreas

How is the diagnosis made?
Plain abdominal film revealing "double bubble," with one air bubble in the stomach and the other in the duodenum

What is the treatment?
Duodenoduodenostomy or duodenojejunostomy

What are the associated abnormalities?
Between 50% and 70% have cardiac, renal, or other gastrointestinal defects; 30% have trisomy 21

JEJUNAL AND ILEAL ATRESIA

What is it?
Obstruction from atresia or stenosis resulting from a late mesenteric vascular accident caused by intrauterine volvulus, malrotation, internal hernia, intussusception, or strangulation in an abdominal wall defect

What are the signs?
Bilious vomiting, abdominal distention, failure to pass meconium (possibly), 3 to 4 air-fluid bubbles on plain films, jaundice (40%), microcolon from disuse, history of polyhydramnios (35%)

What is the primary treatment?
NG tube, fluid resuscitation

What is the definitive treatment?
Surgical resection of atretic loop with reanastomosis, with possible tapering of dilated proximal loop

MECONIUM ILEUS

What is it?	Intestinal obstruction from solid meconium concretions
What is the incidence?	Occurs in about 15% of infants with CF
What percentage of patients with meconium ileus have CF?	More than 95%
What are the signs/symptoms?	Bilious vomiting, abdominal distention, failure to pass meconium, Neuhauser's sign, peritoneal calcifications
What is Neuhauser's sign?	A.K.A. "soap bubble" sign: ground glass appearance in the RLQ on AXR from viscous meconium mixing with air
How is the diagnosis made?	Family history of CF, plain abdominal films showing significant dilation of similar-sized bowel loops, but few if any air-fluid levels, BE may demonstrate "microcolon" and inspissated meconium pellets in the terminal ileum
What is the treatment?	Nonoperative clearance of meconium using Gastrografin enema, which is hypertonic and therefore draws fluid into lumen, separating meconium pellets from bowel wall (60% success rate)
What is the surgical treatment?	If enema is unsuccessful, then enterotomy with intraoperative catheter irrigation using acetylcysteine (Mucomyst)
What is the long-term medical treatment?	Pancreatic enzyme replacement
What is cystic fibrosis (CF)?	Inherited disorder of epithelial Cl^- transport defect affecting sweat glands, airways, and GI tract (pancreas, intestine); diagnosed by sweat test (elevated levels of NaCl > 60 mEq/liter) and genetic testing
What is DIOS?	**D**istal **I**ntestinal **O**bstruction **S**yndrome = intestinal obstruction in older patients

with CF from inspissated luminal contents

MECONIUM PERITONITIS

What is it?

A sign of **intrauterine** bowel perforation; sterile meconium leads to an intense local inflammatory reaction with eventual formation of calcifications

What are the signs?

Calcifications on plain films

MECONIUM PLUG SYNDROME

What is it?

Colonic obstruction from unknown factors that dehydrate meconium, forming a "plug"

What are the signs/ symptoms?

Abdominal distention and **failure to pass meconium within first 24 hours of life;** plain films demonstrate many loops of distended bowel and air-fluid levels

What is the treatment?

Contrast enema is both diagnostic and therapeutic; it demonstrates "microcolon" to the point of dilated colon (usually in transverse colon) and reveals copious intraluminal material.

What is the major differential diagnosis?

Hirschsprung's disease

Is meconium plug highly associated with CF?

No; less than 5% of patients have CF, in contrast to meconium ileus, in which nearly all have CF (95%)

ANORECTAL MALFORMATIONS

What are they?

Malformations of the distal GI tract in the general categories of anal atresia, imperforate anus, and rectal atresia

IMPERFORATE ANUS

What is it?

Congenital absence of normal anus (complete absence or fistula)

Define a "high" imperforate anus.	Rectum patent to level above puborectalis sling
Define "low" imperforate anus.	Rectum patent to below puborectalis sling
Which type is much more common in women?	Low
What are the associated anomalies?	**V**ertebral abnormalities, **A**nal abnormalities, **TE** fistulas, **R**adial/**R**enal abnormalities, **L**umbar abnormalities (**VACTERL;** most commonly TE fistula)
What are the signs/ symptoms?	No anus, fistula to anal skin or bladder, UTI, fistula to vagina or urethra, bowel obstruction, distended abdomen, hyperchloremic acidosis
How is the diagnosis made?	Physical exam, the classic Cross table "invertogram" plain x-ray to see level of rectal gas (not very accurate), perineal ultrasound
What is the treatment of the following conditions:	
Low imperforate anus with anal fistula?	Dilatation of anal fistula and subsequent anoplasty
High imperforate anus?	Diverting colostomy and mucus fistula; neoanus is usually made at 1 year of age

HIRSCHSPRUNG'S DISEASE

What is it also known as?	Aganglionic megacolon
What is it?	Neurogenic form of intestinal obstruction in which obstruction results from inadequate relaxation and peristalsis; absence of normal ganglion cells of the rectum and colon
What are the associated risks?	Family history; 5% chance of having a second child with the affliction
What is the male to female ratio?	4:1

What is the anatomic location?	Aganglionosis begins at the anorectal line and involves rectosigmoid in 80% of cases (10% have involvement to splenic flexure, and 10% have involvement of entire colon).
What are the signs/ symptoms?	Abdominal distention and bilious vomiting; more than 95% present with failure to pass meconium in the first 24 hours; can also present later with constipation, diarrhea, and decreased growth
What is the classic history?	Failure to pass meconium in the first 24 hours of life
What is the differential diagnosis?	Meconium plug syndrome, meconium ileus, sepsis with adynamic ileus, colonic neuronal dysplasia, hypothyroidism, maternal narcotic abuse, maternal hypermagnesemia (tocolysis)
What imaging studies should be ordered?	**AXR:** reveals dilated colon **Unprepared barium enema:** reveals constricted aganglionic segment with dilated proximal segment, but this picture may not develop for 3 to 6 weeks; BE will also demonstrate retention of barium for 24 to 48 hours (normal evacuation = 10 to 18 hours)
What is needed for definitive diagnosis?	**Rectal biopsy:** for definitive diagnosis, submucosal suction biopsy is adequate in 90% of cases; otherwise, full-thickness biopsy should be performed to evaluate Auerbach's plexus
What is the "colonic transition zone"?	The transition (taper) from aganglionic small colon into the large dilated normal colon seen on BE
What is the initial treatment?	In neonates, a colostomy proximal to the transition zone prior to correction, to allow for pelvic growth and dilated bowel to return to normal size
What is a "leveling" colostomy?	The colostomy performed for Hirschsprung's disease at the level of normally

innervated ganglion cells as ascertained on frozen section intraoperatively

Describe the following procedures:

Swenson

Primary anastomosis between the anal canal and healthy bowel (rectum removed)

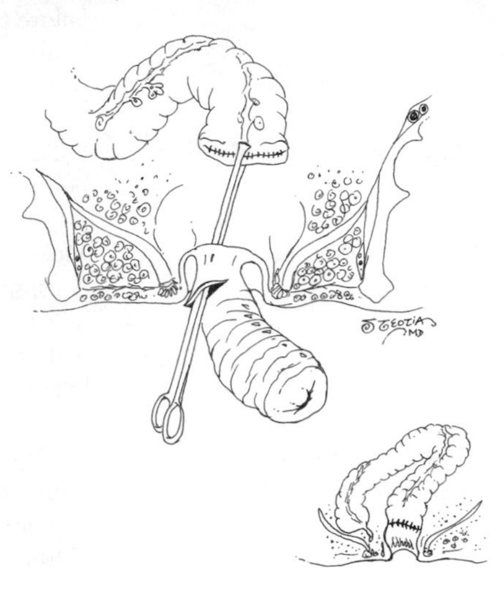

Duhamel

The anterior, aganglionic region of the rectum is preserved and anastomosed to a posterior portion of healthy bowel; a functional rectal pouch is thereby created (**think:** duha = dual barrels side by side)

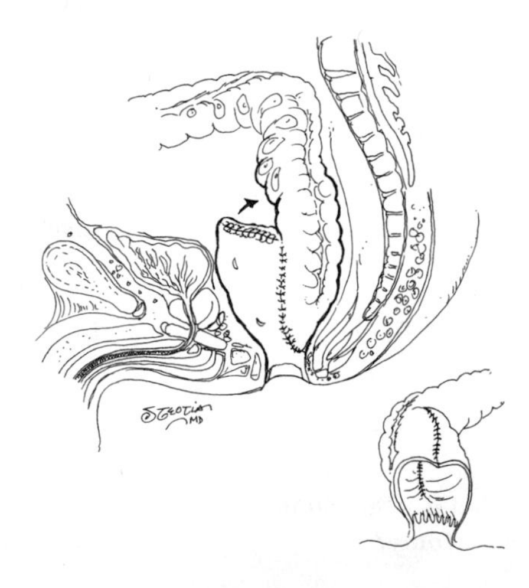

Soave — (A.K.A. endorectal pull-through); this procedure involves bringing proximal normal colon through the aganglionic rectum, which has been stripped of its mucosa but otherwise present (think: **soave** = **save** the rectum, lose the mucosa)

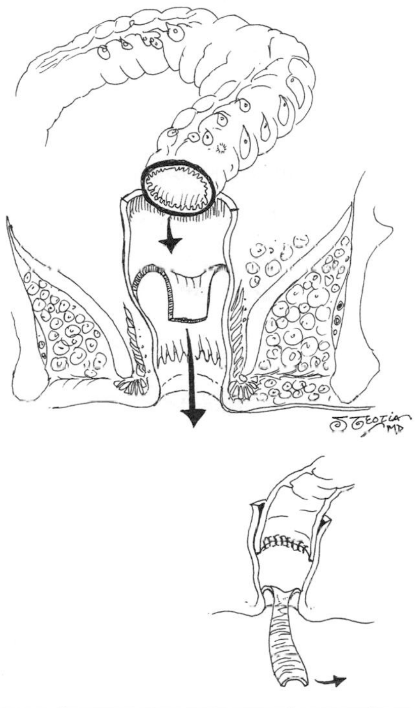

What is the new trend in surgery for Hirschsprung's disease? — No colostomy, remove aganglionic colon (as confirmed on frozen section) and perform pull-through anastomosis at the same time (Boley modification)

What is the prognosis? — Overall survival rate > 90%; > 96% of patients continent; postoperative symptoms improve with age

MALROTATION AND MIDGUT VOLVULUS

What is it? — Failure of the normal bowel rotation, with resultant abnormal intestinal attachments and anatomic positions

Where is the cecum? — With malrotation, the cecum usually ends up in the RUQ

What are Ladd's bands?

Fibrous bands that extend from the abnormally placed cecum in the RUQ, often crossing over the duodenum and causing obstruction

What is the usual age at onset?

One-third are present by 1 week of age, three-fourths by 1 month of age, and 90% by 1 year of age.

What is the usual presentation?

Sudden onset of bilious vomiting (**bilious vomiting in an infant is malrotation until proven otherwise!**)

How is the diagnosis made?

Upper GI contrast study showing cut off in duodenum; BE showing abnormal position of cecum in the upper abdomen

What are the possible complications?

Volvulus with midgut infarction, leading to death or necessitating massive enterectomy (**rapid diagnosis is essential!**)

What is the treatment?

IV antibiotics and fluid resuscitation with LR, followed by emergent laparotomy with Ladd's procedure; second-look laparotomy if bowel is severely ischemic in 24 hours to determine if remaining bowel is viable

What is the Ladd's procedure?

1. **Counterclockwise** reduction of midgut volvulus
2. Splitting of Ladd's bands
3. Division of peritoneal attachments to the cecum, ascending colon
4. Appendectomy

How is the volvulus reduced?

Rotation of the bowel in a counterclockwise direction

Where is the cecum after reduction?

In the LLQ

What is the cause of bilious vomiting in an infant until proven otherwise?

Malrotation with midgut volvulus

OMPHALOCELE

What is it?

Defect of abdominal wall at umbilical ring; sac **covers** extruded viscera

How is it diagnosed prenatally?

It may be seen on **fetal** U/S after 13 weeks' gestation, with elevated maternal AFP.

What comprises the "sac"?

Peritoneum and amnion

What organ is often found protruding from an omphalocele, but is almost never found with a gastroschisis?

The liver

What is the incidence?

Approximately 1 in 5000 births

How is the diagnosis made?

Prenatal U/S

What are the possible complications?

Malrotation of the gut, anomalies

What is the treatment?

1. NG tube for decompression
2. IV fluids
3. Prophylactic antibiotics
4. Surgical repair of the defect

What is the treatment of a small defect (< 2 cm)?

Closure of abdominal wall

What is the treatment of a medium defect (2–10 cm)?

Removal of outer membrane and placement of a silicone patch to form a "silo," temporarily housing abdominal contents; the silo is then slowly decreased in size over 4 to 7 days, as the abdomen accommodates the viscera; then the defect is closed

What is the treatment of large defects (> 10 cm)?

Skin flaps or treatment with Betadine spray, mercurochrome, or silver sulfadiazine (Silvadene) over the defect; this allows an eschar to form, which epithelializes over time, allowing opportunity for future repair months to years later

What are the associated abnormalities?

50% of cases occur with often severe abnormalities of the GI tract, cardiovascular system, GU tract, musculoskeletal system, CNS, and chromosomes.

Of what "pentalogy" is omphalocele a part?	Pentalogy of Cantrell
What is the pentalogy of Cantrell?	"D COPS": **D**iaphragmatic defect (hernia) **C**ardiac abnormality **O**mphalocele **P**ericardium malformation/absence **S**ternal cleft

GASTROSCHISIS

What is it?	Defect of abdominal wall; sac does not cover extruded viscera
How is it diagnosed prenatally?	Possible at fetal ultrasound after 13 weeks' gestation, elevated maternal AFP
Where is the defect?	Lateral to the umbilicus (right > left)
On what side of the umbilicus is the defect found?	The right (think: right = gastroschisis)
What is the usual size of the defect?	Between 2 and 4 cm
What are the possible complications?	Thick edematous peritoneum from exposure to amnionic fluid; malrotation of the gut Other complications include hypothermia; hypovolemia from third-spacing; sepsis; and metabolic acidosis from hypovolemia and poor perfusion, NEC, prolonged ileus
How is the diagnosis made?	Prenatal U/S
What is the treatment?	Primary—NG tube decompression, IV fluids (D10 LR), and IV antibiotics Definitive—surgical reduction of viscera and abdominal closure; may require staged closure with silo
What is a "silo"?	Silastic silo is a temporary housing for external abdominal contents; silo is slowly tightened over time
What is the prognosis?	More than 90% survival rate

What are the associated anomalies?	Unlike omphalocele, relatively uncommon except for intestinal atresia, which occurs in 10% to 15% of cases
What are the major differences compared with omphalocele?	No membrane coverings Uncommon associated abnormalities

POWER REVIEW OF OMPHALOCELE AND GASTROSCHISIS

What are the differences between omphalocele and gastroschisis in terms of the following characteristics:

Anomalies?	Common in omphalocele (50%), uncommon in gastroschisis
Peritoneal/amnion covering (sac)?	Always with omphalocele, never with gastroschisis
Position of umbilical cord?	On the sac with omphalocele, from skin to the left of the gastroschisis defect
Thick bowel?	Common with gastroschisis, rare with omphalocele (unless sac ruptures)
Protrusion of liver?	Common with omphalocele, almost never with gastroschisis
Large defect?	Omphalocele

APPENDICITIS

What is it?	Obstruction of the appendiceal lumen (fecalith, lymphoid hyperplasia), producing a closed loop with resultant inflammation that can lead to necrosis and perforation
What is its claim to fame?	Most common surgical disease requiring emergency surgery in children
What is the affected age?	Very rare before 3 years of age
What is the usual presentation?	Onset of referred or **periumbilical pain** followed by **anorexia,** nausea, and vomiting; *Note:* unlike gastroenteritis, **pain precedes vomiting;** pain then

migrates to the **RLQ,** where it becomes more intense and localized from local peritoneal irritation
If the patient is hungry and can eat, seriously question the diagnosis of appendicitis.

How is the diagnosis made?	History and physical exam
What are the signs/ symptoms?	Signs of peritoneal irritation may be present—guarding, muscle spasm, rebound tenderness, obturator and Psoas signs; low-grade fever rising to high grade if perforation occurs
What is the differential diagnosis?	Intussusception, volvulus, Meckel's diverticulum, Crohn's disease, ovarian torsion, cyst, tumor, perforated ulcer, pancreatitis, PID, ruptured ectopic pregnancy, mesenteric lymphadenitis
What is the common bacterial cause of mesenteric lymphadenitis?	*Yersinia enterocolitica*
What are the associated lab findings?	Increased WBC ($> 10{,}000$ per mm^3 in $> 90\%$ of cases, with a left shift in most)
What is the role of urinalysis?	To evaluate for possible pyelonephritis or renal calculus, but mild hematuria and pyuria are common in appendicitis because of ureteral inflammation
What is the "hamburger" sign?	Ask patients with suspected appendicitis if they would like a hamburger or favorite food; if they can eat, seriously question the diagnosis.
What radiographic studies may be performed?	Often none; CXR to rule out RML or RLL pneumonia; abdominal films are usually nonspecific, but calcified fecalith is present in 5% of cases; U/S to evaluate for ovarian/gynecologic pathology
What is the treatment?	**Nonperforated**—prompt appendectomy and cefoxitin to avoid perforation **Perforated**—triple antibiotics, fluid resuscitation, and prompt

	appendectomy; all pus is drained and cultures obtained, with postoperative antibiotics continued for 5 to 7 days, ± drain
How long should antibiotics be administered if nonperforated?	24 hours
How long if perforated?	Usually 5 to 7 days or until WBCs are normal and patient is afebrile
If a normal appendix is found upon exploration, what must be examined/ ruled out?	Meckel's diverticulum, Crohn's disease, intussusception, gynecologic disease
What is the approximate risk of perforation?	~ 25% after 24 hours from onset of symptoms ~ 50% by 36 hours ~ 75% by 48 hours

INTUSSUSCEPTION

What is it?	Obstruction caused by bowel telescoping into the lumen of adjacent distal bowel; may result when peristalsis carries a "leadpoint" downstream
What is the usual age at presentation?	Disease of infancy; 60% present from 4 to 12 months of age, 80% by 2 years of age
What is the most common site?	Terminal ileum involving ileocecal valve and extending into ascending colon
What is the most common cause?	Hypertrophic Peyer's patches, which act as a lead point; many patients have prior viral illness
What are the signs/ symptoms?	Alternating lethargy and irritability (colic), bilious vomiting, "currant jelly" stools, RLQ mass on plain abdominal film, empty RLQ on palpation (Dance's sign)
What is the intussuscipiens?	The recipient segment of bowel (think: "recipiens" = intussus "cipiens")

What is the intussusceptum? The leading point or bowel that enters the intussuscipiens

Identify locations 1 and 2 on the following illustration:
1. Intussuscipiens
2. Intussusceptum

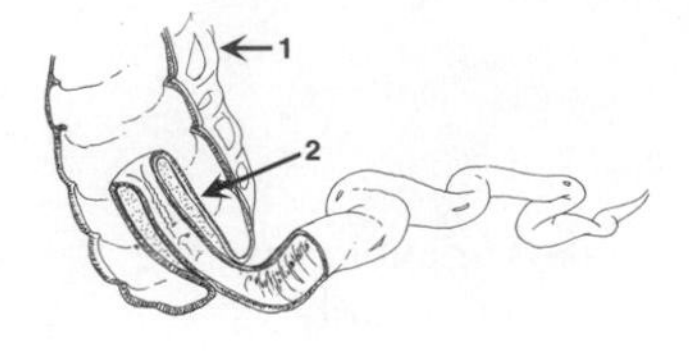

How can the spelling of intussusception be remembered? Intussusception—two "s's," followed by one 's." Think: the United States ship the U.S. = the U.S.S. U.S. (analogous to the ship the U.S.S. Constitution)

What is the treatment? **Air** or barium enema; 85% reduce with hydrostatic pressure (i.e., meter elevation); if unsuccessful, then laparotomy and reduction by "milking" the ileum from the colon should be performed

What are the causes of intussusception in older patients? Meckel's diverticulum, polyps, and tumors, all of which act as a lead point

MECKEL'S DIVERTICULUM

What is it? Remnant of the omphalomesenteric duct/vitelline duct, which connects the yolk sac with the primitive midgut in the embryo

What is the usual location? Between 45 and 90 cm proximal to the ileocecal valve on the antimesenteric border of the bowel

What is the major differential diagnosis? Appendicitis

Is it a true diverticulum? Yes; all layers of the intestine are found in the wall.

What is the incidence? 2% of the population at autopsy, but more than 90% of these are asymptomatic

What is the gender ratio?

Two to three times more common in males

What is the usual age at onset of symptoms?

Most frequently in the first 2 years of life, but can occur at any age

What are the possible complications?

Intestinal hemorrhage (painless)—50%
- Accounts for 50% of all lower GI bleeding in patients younger than 2 years; bleeding results from ectopic gastric mucosa secreting acid → ulcer → bleeding

Intestinal obstruction—25%
- Most common complication in adults; includes volvulus and intussusception

Inflammation (± perforation)—20%

What percentage of cases have heterotopic tissue?

More than 50%; usually gastric mucosa (85%), but duodenal, pancreatic, and colonic mucosa have been described

What is the most common ectopic tissue in a Meckel's diverticulum?

Gastric mucosa

What other pediatric disease entity can also present with GI bleeding secondary to ectopic gastric mucosa?

Enteric duplications

What is the most common cause of lower GI bleeding in children?

Meckel's diverticulum with ectopic gastric mucosa

What is the "rule of 2s"?

2% are symptomatic.
Found about **2 feet** from ileocecal valve
Found in **2%** of the population
Most symptoms occur before age **2**.
One of **2** will have ectopic tissue.
Most diverticula are about **2** inches long.
Male:female ratio = 2:1

What is a Meckel's scan?

Scan for ectopic gastric mucosa in Meckel's diverticulum; uses technetium **pertechnetate** IV, which is preferentially taken up by gastric mucosa

NECROTIZING ENTEROCOLITIS

What is it also known as?
NEC

What is it?
Necrosis of intestinal mucosa often with bleeding; may progress to transmural intestinal necrosis, shock/sepsis, and death

What are the predisposing conditions?
PREMATURITY
Stress: shock, hypoxia, RDS, apneic episodes, sepsis, exchange transfusions, PDA and cyanotic heart disease, hyperosmolar feedings, polycythemia, indomethacin

What is the pathophysiologic mechanism?
Probable splanchnic vasoconstriction with decreased perfusion, mucosal injury, and probable bacterial invasion

What is its claim to fame?
Most common cause of emergent laparotomy in the neonate

What are the signs/ symptoms?
Abdominal distention, vomiting, heme positive or gross rectal bleeding, fever or hypothermia, jaundice, abdominal wall erythema (consistent with perforation and abscess formation)

What are the radiographic findings?
Fixed, dilated intestinal loops; pneumatosis intestinalis (air in the bowel wall); free air; and portal vein air (sign of advanced disease)

What are the lab findings?
Low hematocrit, glucose, and platelets

What is the treatment?
Most are managed medically:
1. Cessation of feedings
2. OG tube
3. IV fluids
4. IV antibiotics
5. Ventilator support, as needed

What are the surgical indications?
Free air in abdomen revealing perforation, and positive peritoneal tap revealing transmural bowel necrosis

What is an option for bowel perforation in < 1000 gram NEC patients?
Placement of percutaneous drain (without laparotomy!)

Is portal vein gas or pneumatosis intestinalis alone an indication for operation with NEC?
No

What are the indications for peritoneal tap?
Severe thrombocytopenia, distended abdomen, abdominal wall erythema, unexplained clinical downturn

What are the possible complications?
Occur commonly and include further bowel necrosis, gram-negative sepsis, DIC, wound infection, cholestasis, short bowel syndrome, and strictures
Long-term complications: SBO

What is the prognosis?
>80% overall survival rate

BILIARY TRACT

What is "physiologic jaundice"?
Hyperbilirubinemia in the first 2 weeks of life from inadequate conjugation of bilirubin

What enzyme is responsible for conjugation of bilirubin?
Glucuronyl transferase

How is hyperbilirubinemia from "physiologic jaundice" treated?
UV light

What is Gilbert's syndrome?
Partial deficiency of glucuronosyl-transferase, leading to intermittent asymptomatic jaundice in the second or third decade of life

What is Crigler-Najjar syndrome?
Rare genetic absence of glucuronosyl-transferase activity, causing unconjugated hyperbilirubinemia, jaundice, and death from kernicterus (usually within the first year)

BILIARY ATRESIA

What is it?
Obliteration of extrahepatic biliary tree

What is the incidence?
One in 16,000 births

What are the signs/ symptoms?
Persistent jaundice (normal physiologic jaundice resolves in <2 weeks),

hepatomegaly, splenomegaly, ascites and other signs of portal hypertension, acholic stools, biliuria

What are the lab findings?

Mixed jaundice is always present (i.e., both direct and indirect bilirubin increased), with an elevated serum alkaline phosphatase level.

What is the "rule of 5s" of indirect bilirubinemia?

Bizarre: with progressive hyperbilirubinemia, jaundice progresses by levels of 5 from the head to toes: 5 mg/dl = jaundice of head, 10 mg/dl = jaundice of trunk, 15 mg/dl = jaundice of leg/feet

What is the differential diagnosis?

Neonatal hepatitis (TORCH); biliary hypoplasia

How is the diagnosis made?

1. U/S to rule out choledochal cyst and to examine extrahepatic bile ducts and gallbladder
2. HIDA scan—shows no excretion into the GI tract (with phenobarbital preparation)
3. Operative cholangiogram and liver biopsy

What is the treatment?

Early laparotomy by 2 months of age with a modified form of the Kasai hepatoportoenterostomy

How does a Kasai work?

The anastomosis of the porta hepatis and the small bowel allows drainage of bile via many microscopic bile ducts in the fibrous structure of the porta hepatis.

What if the Kasai fails?

Revise or liver transplantation

What are the possible postoperative complications?

Cholangitis (manifested as decreased bile secretion, fever, leukocytosis, and recurrence of jaundice), progressive cirrhosis (manifested as portal hypertension with bleeding varices, ascites, hypoalbuminemia, hypothrombinemia, and fat-soluble vitamin K, A, D, E deficiencies)

What are the associated abnormalities?

Between 25% and 30% have other anomalies, including annular pancreas, duodenal atresia, malrotation, polysplenic syndrome, situs inversus, and preduodenal portal vein; 15% have congenital heart defects.

CHOLEDOCHAL CYST

What is it?

Cystic enlargement of bile ducts; most commonly arises in extrahepatic ducts, but can also arise in intrahepatic ducts

What is the usual presentation?

50% present with intermittent jaundice, RUQ mass, and abdominal pain; may also present with pancreatitis.

What are the possible complications?

Cholelithiasis, cirrhosis, carcinoma, and portal HTN

What are the anatomic variants:

I?

Dilation of common hepatic and common bile duct, with cystic duct entering the cyst; most common type (90%)

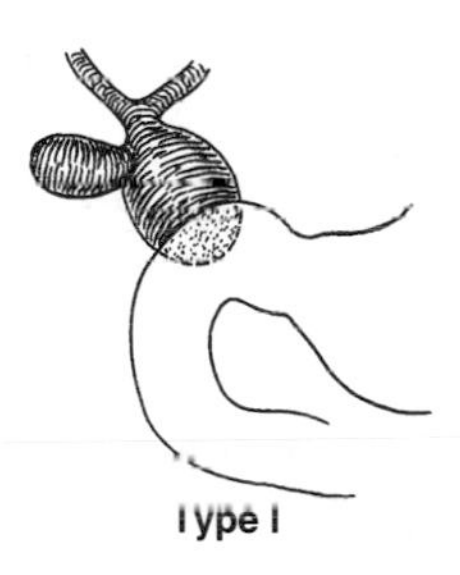
Type I

II?

Lateral saccular cystic dilation

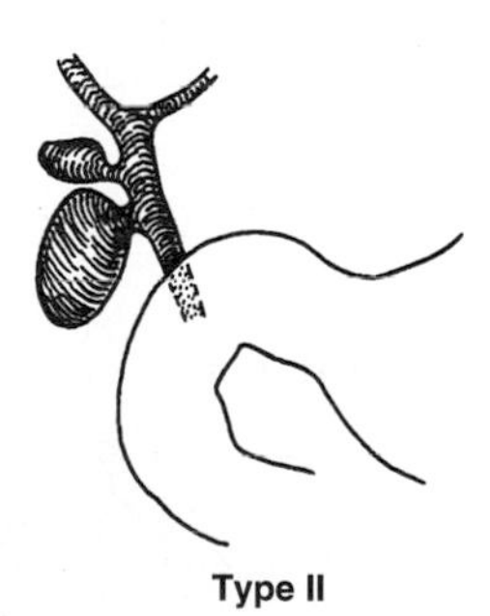
Type II

III? Choledochocele represented by an intradoudenal cyst

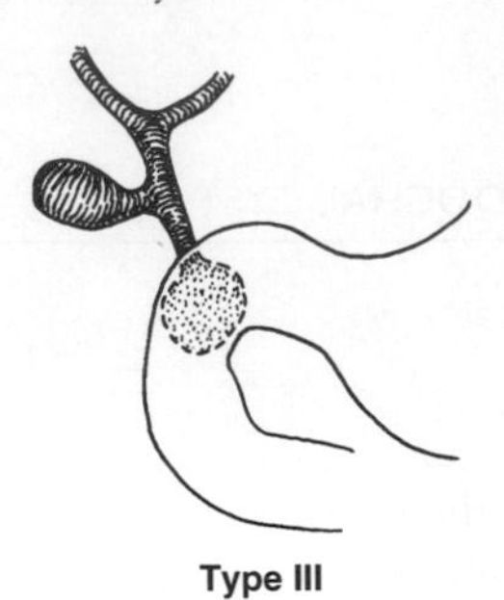

Type III

IV? Multiple extrahepatic cysts, intrahepatic cysts, or both

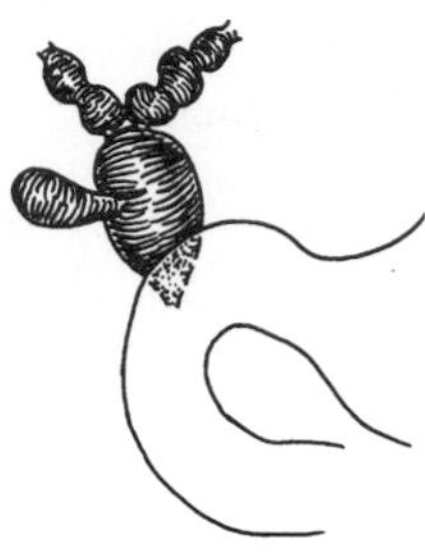

Type IV

V? Single or multiple intrahepatic cysts

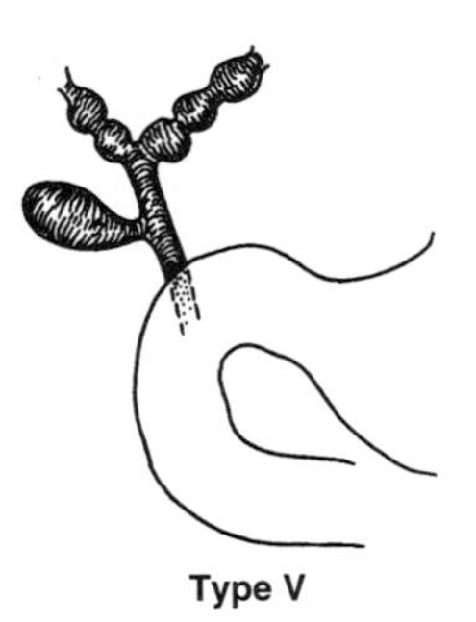

Type V

How is the diagnosis made? U/S

What is the treatment? Operative cholangiogram to clarify pathologic process and delineate the pancreatic duct, followed by complete resection of the cyst and a Roux-en-Y hepatojejunostomy

What condition are these patients at increased risk of developing?	**Cholangiocarcinoma** often arises in the cyst; therefore, treat by complete prophylactic resection of the cyst.

CHOLELITHIASIS

What is it?	The formation of gallstones
What are the common causes in children?	The etiology differs somewhat from that of adults; the most common cause is cholesterol stones, but there is an increased percentage of pigmented stones from hemolytic disorders.
What is the differential diagnosis?	Hereditary spherocytosis, thalassemia, pyruvate kinase deficiency, sickle-cell disease, cystic fibrosis, long-term parenteral nutrition, idiopathic
What are the associated risks?	Use of oral contraceptives, teenage, positive family history
What is the treatment?	Cholecystectomy is recommended for all children with gallstones.

ANNULAR PANCREAS

What is an annular pancreas?	Congenital pancreatic abnormality with complete encirclement of the duodenum by the pancreas
What are the symptoms of annular pancreas?	Duodenal obstruction
What is the treatment of annular pancreas?	Duoduodenostomy bypass of obstruction (do not resect the pancreas!)

TUMORS

What is the differential diagnosis of pediatric abdominal mass?	Wilms' tumor, neuroblastoma, hernia, intussusception, malrotation with volvulus, mesenteric cyst, duplication cyst, liver tumor (hepatoblastoma/hemangioma), rhabdomyosarcoma, teratoma

WILMS' TUMOR

What is it?	Embryonal tumor of **renal** origin
What is the incidence?	Very rare: 500 new cases in the United States per year
What is the average age at diagnosis?	Usually between 2 and 4 years of age
What are the symptoms?	Usually asymptomatic except for abdominal mass; 20% of patients present with minimal blunt trauma to mass
What are the signs?	Abdominal mass (most do not cross the midline); hematuria (10–15%); HTN in 20% of cases, related to compression of juxtaglomerular apparatus; signs of Beckwith-Wiedemann syndrome
How is the diagnosis made?	Physical exam, abdominal CT with IV contrast to evaluate collecting system, CXR to rule out lung metastases, U/S
Define the stages:	
Stage I	Limited to kidney and completely resected
Stage II	Extends beyond kidney, but completely resected; capsule invasion and perirenal tissues may be involved
Stage III	Residual nonhematogenous tumor after resection
Stage IV	Hematogenous metastases (lung, distal lymph nodes, and brain)
Stage V	Bilateral renal involvement
What are the best indicators of survival?	Stage and histologic subtype of tumor; 85% of patients have favorable histology (FH); 15% have unfavorable histology (UH); overall survival for FH is 90% for all stages
What is the treatment?	Radical resection of affected kidney with evaluation for staging, followed by

chemotherapy (low stages) and radiation (higher stages)

What are the associated abnormalities?

Aniridia, hemihypertrophy, Beckwith-Wiedemann syndrome, neurofibromatosis, horseshoe kidney

What is the Beckwith-Wiedemann syndrome?

Syndrome of:
1. Umbilical defect
2. Macroglossia (big tongue)
3. Gigantism
4. Visceromegaly (big organs) (think **W**ilms' = Beckwith-**W**iedemann)

NEUROBLASTOMA

What is it?

Embryonal tumor of neural crest origin

What are the anatomic locations?

Adrenal medulla—50%
Paraaortic abdominal paraspinal ganglia—25%
Posterior mediastinum—20%
Neck—3%
Pelvis—3%

With which type of tumor does a patient with Horner's syndrome present?

Neck, superior mediastinal tumors

What is the incidence?

One in 7,000 to 10,000 live births; most common solid malignant tumor of infancy; most common solid tumor in children outside the CNS

What is the average age at diagnosis?

Approximately 50% are diagnosed by 2 years of age
Approximately 90% are diagnosed by 8 years of age

What are the symptoms?

Vary by tumor location—anemia, failure to thrive, weight loss, and poor nutritional status with advanced disease

What are the signs?

Asymptomatic abdominal mass (palpable in 50% of cases), respiratory distress (mediastinal tumors), Horner's syndrome (upper chest or neck tumors), proptosis (with orbital metastases), subcutaneous tumor nodules, HTN (20–35%)

How is the diagnosis made?
Physical exam; 24-hour urine to measure VMA, HVA, and metanephrines (elevated in > 85%); plain x-rays (may show calcifications); CXR; CT; MIBG scan (I-Metaiodobenzylguanidine as used in pheochromocytoma); and bone marrow biopsy to rule out metastases, ferritin, neuron-specific enolase, N-*myc* oncogene, DNA ploidy

What is the difference in position of tumors in neuroblastoma versus Wilms' tumors?
Neuroblastoma may cross the midline, but Wilms' tumors do so only rarely.

What is the treatment?
Depends on staging

Define the stages:

Stage I
Tumor is confined to organ of origin.

Stage II
Tumor extends beyond organ of origin **but not** across the midline.

Stage III
Tumor extends **across the midline**.

Stage IV
Metastatic disease is found.

Stage IVS
Localized primary tumor does not cross the midline, but **remote disease** is confined to the liver, subcutaneous tissues, and bone marrow.

What is the treatment of each stage:

Stage I?
Surgical resection

Stage II?
Resection and chemotherapy

Stage III?
Resection and chemotherapy

Stage IV?
Resection and chemotherapy, with or without radiation therapy

What is the survival rate of each stage:

Stage I?
Approximately 90%

Stage II?
Approximately 80%

Stage III?
Approximately 40%

Stage IV? Approximately 15%

Stage IVS? Survival rate is more than 80%! *Note:* these tumors are basically stage I or II with metastasis to liver, subcutaneous tissue, or bone marrow; most of these patients, if younger than 1 year of age, have a spontaneous cure. (think: stage IV S = Special condition)

What are the laboratory prognosticators? Aneuploidy is favorable! The lower the number of N-*myc* oncogene copies, the better the prognosis.

Which oncogene is associated with neuroblastoma? N-*myc* oncogene
Think: **N**-*myc* = **N**euroblastoma

RHABDOMYOSARCOMA

What is it? Highly malignant **striated muscle** sarcoma

What is its claim to fame? Most common sarcoma in children

What are the most common sites?
1. Head and neck (40%)
2. GU tract (20%)
3. Extremities (20%)

Other sites: abdomen, anus, retroperitoneum, pelvis, thorax

What are the signs/symptoms? Mass

How is the diagnosis made? Tissue biopsy, CT, MRI, bone marrow, plain x-rays

What is the treatment? Surgical excision, chemotherapy, and radiation therapy

HEPATOBLASTOMA

What is it? Malignant tumor of the liver (derived from embryonic liver cells)

What is the average age at diagnosis? Presents in the first 3 years of life

What is the male to female ratio? 2:1

How is the diagnosis made?

Physical exam—abdominal distention; RUQ mass that moves with respiration
Elevated serum α-fetoprotein and ferritin (can be used as tumor markers)
CT scan of abdomen, which often predicts resectability

What percentage will have an elevated α-fetoprotein level?

Approximately 90%

What is the treatment?

Resection by lobectomy or trisegmentectomy is the treatment of choice; large tumors may require preoperative chemotherapy and **subsequent** hepatic resection.

What is the overall survival rate?

Approximately 50%

What is the major difference in age presentation between hepatoma and hepatoblastoma?

Hepatoblastoma presents at younger than 3 years of age; hepatoma presents at older than 3 years of age and in adolescents.

PEDIATRIC TRAUMA

What is the leading cause of death in pediatric patients?

Trauma

How are the vast majority of splenic and liver injuries treated in children?

Observation (i.e., nonoperatively)

What is the role of DPL in children?

Much less than with adults because most centers go to the CT scanner to evaluate the abdomen

What is a common simulator of peritoneal signs in the blunt pediatric trauma victim?

Gastric distention (place an NG tube)

What is the 20–20-10 rule for fluid resuscitation of the unstable pediatric trauma patient?

Fluid resuscitation in the unstable pediatric patient: first give a 20 cc/kg LR bolus followed by a second bolus of 20 cc/kg LR bolus if needed. If the patient is still unstable after the second LR bolus, then administer a 10cc/kg bolus of **blood**

What CT scan findings suggest small bowel injury?	Free fluid with **no** evidence of liver or spleen injury, free air, contrast leak, bowel thickening, mesentery streaking
What is the treatment for duodenal hematoma?	Observation with NGT and TPN

OTHER PEDIATRIC SURGERY QUESTIONS

What is bilious vomiting in an infant?	Malrotation, until proven otherwise! (About 90% of patients with malrotation present before the first year of life.)
What does TORCHES stand for?	Nonbacterial fetal and neonatal infections: **T**oxoplasmosis, **R**ubella, **C**ytomegalovirus (CMV), **H**erpes, **S**yphilis
What is the common pediatric sedative?	Chloral hydrate
What are the contraindications to circumcision?	Hypospadias, etc., because the foreskin might be needed for future repair of the abnormality
When should an umbilical hernia be repaired?	After 4 years of age; otherwise observe, because most close spontaneously; repair before school age if it persists
What is the cancer risk in the cryptorchid testicle?	More than ten times the normal testicular cancer rate
When should orchidopexy be performed?	All patients with undescended testicle undergo orchidopexy after 1 year of age
What are the signs of child abuse?	Cigarette burns, rope burns, scald to posterior thighs and buttocks, multiple fractures/old fractures, genital trauma, delay in accessing health care system
What is the treatment of child abuse?	**Admit the patient** to the hospital.
What is Dance's sign?	Empty RLQ in patients with ileocecal intussusception
What is the treatment of hemangioma?	Observation, because most regress spontaneously

What are the indications for operation in hemangiomas?
Severe thrombocytopenia, congestive heart failure, functional impairment (vision, breathing)

What are treatment options for hemangiomas?
Steroids, radiation, surgical resection, angiographic embolization

What is the most common benign liver tumor in children?
Hemangioma

What is Eagle-Barrett's syndrome?
A.K.A. prune belly; congenital inadequate abdominal musculature (very lax and thin)

What are the most common cancers in children?
1. Leukemia
2. CNS tumors
3. Lymphomas

What is the most common solid neoplasm in infants?
Neuroblastoma

What is the most common solid tumor in children?
CNS tumors

What syndrome must you consider in the patient with abdominal pain, hematuria, history of joint pain, and a purpuric rash?
Henoch-Schönlein syndrome; patient may also have melena (50%) or at least guaiac-positive stools (75%)

What is Apley's law?
The farther a chronically recurrent abdominal pain is from the umbilicus, the greater is the likelihood of an organic cause for the pain.

What is the most common cause of SBO in children?
Hernias

What is a patent urachus?
Persistence of the urachus, a communication between the bladder and umbilicus; presents with urine out of the umbilicus and recurrent UTIs

What is a "Replogle tube"?
10 French sump pump NG tube for babies (originally designed by Dr. Replogle for suction of the esophageal blind pouch of esophageal atresia)

What are "A's and B's"?
Apnea and **B**radycardia episodes in babies

What is the "Double Bubble" sign on AXR?
Gastric bubble and **duodenal bubble** on AXR; seen with duodenal obstruction (web, annular pancreas, malrotation with volvulus, duodenal atresia, etc.)

What is Poland's syndrome?
Absence of pectoralis major muscle
Absence of pectoralis minor muscle
Often associated with ipsilateral hand malformation
Nipple/breast/right-breast hypoplasia

What is the treatment of ATYPICAL mycobacterial lymph node infection
Surgical removal of the node

What chromosomal abnormality is associated with duodenal web/atresia/ stenosis?
Trisomy 21

POWER REVIEW

What is the usual age at presentation of the following conditions:

Pyloric stenosis?
From 2 weeks to 2 months of age

Intussusception?
From 4 months to 2 years of age (>80%)

Wilms' tumor?
Between 1 and 4 years of age

Malrotation?
Birth to 1 year of age (>85%)

Neuroblastoma?
Approximately 50% present by 2 years of age, and more than 80% present by 8 years of age

Hepatoblastoma?
Younger than 3 years of age

Appendicitis?
Older than 3 years of age

65

Plastic Surgery

Define the following terms:

Blepharoplasty
Eyelid surgery—removing excess skin/fat

Face lift
Removal of excess facial skin via hairline/chin/ear incisions

FTSG
Full **T**hickness **S**kin **G**raft

Langer's lines
The natural direction/alignment of connective tissue in the dermis (e.g., transverse lines across the abdomen); incisions perpendicular to Langer's lines result in larger scars than incision parallel to the lines

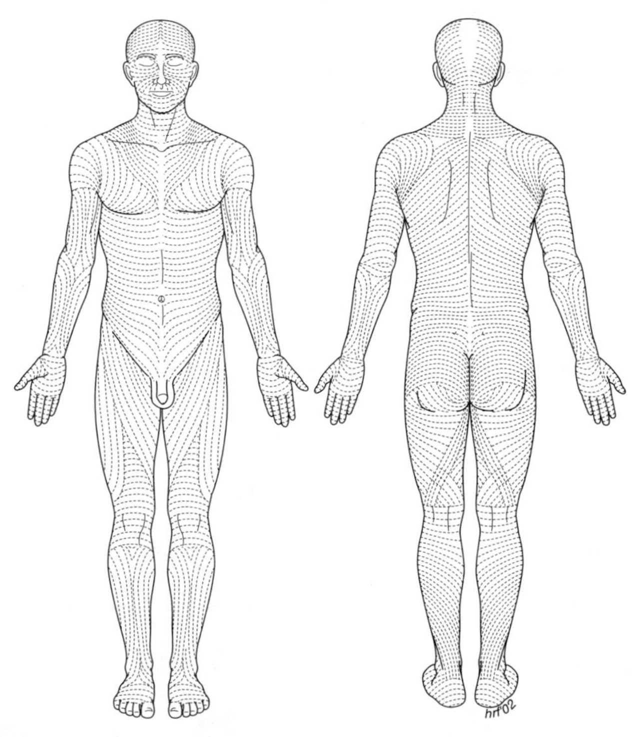

Mammoplasty Breast surgery (reduction/augmentation)

Polydactyly Extra fingers

Rhinoplasty Nose surgery, after trauma or cosmetic

STSG **S**plit **T**hickness **S**kin **G**raft

Syndactyly Webbed fingers

WOUND HEALING

What are the phases of wound healing?

1. Inflammation
2. Epithelialization
3. Fibroplasia
4. Contraction

What is a memory aid for the phases of wound healing? "**I**n **E**very **F**resh **C**ut" = **I.E.F.C.** = **I**nflammation, **E**pithelialization, **F**ibroplasia, **C**ontraction

What are the actions of the following phases:

Inflammation? Vasoconstriction followed by vasodilation, capillary leak

Epithelialization? Epithelial coverage of wound

Fibroplasia? Fibroblasts and accumulation of collagen, elastin, and reticulin

Wound contraction? Myofibroblasts contract wound

What is the maximal contraction of wound in mm/day? Less than 0.75 mm/day

EPITHELIALIZATION

What degree of bacterial contamination prevents epithelialization? More than 100,000 organisms/gm tissue (10^5)

What structures does the epithelium grow in from superficial burns/wounds? Epithelial lining of sweat glands and hair follicles

In full-thickness burns? From wound margins, grows in less than 1 cm from wound edge because no sweat glands or hair remains; this epithelium has no underlying dermis

What malignant ulcer is associated with a long-standing scar/burn?

Marjolin's ulcer (A.K.A. burn scar carcinoma

WOUND CONTRACTION

What are myofibroblasts?

Specialized fibroblasts that behave like smooth muscle cells to pull the wound edges together following granulation

Which contracts more: an STSG or an FTSG?

An STSG contracts up to 41% in surface area, whereas an FTSG contracts little, if at all.

What is granulation tissue?

Within 4 to 6 days after an open wound, development of capillary beds and fibroblasts provides a healthy base for epithelial growth from wound edges; this tissue also resists bacterial infection.

Name the local factors that impair wound healing.

Hematoma, seroma, infection, tight sutures, tight wrap

What generalized conditions inhibit wound healing?

Anemia
Malnutrition
Steroids
Cancer
Radiation
Hypoxia
Sepsis

What helps wound healing in patients taking steroids?

Vitamin A is thought to counteract the deleterious effect of steroids on wound healing.

When does a wound gain more than 80% of its maximal tensile strength?

After approximately 6 weeks

Define the following terms:

Laceration

Torn/mangled/cut wound

Abrasion

Superficial skin removal

Contusion

Bruise without a break in the skin

Keloid	Proliferative scar, progressively enlarging scar
Why not clean lacerations with Betadine?	Betadine is harmful to and inhibits normal healthy tissue.
What is the best way to clean out a laceration?	H_2O irrigation

SKIN GRAFTS

What is an STSG?	Split thickness: includes the epidermis and a variable amount of the dermis
How thick is it?	Between 12/1000 and 18/1000 of an inch (Think 12–18 = teenager.)
What is an FTSG?	Full thickness: includes the entire epidermis and dermis
What are the prerequisites for a skin graft to take?	The bed must be vascularized; a graft to a bone or tendon will not take. Bacteria must be less than 100,000. Shearing motion and fluid beneath the graft must be minimized.
What is a better bed for a skin graft: fascia or fat?	Fascia (much better blood supply)
How to increase surface area of an STSG?	Mesh it 2:1 or 4:1 (also allows for blood/serum to be removed from underneath the graft)

FLAPS

Where does a random skin flap get its blood supply?	From the dermal-subdermal plexus
Where does an axial skin flap get its blood supply?	It is vascularized by direct cutaneous arteries.
Name some axial flaps and their arterial supply.	Forehead flap—superficial temporal artery; often used for intraoral lesions Deltopectoral flap—second, third, and fourth anterior perforators of the internal mammary artery; often used for head and neck wounds Groin flap—superficial circumflex iliac

artery; allows coverage of hand and forearm wounds

What is a "free flap"?

A flap separated from all vascular supply that requires microvascular anastomosis (microscope)

What is a TRAM flap?

Transverse **R**ectus **A**bdominis **M**yocutaneous flap
(see Chapter 53)

What is a "Z-plasty"?

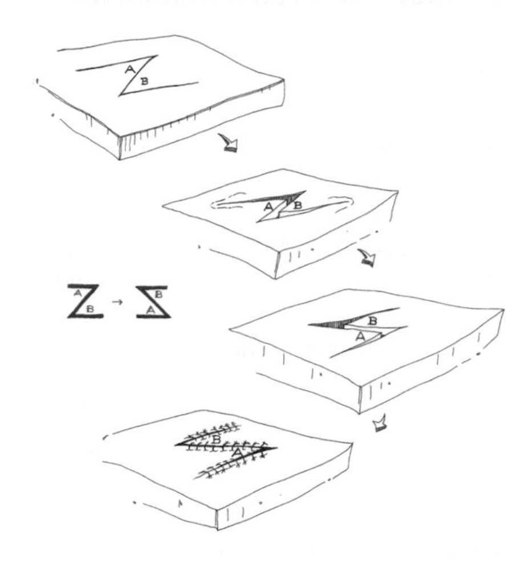

HANDS

Who operates on hands?

Plastic surgeons **and** orthopaedic surgeons

What are the bones of the hand?

Phalanges (fingers)
Metacarpal bones
Carpal bones

What is the distal finger joint?

Distal interphalangeal (DIP) joint

What is the middle finger joint?

Proximal interphalangeal (PIP) joint

What is the proximal finger joint?

Metacarpal phalangeal (MP) joint

What name is given to the "intrinsic" hand muscles?

Lumbricals

Where is "no man's land"?
The zone extending from the distal palmar crease to just beyond the PIP joint

What is the significance of the "no man's land"?
The flexor digitorum superficialis tendon and the flexor digitorum profundus tendon are ensheathed together; a hand expert needs to repair these injuries.

SENSORY SUPPLY TO THE HAND

What is the ulnar nerve distribution?

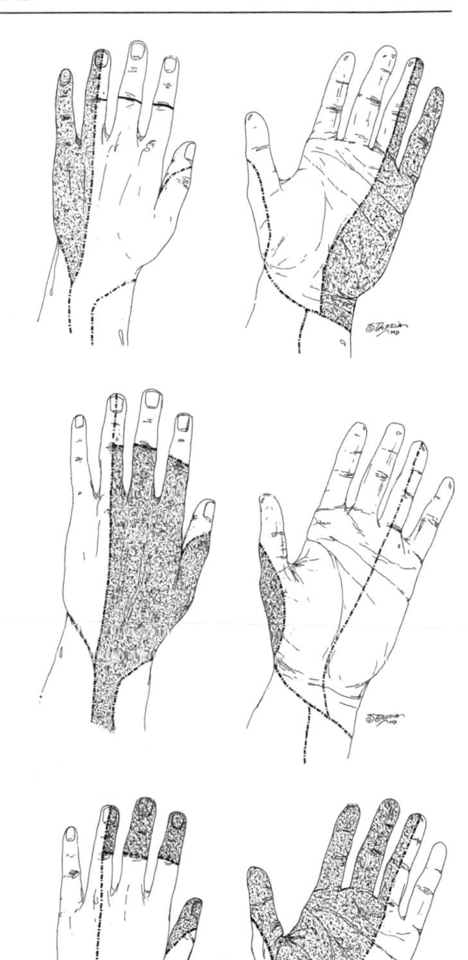

What is the radial nerve distribution?

What is the median nerve distribution?

How can the radial nerve motor function be tested?

1. Wrist and MCP extension
2. Abduction and extension of thumb

How can the ulnar nerve motor function be tested?

1. Spread fingers apart against resistance.
2. Check ability to cross index and middle fingers.

How can the median nerve function be tested?

1. Touch the thumb to the pinky (distal median nerve).
2. Squeeze examiner's finger (proximal median nerve).

How can the flexor digitorum *profundus* apparatus be tested?

Check isolated flexion of the finger DIP joint.

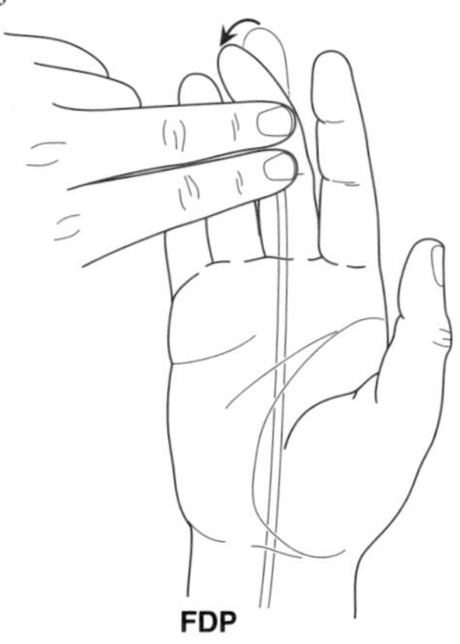

How can the flexor digitorum *superficialis* apparatus be tested?

Check isolated flexion of the finger at the MP joint.

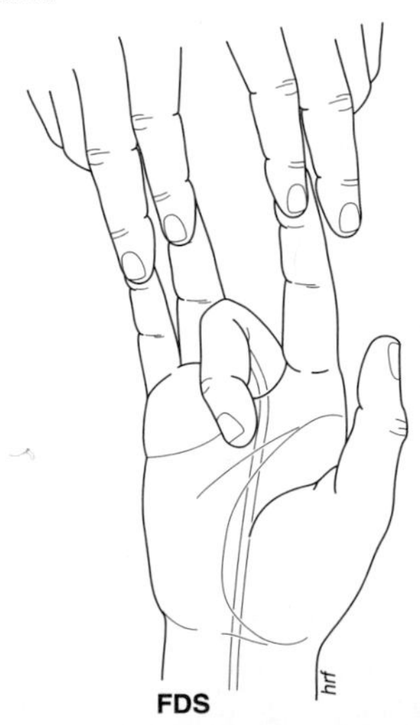

Where do the digital arteries run?	On medial and lateral sides of the digit
What hand laceration should be left unsutured?	Lacerations from human bites or animal bites
Should a clamp ever be used to stop a laceration bleeder?	**No;** use pressure and then tourniquet for definitive repair if bleeding does not cease because **nerves run with blood vessels!**
What is a felon?	Infection in **the tip** of the finger pad (**think:** felon = fingerprints = infection in pad); treat by incision and drainage
What is a paronychia?	Infection on the **side** of the finger nail (nail fold); treat by incision and drainage
What is tenosynovitis?	Tendon sheath infection
What are Kanavel's signs?	Four signs of tenosynovitis: 1. Affected finger held in slight flexion 2. Pain over volar aspect of affected finger tendon upon palpation 3. Swelling of affected finger 4. Pain on passive extension of affected finger
Most common bacteria in tenosynovitis and paronychia?	*Staphylococcus aureus*
How are human and animal hand bites treated?	Debridement/irrigation/administration of antibiotics; leave wound open
What unique bacteria are found in human bites?	*Eikenella corrodens*
What unique bacteria are found in dog and cat bites?	*Pasteurella multocida*
What is the most common hand/wrist tumor?	Ganglion cyst
What is an extremely painful type of subungual tumor?	Glomus tumor

What is a "boxer's fracture"?

Fracture of the fourth or fifth metacarpal

What is the classic deformity resulting from laceration of the extensor tendon over the DIP joint?

Mallet finger

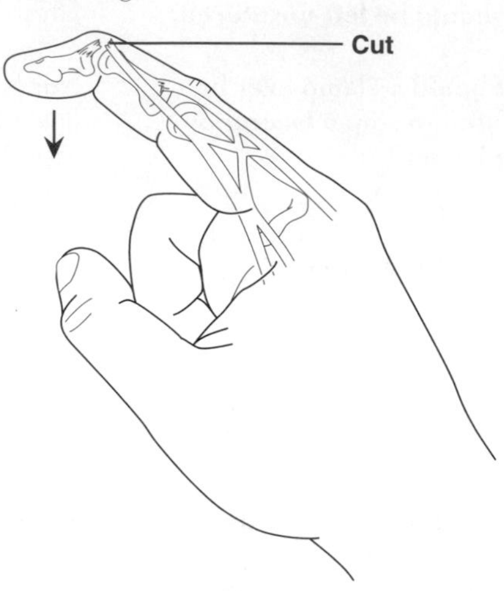

What is the classic deformity resulting from laceration of the extensor tendon over the PIP joint?

Boutonniere deformity

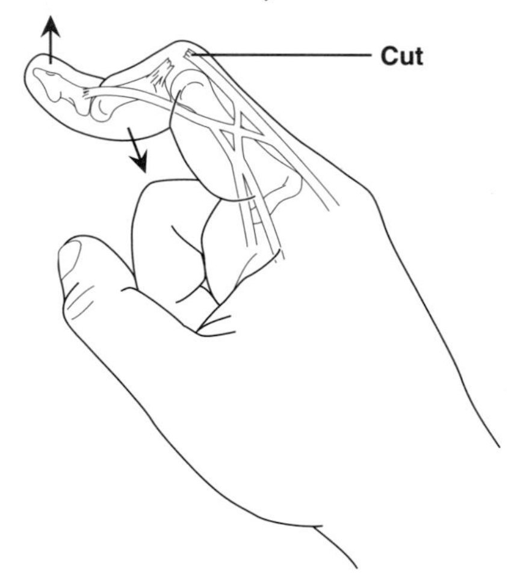

Which fracture causes pain in the "anatomic snuffbox"?

Scaphoid fracture; often not seen on x-ray at presentation, usually seen at a later date (2 weeks) on x-ray
Can result in avascular necrosis
Place in a cast if clinically suspected, regardless of x-ray findings.

What is the "safe position" of hand splinting?

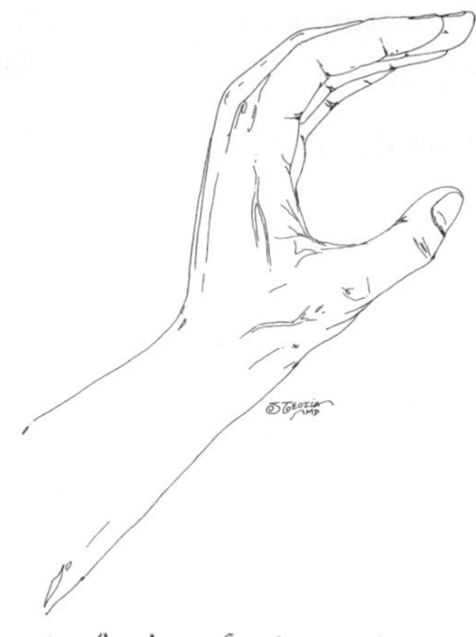

What is Dupuytren's contracture?

Fibrosis of palmar fascia, causing contracture of and inability to extend digits

What is Gamekeeper's thumb?

Injury to the ulnar collateral ligament of the thumb

How should a subungual (i.e., under the nail) hematoma be treated?

Release pressure by burning a hole in the nail (use hand-held disposable battery-operated coagulation probe).

What is a "Bible" cyst?

Ganglion cyst—they used to be treated by a good whack from a Bible!

CARPAL TUNNEL SYNDROME

What is it?

Compression of the median nerve in the carpal tunnel

What is the most common cause?

Synovitis

What are other causes?

MEDIAN TRAPS:

M = **M**edian artery (persistent)
E = **E**dema of pregnancy
D = **D**iabetes
I = **I**diopathic
A = **A**cromegaly
N = **N**eoplasm (e.g. ganglioneuroma)

T = **T**hyroid (myxedema)
R = **R**heumatoid arthritis
A = **A**myloid
P = Pneumatic drill usage
S = SLE

What are symptoms?
Pain and numbness in the median nerve distribution

What are signs?
Tinel's sign (symptoms with percussion over median nerve), Phalen's test (symptoms with flexion of wrists, thenar atrophy)

What is the work-up?
EMG, nerve conduction study

What is initial treatment?
Nonoperative + night wrist splint, vitamin B_6, NSAIDs, steroid injections

What are indications for surgery?
Refractory symptoms, thenar atrophy, thenar weakness

What surgery is performed?
Release transverse carpal ligament

66

Otolaryngology: Head and Neck Surgery

Define:

Anosmia	Inability to **smell**
Otorrhea	Fluid discharge from ear
Dysphagia	Difficulty swallowing
Odynophagia	Painful swallowing
Globus	Sensation of a "lump in the throat"

ANATOMY

Define the cranial nerves:

I	Olfactory nerve
II	Optic nerve
III	Oculomotor nerve
IV	Trochlear nerve
V	Trigeminal nerve
VI	Abducens nerve
VII	Facial nerve
VIII	Vestibulocochlear nerve
IX	Glossopharyngeal nerve
X	Vagus nerve
XI	Accessory nerve
XII	Hypoglossal nerve

Define motor/sensory actions of the following cranial nerves:	
I	Smell
II	Sight (**sensory pupil reaction**)
III	Eyeball movement, pupil sphincter, ciliary muscle (**motor pupil reaction**)
IV	Superior oblique muscle movement
V	Sensory: face, teeth, sinuses, cornea Motor: chewing (masseter muscle)
VI	Lateral rectus muscle (lateral gaze)
VII	Motor: facial muscles, lacrimal/sublingual/submandibular glands Sensory: anterior tongue/soft palate, taste
VIII	Hearing, positioning
IX	Motor: stylopharyngeus, parotid, pharynx Sensory: posterior tongue, pharynx, middle ear
X	Motor: vocal cords, heart, bronchus, GI tract Sensory: bronchus, heart, GI tract, larynx, ear
XI	Motor: trapezius muscle, sternocleidomastoid muscle
XII	Motor: tongue, strap muscles (ansa cervicalis branch)
What are the three divisions of the trigeminal nerve (cranial nerve V)?	1. Ophthalmic 2. Maxillary 3. Mandibular
What happens when the hypoglossal nerve (cranial nerve XII) is cut?	When the patient sticks out the tongue, it deviates to the same side as the injury (wheelbarrow effect).
Name the duct of the submandibular gland.	Wharton's duct

Name the duct of the parotid gland.

Stensen's duct

What is the source of blood supply to the nose?

1. Internal carotid artery: anterior and posterior ethmoidal arteries via ophthalmic artery
2. External carotid artery: superior labial artery (via facial artery) and sphenopalatine artery (via internal maxillary artery)

Name the three bones that make up the posterior nasal septum.

1. Ethmoid (perpendicular plate)
2. Vomer (Latin for plow)
3. Palatine (some also include maxillary crest)

Name the seven bones of the bony eyeball orbit.

1. Frontal
2. Zygoma
3. Maxillary
4. Lacrimal
5. Ethmoid
6. Palatine
7. Sphenoid

Which sinus is fully formed at birth?

Ethmoid sinus

Name the four strap muscles.

T.O.S.S.:
1. Thyrohyoid
2. Omohyoid
3. Sternothyroid
4. Sternohyoid

Which muscle crosses the external and internal carotid arteries?

Digastric muscle

In a neck incision, what is the first muscle incised?

Platysma

Which nerve supplies the strap muscles?

Ansa cervicalis (XII)

Which nerve runs with the carotid in the carotid sheath?

Vagus

Which nerve crosses the internal carotid artery at approximately 1 to 2 cm above the bifurcation?

Hypoglossal nerve

Name the three auditory ossicle bones.
1. Malleus (hammer)
2. Incus (anvil)
3. Stapes (stirrup)

What comprises the middle ear?
Eustachian tube, ossicle bones, tympanic membrane ("ear drum"), mastoid air cell

What comprises the inner ear?
Cochlea, semicircular canals, internal auditory canal

EAR

OTITIS EXTERNA (SWIMMER'S EAR)

What is it?
Generalized infection involving the external ear canal and often the tympanic membrane

What is the usual cause?
Prolonged water exposure and damaged squamous epithelium of the ear canal (i.e., swimming, hearing aid use)

What are the typical pathogens?
Most frequently *Pseudomonas;* may be *Proteus, Staphylococcus,* occasionally *Escherichia coli,* fungi (*Aspergillus, Candida*), or virus (herpes zoster or herpes simplex)

What are the signs/ symptoms?
Ear pain (otalgia); swelling of external ear, ear canal, or both; erythema; pain on manipulation of the auricle; debris in canal; otorrhea

What is the treatment?
Most importantly, keep the ear dry; mild infections respond to cleaning and dilute acetic acid drops. Most infections require complete removal of all debris and topical antibiotics with or without hydrocortisone (antiinflammatory); consider antifungal drops for otomycosis.

MALIGNANT OTITIS EXTERNA (MOE)

What is it?
Fulminant **bacterial** otitis externa

Is it malignant cancer?
NO!

Who is affected?
Most common scenario: an elderly patient with poorly controlled diabetes (other

forms of immunosuppression do not appear to predispose patients to MOE)

What are the causative organisms?

Usually *Pseudomonas aeruginosa*

What is the classic feature?

A nub of granulation tissue on the floor of the external ear canal at the bony–cartilaginous junction

What are the other signs/ symptoms?

Severe ear pain, excessive purulent discharge, and usually **exposed bone**

What are the diagnostic tests?

1. CT scan: shows erosion of bone, inflammation
2. Technetium-99 scan: temporal bone inflammatory process
3. Gallium-tagged white blood cell scan: to follow and document resolution

What are the complications?

Invasion of surrounding structures to produce a cellulitis, osteomyelitis of temporal bone, mastoiditis; later, a facial nerve palsy, meningitis, or brain abscess

What is the treatment?

Control of diabetes, meticulous local care with extensive debridement, hospitalization and IV antibiotics (anti-*Pseudomonas:* usually an aminoglycoside plus a penicillin)

TUMORS OF THE EXTERNAL EAR

What are the most common types?

Squamous cell most common; occasionally, basal cell carcinoma or melanoma

From what location do they usually arise?

The auricle, but occasionally from the external canal

What is the associated risk factor?

Excessive sun exposure

What is the treatment of the following conditions:

Cancers of the auricle?

Usually wedge excision

Extension to the canal?

May require excision of the external ear canal or partial temporal bone excision

Middle ear involvement? Best treated by en bloc temporal bone resection and lymph node dissection

TYMPANIC MEMBRANE (TM) PERFORATION

What is the etiology? Usually the result of trauma (direct or indirect) or secondary to middle ear infection; often occurs secondary to slap to the side of the head (compression injury)

What are the symptoms? Pain, conductive hearing loss, tinnitus

What are the signs? Bleeding from the ear, clot in the meatus, visible tear in the TM

What is the treatment? Keep dry; use systemic antibiotics if there is evidence of infection or contamination

What is the prognosis? Most (90%) heal spontaneously, though larger perforations may require surgery (e.g., fat plug, temporalis fascia tympanoplasty).

CHOLESTEATOMA

What is it? An epidermal inclusion cyst of the middle ear or mastoid, containing desquamated keratin debris; may be acquired or congenital

What are the causes? Negative middle ear pressure from eustachian tube dysfunction (primary acquired; typically in attic) or direct growth of epithelium through a TM perforation (secondary acquired)

What other condition is it often associated with? Chronic middle ear infection

What is the usual history? Chronic ear infection with chronic, malodorous drainage

What is the appearance? Grayish-white, shiny keratinous mass behind or involving the TM; often described as a "pearly" lesion

What are the associated problems?

Ossicular erosion, producing conductive hearing loss; also, local invasion resulting in:

- Vertigo/sensorineural hearing loss
- Facial paresis/paralysis
- CNS dysfunction/infection

What is the treatment?

Surgery (tympanoplasty/mastoidectomy) aimed at eradication of disease and reconstruction of the ossicular chain

BULLOUS MYRINGITIS

What is it?

A vesicular infection of the TM and adjacent deep canal

What are the causative agents?

Unknown; viral should be suspected because of frequent association with viral URI (in some instances, *Mycoplasma pneumoniae* has been cultured)

What are the symptoms?

Acute, severe ear pain; low-grade fever; and bloody drainage

What are the findings on otoscopic examination?

Large, reddish blebs on the TM, wall of the meatus, or both

Is hearing affected?

Not usually; occasional reversible sensorineural loss

What is the treatment?

Oral antibiotics (erythromycin if *Mycoplasma* is suspected); topical analgesics may be used, with resolution of symptoms usually occurring in 36 hours

ACUTE SUPPURATIVE OTITIS MEDIA (OM)

What is it?

A bacterial infection of the middle ear, often following a viral URI; may be associated with a middle ear effusion

What is the cause?

Dysfunction of the eustachian tube that allows bacterial entry from nasopharynx; often associated with an occluded eustachian tube, although it is uncertain whether this is a cause or a result of the infection

What are the predisposing factors?

Young age, male gender, bottle feeding, crowded living conditions (i.e., day care), cleft palate, Down's syndrome, cystic fibrosis

What is the etiology?

1. *Streptococcus pneumoniae* (one-third of cases)
2. *Haemophilus influenzae*
3. *Moraxella catarrhalis*
4. *Staphylococcus*
5. β-hemolytic strep
6. *Pseudomonas aeruginosa*
7. Viral/no culture

What is the etiology in infants younger than 6 months?

1. *Staphylococcus aureus*
2. *E. coli*
3. *Klebsiella*

What are the symptoms?

Otalgia, fever, decreased hearing, infant pulls on ear, increased irritability; as many as 25% of patients are asymptomatic

What are the signs?

Early, redness of the TM; later, TM bulging with loss of the normal landmarks; finally, impaired TM mobility on pneumatic otoscopy

If pain disappears instantly what may have happened?

TM perforation!

What are the complications?

TM perforation, acute mastoiditis, meningitis, brain abscess, extradural abscess, labyrinthitis; if recurrent or chronic, OM may have adverse effects on speech and cognitive development as a result of decreased hearing

What is the treatment?

10-day course of antibiotics; amoxicillin is the first-line agent; if the patient is allergic to PCN, trimethoprim-sulfamethoxazole or erythromycin should be administered

What is the usual course?

Symptoms usually resolve in 24 to 36 hours.

What are the indications for myringotomy and PE tube placement?

1. Persistent middle ear effusion over 3 months
2. Debilitated or immunocompromised patient

3. More than three episodes over 6 months (especially if bilateral)

What is a PE tube?

Pneumatic **E**qualization tube (tube placed across tympanic membrane)

What is a Bezold's abscess?

Abscess behind the superior attachment of the sternocleidomastoid muscle resulting from extension of a mastoiditis infection

What are causes of chronic otitis media?

Mixed, *S. aureus, P. aeruginosa*

What are the signs/ symptoms of chronic otitis media?

Otorrhea and hearing loss

OTOSCLEROSIS

What is it?

A genetic disease characterized by abnormal spongy and sclerotic bone formation in the temporal bone around the footplate of the stapes, thus preventing its normal movement

What is the inheritance pattern?

Autosomal dominant with incomplete one-third penetrance

What are the symptoms?

Painless, progressive hearing loss (may be unilateral or bilateral), tinnitus

What is the usual age of onset?

Second through fourth decade

How is the diagnosis made?

Normal TM with conductive hearing loss and no middle-ear effusion (though may be mixed or even sensorineural if bone of cochlea is affected)

What is Schwartze's sign?

Erythema around the stapes from hypervascularity of new bone formation

What is the treatment?

Frequently surgical (stapedectomy with placement of prosthesis), hearing aids, or observation; sodium fluoride may be used if a sensorineural component is present or for preoperative stabilization

FACIAL NERVE PARALYSIS

How is the defect localized?

Supranuclear—paralysis of lower face only, forehead muscles are spared because of bilateral corticobulbar supply
Intratemporal bone—paralysis of upper and lower face, decreased tearing, altered taste, absent stapedius reflex
Distal to stylomastoid foramen—paralysis of facial muscles only

What are the causes?

Usually from lesions of the nerve within its course through the temporal bone:
- Bell's palsy
- Trauma
- Cholesteatoma with erosion of facial canal
- Tumor (carcinoma, glomus jugulare)
- Herpes zoster inflammation of geniculate ganglion (Ramsey-Hunt syndrome)
- Peripheral lesions are usually parotid gland tumors or facial laceration.

What is the most common cause of bilateral facial nerve palsy?

Lyme disease (*Borrelia burgdorferi*)

BELL'S PALSY

What is it?

Sudden onset, unilateral facial weakness or paralysis in absence of CNS, ear, or cerebellopontine angle disease (i.e., no identifiable cause)

What is the clinical course?

Acute onset, with greatest muscle weakness reached within 3 weeks

What is the incidence?

Most common cause of **unilateral** facial weakness/paralysis

What is the pathogenesis?

Unknown; most widely accepted hypothesis is viral etiology (herpes virus); ischemic and immunologic factors are also implicated

What is the common preceding event?

URI

What are the signs/ symptoms?

Pathology is related to swelling of the facial nerve; may present with total facial paralysis, altered lacrimation, increased tearing on affected side, change in taste if region above chorda tympani is affected, dry mouth, and hyperacusis.

What is the treatment?

Usually none is required, as most cases resolve spontaneously in 1 month; protect eye with drops and tape closed as needed; most otolaryngologists advocate steroids and acyclovir. Surgical decompression of CN VII is indicated if paralysis progresses or tests indicate deterioration.

What is the prognosis?

Overall, 90% of patients recover completely; if paralysis is incomplete, 95% to 100% will recover without sequelae.

SENSORINEURAL HEARING LOSS

What is it?

Hearing loss from a lesion occurring in the cochlea or acoustic nerve rather than the external or middle ear

What are the symptoms?

Distortion of hearing, impaired speech discrimination, tinnitus

What are the signs?

Air conduction is better than bone conduction (positive Rinne test), Weber lateralizes to the side without the defect; audiogram varies, but most commonly shows greatest loss in high-frequency tones.

What are the causes?

Aging (presbycusis)—leading cause
Acoustic injury from sudden or prolonged exposure to loud noises
Perilymph fistula
Congenital (TORCH: maternal toxoplasmosis, rubella, CMV, herpes, and syphilis)
Ménière's disease
Drug/toxin-induced (antibiotics, especially aminoglycosides; aspirin; quinine; anticancer medications such as cisplatin; loop diuretics)
Acoustic neuroma

Pseudotumor cerebri
CNS disease (e.g., meningitis, multiple sclerosis)
Endocrine disorders (e.g., diabetes, hypothyroid)
Sarcoidosis
Metabolic disorders (e.g., hyperlipoproteinemia, chronic renal failure)

What is the most common cause in children?

Meningitis (bacterial)

What is the treatment?

Treatment of underlying cause, hearing aids, lip reading, cochlear implant

VERTIGO

What is it?

The sensation of head/body movement, or movement of surroundings (usually rotational)

What is the cause?

Asymmetric neuronal activity between right and left vestibular systems

What is the history of:

Peripheral vertigo?

Severe vertigo, nausea, vomiting, always accompanied by horizontal or rotatory nystagmus (fast component almost always to side opposite disease), other evidence of inner ear disease (tinnitus, hearing loss); frequently associated with a previously operated ear, a chronic draining ear, barotrauma, or abdominal or head trauma

Central vertigo?

Found in brainstem or cerebellum: insidious onset, less intense and more subtle sensation of vertigo; difficulty describing the symptoms; occasionally, vertical nystagmus

What are the steps in diagnostic evaluation?

Depends on probability of central versus peripheral; careful neurologic and otologic examinations are required
May need FTA/VDRL (syphilis), temporal bone scans/CT/MRI, ENG, position testing, audiometric testing

What is the most common etiology?

Benign paroxysmal positional vertigo (BPPV); history of brief spells of severe vertigo with specific head positions

What is the differential diagnosis?

Central: vertebral basilar insufficiency (often in older patients with DJD of spine), Wallenberg syndrome, MS, epilepsy, migraine
Peripheral: BPPV, motion sickness, syphilis, Ménière's disease, vestibular neuronitis, labyrinthitis, acoustic neuroma, syphilis, perilymph fistula

What is Tullio's phenomenon?

Induction of vertigo by loud noises
Classically result of otosyphilis

MÉNIÈRE'S DISEASE

What is it?

Disorder of the membranous labyrinth, causing fluctuating sensorineural hearing loss, episodic vertigo, nystagmus, tinnitus, and aural fullness, N/V

What is the classic triad?

Hearing loss, tinnitus, vertigo (H, T, V)

What is the pathophysiology?

Obscure, but most experts believe excessive production/defective resorption of endolymph.

What is the treatment?

Primarily medical: salt restriction, diuretics (thiazides), antinausea agents; occasionally diazepam is added; 80% of patients respond to medical management, antihistamines
Surgery is offered to those who fail medical treatment or who have incapacitating vertigo (60% to 80% effective).

GLOMUS TUMORS

What are they?

Benign, slow-growing tumors arising in glomus bodies found in the adventitial layer of blood vessels; often associated with cranial nerves IX and X in the middle ear

What is the usual location?

Middle ear, jugular bulb, course of CN IX to XII

How common are they? Most common benign tumor of the temporal bone

What is the treatment? Surgical resection, radiation therapy for poor operative candidates or for recurrences

NOSE AND PARANASAL SINUSES

EPISTAXIS

What is it? Bleeding from the nose

What are the predisposing factors? Trauma, "nose picking," sinus infection, allergic or atrophic rhinitis, blood dyscrasias, tumor, environmental extremes (hot, dry climates, winters)

What is the usual cause? Rupture of superficial mucosal blood vessels (Kiesselbach's plexus if anterior, sphenopalatine artery if posterior)

What is the most common type? Anterior (90% of all epistaxis); usually the result of trauma

Which type is more serious? Posterior; usually occurs in the elderly or is associated with a systemic disorder (hypertension, tumor, arteriosclerosis)

What is the treatment? Direct pressure; if this fails, proceed to anterior nasal packing with gauze strips, followed if necessary by posterior packing with Foley catheter or lamb's wool; packs must be removed in less than 5 days to prevent infectious complications

What is the treatment of last resort? Ligation or embolization of the sphenopalatine artery (posterior) or ethmoidal artery (anterior) (think, alphabetically = sphenopalatine = posterior and ethmoid = anterior)

What infectious disease syndrome is seen with nasal packing? Toxic shock syndrome: fever, shock, **rash** caused by exotoxin from *Staphylococcus aureus*

What is the treatment? Supportive with removal of nasal packing, IV hydration, oxygen, and anti-staphylococcal antibiotics

ACUTE RHINITIS

What is it?	Inflammation of nasal mucous membrane
What is the most common cause?	URI infection; rhinovirus is the most common agent in adults (other nonallergic causes: nasal deformities and tumors, polyps, atrophy, immune diseases, vasomotor problems)

ALLERGIC RHINITIS

What are the symptoms?	Nasal stuffiness; watery rhinorrhea; paroxysms of morning sneezing; and itching of nose, conjunctiva, or palate
How is the condition characterized?	Early onset (before 20 years of age), familial tendency, other allergic disorders (eczema, asthma), elevated serum IgE, eosinophilia on nasal smear
What are the findings on physical examination?	Pale, boggy, bluish nasal turbinates coated with thin, clear secretions; in children, a transverse nasal crease sometimes results from repeated "allergic salute"
What is the treatment?	Allergen avoidance, antihistamines, decongestants; steroids or sodium cromylate in severe cases; desensitization via allergen immunotherapy is the only "cure"

ACUTE SINUSITIS

What is the typical history?	Previously healthy patient with unrelenting progression of a viral URI or allergic rhinitis beyond the normal 5- to 7-day course
What are the symptoms?	Periorbital pressure/pain, nasal obstruction, nasal/postnasal mucopurulent discharge, fatigue, fever, headache
What are the signs?	Tenderness over affected sinuses, pus in the nasal cavity; may also see reason for obstruction (septal deviation, spur, tight osteomeatal complex); transillumination is unreliable

What is the pathophysiology? Thought to be secondary to decreased ciliary action of the sinus mucosa and edema causing obstruction of the sinus ostia, lowering intrasinus oxygen tension and predisposing patients to bacterial infection

What are the causative organisms? Up to 50% of patients have negative cultures and cause is presumably (initially) viral; pneumococcus, S. *aureus*, group A streptococci, and *H. influenzae* are the most common bacteria cultured.

What is the treatment? 14-day course of antibiotics (penicillin G, amoxicillin, Ceclor, and Augmentin are commonly used), topical and systemic decongestants, and saline nasal irrigation

CHRONIC SINUSITIS

What is it? Infection of nasal sinuses lasting longer than 4 weeks, or pattern of recurrent acute sinusitis punctuated by brief asymptomatic periods

What is the pathology? Permanent mucosal changes secondary to inadequately treated acute sinusitis, consisting of mucosal fibrosis, polypoid growth, and inadequate ciliary action, hyperostosis (increased bone density on CT scan)

What are the symptoms? Chronic nasal obstruction, postnasal drip, mucopurulent rhinorrhea, low-grade facial and periorbital pressure/pain

What are the causative organisms? Usually anaerobes (such as *Bacteroides, Veillonella, Rhinobacterium*); also *H. influenzae, Streptococcus viridans, Staphylococcus aureus, Staphylococcus epidermidis*

What is the treatment? Medical management with decongestants, mucolytics, topical steroids, and antibiotics; if this approach fails, proceed to endoscopic or external surgical intervention

What is FESS? **F**unctional **E**ndoscopic **S**inus **S**urgery

What are the complications of sinusitis?

Orbital cellulitis (if ethmoid sinusitis), meningitis, epidural or brain abscess (frontal sinus), cavernous sinus thrombosis (ethmoid or sphenoid), osteomyelitis (A.K.A. Pott's puffy tumor if frontal)

CANCER OF THE NASAL CAVITY AND PARANASAL SINUSES

What are the usual locations?

Maxillary sinus (two-thirds)
Nasal cavity
Ethmoid sinus
Rarely in frontal or sphenoid sinuses

What are the associated cell types?

Squamous cell (80%)
Adenocellular (15%)
Uncommon: sarcoma, melanoma

What rare tumor arises from olfactory epithelium?

Esthesioneuroblastoma; usually arises high in the nose (cribriform plate) and is locally invasive

What are the signs/symptoms?

Early—nasal obstruction, blood-tinged mucus, epistaxis
Late—localized pain, cranial nerve deficits, facial/palate asymmetry, loose teeth

How is the diagnosis made?

CT can adequately identify extent of the disease and local invasion. MRI is often also used to evaluate soft-tissue disease.

What is the treatment?

Surgery with or without x-ray therapy

What is the prognosis?

5-year survival for T1 or T2 lesions approaches 70%.

JUVENILE NASOPHARYNGEAL ANGIOFIBROMA

What is it?

The most commonly encountered vascular mass in the nasal cavity; locally aggressive but nonmetastasizing

What is the usual history?

Adolescent boys who present with nasal obstruction, recurrent massive epistaxis, possibly anosmia

What is the usual location?

Site of origin is the roof of the nasal cavity at the superior margin of sphenopalatine foramen

Into what can the mass transform?
Fibrosarcoma (rare cases reported)

How is the diagnosis made?
Carotid arteriography, CT; biopsy is contraindicated secondary to risk of uncontrollable hemorrhage

What are indications for biopsy?
None!

What is the treatment?
Surgery via lateral rhinotomy or sublabial maxillotomy with bleeding controlled by internal maxillary artery ligation or preoperative embolization, in the setting of hypotensive anesthesia; preoperative irradiation has also been used to shrink the tumor

ORAL CAVITY AND PHARYNX

PHARYNGOTONSILLITIS

What is it?
Acute or chronic infection of the nasopharynx or oropharynx and/or Waldeyer's ring of lymphoid tissue (consisting of palatine, lingual, and pharyngeal tonsils and the adenoids)

What is the etiology?
Acute attacks can be viral (adenovirus, enterovirus, coxsackievirus, Epstein-Barr virus in infectious mononucleosis) or bacterial (group A β-hemolytic streptococci are the leading bacterial agent); chronic tonsillitis often with mixed population, including streptococci, staphylococci, and *M. catarrhalis*

What are the symptoms?
Acute—Sore throat, fever, local lymphadenopathy, chills, headache, malaise
Chronic—Noisy mouth breathing, speech and swallowing difficulties, apnea, halitosis

What are the signs?
Viral—Injected tonsils and pharyngeal mucosa; exudate may occur, but less often than with bacterial tonsillitis
Bacterial—Swollen, inflamed tonsils with white-yellow exudate in crypts and on surface; cervical adenopathy

How is the diagnosis made?	CBC, throat culture, monospot test
What are the possible complications?	Peritonsillar abscess (quinsy), retropharyngeal abscess (causing airway compromise), rheumatic fever, poststreptococcal glomerulonephritis (with β-hemolytic streptococci)
What is the treatment?	Viral—Symptomatic → acetaminophen, warm saline gargles, anesthetic throat spray Bacterial—10 days PCN (erythromycin if PCN-allergic)
What are the indications for tonsillectomy?	Sleep apnea/cor pulmonale secondary to airway obstruction, suspicion of malignancy, hypertrophy causing malocclusion, peritonsillar abscess, recurrent acute or chronic tonsillitis
What are the possible complications?	Acute or delayed hemorrhage

PERITONSILLAR ABSCESS

What is the clinical setting?	Inadequately treated recurrent acute or chronic tonsillitis
What is the associated microbiology?	Mixed aerobes and anaerobes (which may be PCN-resistant)
What is the site of formation?	Begins at the superior pole of the tonsil
What are the symptoms?	Severe throat pain, drooling dysphagia, odynophagia, trismus, cervical adenopathy, fever, chills, malaise
What is the classic description of voice?	"Hot-potato voice"
What are the signs?	Bulging, erythematous, edematous tonsillar pillar; swelling of uvula and displacement to contralateral side
What is the treatment?	IV antibiotics and surgical evacuation by incision and drainage; most experts recommend tonsillectomy after resolution of inflammatory changes

CANCER OF THE ORAL CAVITY

What is the usual cell type?
Squamous cell (>90% of cases)

What are the most common sites?
Lip, tongue, floor of mouth, gingiva, cheek, and palate

What is the etiology?
Linked to smoking, alcohol, and smokeless tobacco products (alcohol and tobacco together greatly increase the risk)

What is the frequency of the following conditions:

Regional metastasis?
About 30%

Second primary?
About 25%

Nodal metastasis?
Depends on size of tumor and ranges from 10% to 60%, usually to jugular and **jugulodigastric nodes, submandibular nodes**

Distant metastasis?
Infrequent

How is the diagnosis made?
Full history and physical examination, dental assessment, Panorex or bone scan if mandible is thought to be involved, CT/MRI for extent of tumor and nodal disease, FNA (often U/S guided)

What is the treatment?
Radiation, surgery, or both for small lesions; localized lesions can usually be treated surgically; larger lesions require combination therapy, possible mandibulectomy and neck dissection

What is the prognosis?
Depends on stage and site:
- Tongue: 20% to 70% survival
- Floor of mouth: 30% to 80% survival

Most common cause of death in successfully treated head and neck cancer is development of a second primary (occurs in 20% to 40% of cases).

SALIVARY GLAND TUMORS

What is the frequency of gland involvement?
Parotid gland (80%)
Submandibular gland (15%)
Minor salivary glands (5%)

What is the potential for malignancy?

Greatest in **minor salivary gland** tumors (80% are malignant) and least in parotid gland tumors (80% are benign); the smaller the gland, the greater the likelihood of malignancy

How do benign and malignant tumors differ in terms of history and physical examination?

Benign—mobile, nontender, no node involvement or facial weakness
Malignant—painful, fixed mass with evidence of local metastasis and facial paresis/paralysis

What is the diagnostic procedure?

FNA; never perform excisional biopsy of a parotid mass. Superficial parotidectomy is the procedure of choice for benign lesions of the lateral lobe.

What is the treatment?

Involves adequate surgical resection, sparing facial nerve if possible, neck dissection for node-positive necks
Postoperative radiation therapy if high-grade cancer, recurrent cancer, residual disease, invasion of adjacent structures, any T3 or T4 parotid tumors

What is the most common benign salivary tumor?

Pleomorphic adenoma (benign mixed tumor) accounts for two-thirds of total (think: **P**leomorphic = **P**opular)

What is the usual location?

Parotid gland

What is the clinical course?

They are well-delineated and slow growing.

What is the second most common benign salivary gland tumor?

Warthin's tumor (1% of all salivary gland tumors)

What is the usual location?

95% are found in parotid; 3% are bilateral.

Describe the lesion.

Slow-growing, cystic mass is usually located in the tail of the superficial portion of the parotid; it rarely becomes malignant.

What is the most common malignant salivary tumor?

Mucoepidermoid carcinoma (10% of all salivary gland neoplasms) Think: **M**ucoepidermoid = **M**alignant

	Most common parotid malignancy Second most common submandibular gland malignancy
What is the second most common malignant salivary tumor in adults?	Adenoid cystic carcinoma Less than 10% of all salivary gland neoplasms Most common malignancy in submandibular and minor salivary glands Second most common malignancy in parotid Tends to have perineural invasion

LARYNX ANATOMY

Define the three parts.	1. Glottis: begins halfway between the true and false cords (in the ventricle) and extends inferiorly 1.0 cm below the edge of the vocal folds 2. Supraglottis: extends from superior glottis to superior border of hyoid and tip of epiglottis 3. Subglottis: extends from lower border of glottis to inferior edge of cricoid cartilage
Innervation?	Via the vagus nerve: superior laryngeal and recurrent laryngeal nerves; superior laryngeal supplies sensory to supraglottis and motor to inferior constrictor and cricothyroid muscle; recurrent laryngeal supplies sensory to glottis and subglottis and motor to all remaining intrinsic laryngeal muscles

CROUP (LARYNGOTRACHEOBRONCHITIS)

What is it?	A viral infection of the larynx and trachea, generally affecting children (boys > girls)
What is the usual cause?	Parainfluenza virus (think: crou**P** = **P**arainfluenza)
What age group is affected most?	6 months to 3 years of age
Is the condition considered seasonal?	Yes; outbreaks most often occur in autumn.

What are the precipitating events? Usually preceded by URI

What is the classic symptom? Barking (seal-like), nonproductive cough

What are the other symptoms? Respiratory distress, low-grade fever

What are the signs? Tachypnea, inspiratory retractions, prolonged inspiration, inspiratory stridor, expiratory rhonchi/wheezes

What is the differential diagnosis? Epiglottitis, bacterial tracheitis, foreign body, diphtheria, retropharyngeal abscess, peritonsillar abscess, asthma

How is the diagnosis made? A-P neck x-ray shows classic "steeple sign," indicating subglottic narrowing; ABG may show hypoxemia plus hypercapnia.

What is the treatment? **Keep child calm** (agitation only worsens obstruction); cool mist; steroids; aerosolized racemic EPI may be administered to reduce edema/airway obstruction

What are the indications for intubation? If airway obstruction is severe or child becomes exhausted

What is the usual course? Resolves in 3 to 4 days; secondary bacterial infection (streptococcal, staphylococcal) may require antibiotics

EPIGLOTTITIS

What is it? Severe, rapidly progressive infection of the epiglottis

What is the usual causative agent? *Haemophilus influenzae* type B

What age group is affected? Children 2 to 5 years of age

What are the signs/symptoms? Sudden onset, high fever (40°C); "hot potato" voice; dysphagia (→ drooling); no cough; patient prefers to sit upright, lean forward; patient appears toxic and stridulous

How is the diagnosis made? Can usually be made clinically and does not involve direct observation of the epiglottis (which may worsen obstruction by causing laryngospasm)

What is the treatment? Involves immediate airway support via OR intubation or possibly tracheotomy; medical treatment is comprised of steroids and IV antibiotics *against H. influenzae* (ampicillin + chloramphenicol)

MALIGNANT LESIONS OF THE LARYNX

What is the incidence? Accounts for approximately 2% of all malignancies, more often in males

What is the most common site? Glottis (two-thirds)

What is the second most common type? Supraglottis (one-third)

Which type has the worst prognosis? Subglottic tumors (infrequent)

What are the risk factors? Tobacco, alcohol

What is the pathology? 90% are squamous cell carcinoma.

What are the symptoms? Hoarseness, throat pain, dysphagia, odynophagia, neck mass, (referred) ear pain

SUPRAGLOTTIC LESIONS

What is the usual location? Laryngeal surface of epiglottis

What area is often involved? Pre-epiglottic space

Extension? Tend to remain confined to supraglottic region, though may extend to vallecula or base of tongue

What is the associated type of metastasis? High propensity for nodal metastasis

GLOTTIC LESIONS

What is the usual location? Anterior part of true cords

Extension? May invade thyroid cartilage, cross midline to invade contralateral cord, or invade paraglottic space

What is the associated type of metastasis? Rare nodal metastasis

What is the treatment? Total or supraglottic laryngectomy, depending on location and extent of lesion; neck dissection if nodal involvement
Radiation therapy or surgery is given for early (T1 or T2) lesions. Combination therapy (surgery + radiation) is given for advanced (T3 and T4) disease.

What is the 5-year survival for:

T1 lesions? 90%

T2 lesions? 80%

T3 lesions? 75%

T4 lesions? 30%

NECK MASS

What is the usual etiology in infants? Congenital (branchial cleft cysts, thyroglossal duct cysts)

What is the usual etiology in adolescents? Inflammatory (cervical adenitis is number one), with congenital also possible

What is the usual etiology in adults? Malignancy (squamous is number one), especially if painless and immobile

What is the "80% rule"? In general, 80% of neck masses are **benign** in children; 80% are **malignant** in adults older than 40 years of age.

What are the seven cardinal symptoms of neck masses?

Dysphagia, odynophagia, hoarseness, stridor (signifies upper airway obstruction), globus, speech disorder, referred ear pain (via CN V, IX, or X)

What comprises the workup?

Full head and neck examination, indirect laryngoscopy, CT and MRI to search for hidden primary; FNA for tissue diagnosis; biopsy contraindicated because it adversely affects survival if malignant

What is the differential diagnosis?

Inflammatory: cervical lymphadenitis, cat-scratch disease, infectious mononucleosis, infection in neck spaces
Congenital: thyroglossal duct cyst (midline, elevates with tongue protrusion), branchial cleft cysts (lateral), dermoid cysts (midline submental), hemangioma, cystic hygroma
Neoplastic: primary or metastatic

What is the treatment?

Surgical excision for congenital or neoplastic; two most important procedures for cancer treatment are radical and modified neck dissection

RADICAL NECK DISSECTION

What is involved?

Classically, removal of **nodes** from clavicle to mandible, sternocleidomastoid muscle, **submandibular gland,** tail of **parotid,** internal **jugular vein, digastric muscles, stylohyoid** and **omohyoid muscles, fascia** within the anterior and posterior triangles, CN XI, and cervical plexus sensory nerves

What are the indications?

1. Clinically positive nodes that likely contain metastatic cancer
2. Clinically negative nodes in neck, but high probability of metastasis from a primary tumor elsewhere
3. A fixed cervical mass that is resectable

What are the contraindications?

1. Distant metastasis
2. Fixation to structure that cannot be removed (e.g., carotid artery)
3. Low neck masses

MODIFIED NECK DISSECTION

What are the types:

Type I? Spinal accessory nerve preserved

Type II? Spinal accessory and internal jugular nerves preserved

Type III? Spinal accessory, IJ, and sternocleidomastoid nerves preserved

What are the advantages? Increased postoperative function and decreased morbidity (especially if bilateral), most often used in N0 lesions; these modifications are usually intraoperative decisions based on the location and extent of tumor growth

What are the disadvantages? May result in increased mortality from local recurrence

FACIAL FRACTURES

MANDIBLE FRACTURES

What are the symptoms? Gross disfigurement, pain, **malocclusion,** drooling

What are the signs? Trismus, fragment mobility and lacerations of gingiva, hematoma in floor of mouth

What are the possible complications? Malunion, nonunion, osteomyelitis, TMJ ankylosis

What is the treatment? Open or closed reduction
MMF = maxillomandibular fixation (wiring jaw shut)

MIDFACE FRACTURES

How are they evaluated? Careful physical examination and CT

Classification

Le Fort I? Transverse maxillary fracture above the dental apices, which also traverses the pterygoid plate; palate is mobile, but nasal complex is stable

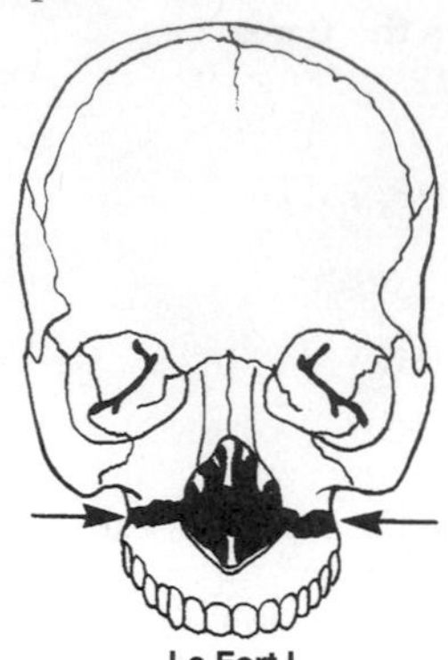
Le Fort I

Le Fort II?

Fracture through the frontal process of the maxilla, through the orbital floor and pterygoid plate; midface is mobile

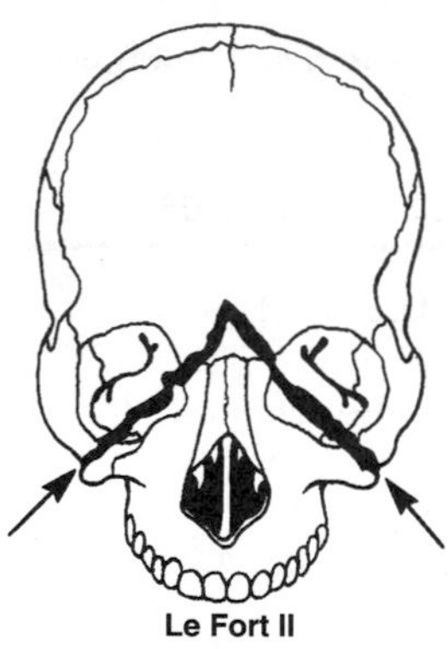
Le Fort II

Le Fort III?

Complete craniofacial separation; differs from II in that it extends through the nasofrontal suture and frontozygomatic sutures

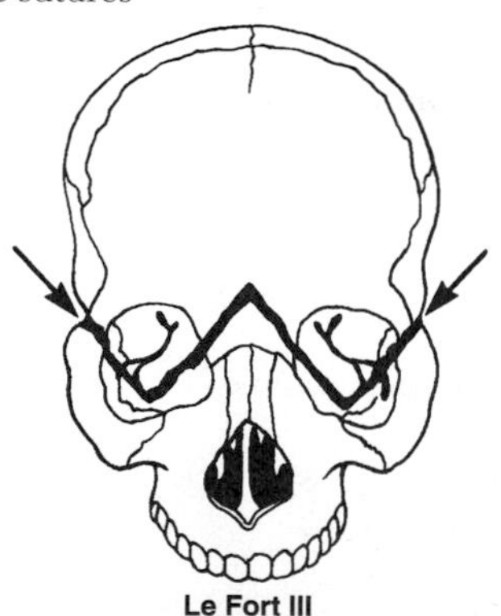
Le Fort III

What is a "tripod" fracture?

Fracture of the zygomatic complex; involves four fractures:

1. Frontozygomatic suture
2. Zygomaticomaxillary suture
3. Inferior orbital rim
4. Zygomaticotemporal suture

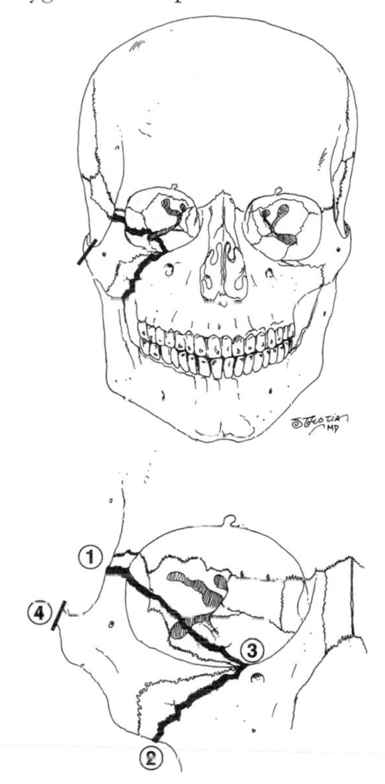

What is a "blowout" fracture?

Orbital fracture with "blowout" of supporting bony structural support of orbital floor; patient has enophthalmos (sunken-in eyeball)

What is "entrapment"?

Orbital fracture with "entrapment" of periorbital tissues within the fracture opening, including entrapment of extraocular muscles; loss of extraocular muscle mobility (e.g., lateral tracking) and diplopia (double vision)

What is a "step off"?

Fracture of the orbit with palpable "step off" of bony orbital rim (inferior or lateral)

Are mandibular fractures usually a single fracture?
No; because the mandible forms an anatomic ring, more than 95% of mandible fractures have more than one fracture site.

What is the best x-ray study for mandibular fractures?
Panorex

What must be ruled out and treated with a broken nose (nasal fracture)?
Septal hematoma; must drain to remove chance of a pressure-induced septal necrosis

ENT WARD QUESTIONS

How can otitis externa be distinguished from otitis media on examination?
Otitis externa is characterized by severe pain upon manipulation of the auricle.

What causes otitis media?
Most cases are caused by pneumococci and *H. influenzae*.

What causes otitis externa?
Pseudomonas aeruginosa

What must be considered in unilateral serous otitis?
Nasopharyngeal carcinoma

What is most the common cause of facial paralysis?
Bell's palsy, which has an unidentified etiology

What is the single most important prognostic factor in Bell's palsy?
Whether the affected muscles are completely paralyzed (if not, prognosis is >95% complete recovery)

What is the most common cause of parotid swelling?
Mumps

What is Heerfordt's syndrome?
Sarcoidosis with parotid enlargement, facial nerve paralysis, and uveitis

Which systemic disease causes salivary gland stones?
Gout

What is the most common salivary gland site of stone formation?
Submandibular gland

What is Mikulicz's syndrome?
Any cause of bilateral enlargement of the parotid, lacrimal, and submandibular glands

What are the three major functions of the larynx?

1. Airway protection
2. Airway/respiration
3. Phonation

What is a cricothyroidotomy?

Emergent surgical airway by incising the cricothyroid membrane

Name the four major indications for a tracheostomy?

1. Prolonged mechanical ventilation (usually > 2 weeks)
2. Upper airway obstruction
3. Poor life-threatening pulmonary toilet
4. Severe obstructive sleep apnea

What is a ranula?

Sublingual retention cyst

What is Frey's syndrome?

Flushing, pain, and diaphoresis in the auriculotemporal nerve distribution initiated by chewing; caused by abnormal regeneration of the sympathetic/ parasympathetic nerves upon cutting the auriculotemporal nerve, usually during a parotidectomy. These parasympathetic fibers, once destined for the parotid gland, find new targets in skin sweat glands. Thus, people sweat when eating.

What is the classic triad of Ménière's disease?

Hearing loss, tinnitus, vertigo

What is the most common posterior fossa tumor and where is it located?

Acoustic neuromas, usually occurring at the cerebellopontine angle

What is the most common site of sinus cancer?

Maxillary sinus

What tumor arises from olfactory epithelium?

Esthesioneuroblastoma

What cell type is most common in head and neck cancer?

Squamous cell

What are the most important predisposing factors to head and neck cancer?

Excessive alcohol use and **tobacco** abuse of any form

What is the most frequent site of salivary gland tumor?

Parotid gland

What is the most common salivary gland neoplasm:	Minor salivary glands (>75% malignant)
Benign?	Pleomorphic adenoma
Malignant?	Mucoepidermoid carcinoma
What is the classic feature of croup?	Barking, seal-like cough
What are the classic features of epiglottitis?	"Hot potato" voice, sitting up, **drooling,** toxic appearance, high fever, **leaning forward**
What comprises the workup of neck mass?	Do **not** biopsy; obtain tissue **via FNA** and complete head and neck examination.
What is Ramsay Hunt's syndrome?	Painful facial nerve paralysis from herpes zoster of the ear
What is the most common malignant neck mass in children, adolescents, and young adults?	Lymphoma
What is the most common primary malignant solid tumor of the head and neck in children?	Rhabdomyosarcoma
Throat pain is often referred to what body area?	**Ear**
What ENT condition is described as "crocodile tears"?	Frey's syndrome!

67 Thoracic Surgery

What does VATS stand for? Video Assisted Thoracic Surgery

THORACIC OUTLET SYNDROME (TOS)

What is it?
Compression of the:
Subclavian artery
Subclavian vein or
Brachial plexus at the superior outlet of the thorax

What are the causes (3)?
1. Various congenital anomalies, including cervical rib or abnormal fascial bands to the first rib, or abnormal anterior scalene muscle
2. Trauma:
   Fracture of clavicle or first rib
   Dislocation of humeral head
   Crush injuries
3. Repetitive motor injuries (baseball pitchers)

What are the symptoms?
Paresthesias (neck, shoulder, arm, hand); 90% in ulnar nerve distribution
Weakness (neural/arterial)
Coolness of involved extremity (arterial)
Edema, venous distension, discoloration (venous)

What is the most common problem seen with TOS?
Neurologic symptoms

Which nerve is most often involved?
Ulnar nerve

What are the signs?
Paget-von Schroetter syndrome—venous thrombosis leading to edema, arm discoloration, and distension of the superficial veins

Weak brachial and radial pulses in the involved arm
Hypesthesia/anesthesia
Occasionally, atrophy in the distribution of the ulnar nerve
Positive Adson maneuver/Tinel's sign
Edema

What is the Adson maneuver?

Evaluates for arterial compromise
Patient:
1. Extends neck (lifts head)
2. Takes a deep breath
3. Turns head toward examined side

Physician:
Monitors radial pulse on examined side
Test finding is positive if the radial pulse decreases or disappears during maneuver.

What is Tinel's test?

Tapping of the supraclavicular fossa producing paresthesias

What is the treatment?

Physical therapy (vast majority of cases)
Decompression of the thoracic outlet by resecting the first rib and cervical rib (if present) if physical therapy fails and as a last resort

CHEST WALL TUMORS

BENIGN TUMORS

What are the most common types?

1. Fibrous rib dysplasia (posterolateral rib)
2. Chondroma (at costochondral junction)
3. Osteochondroma (any portion of rib)

What is the treatment?

Wide excision and reconstruction with autologous or prosthetic grafts

MALIGNANT TUMORS

What are the most common types?

1. Fibrosarcoma
2. Chondrosarcoma
3. Osteogenic sarcoma
4. Rhabdomyosarcoma
5. Myeloma
6. Ewing's sarcoma

What is the treatment? Excision with or without radiation

DISEASES OF THE PLEURA

PLEURAL EFFUSION

What is it? Fluid in the pleural space

What are the causes?

1. Pulmonary infections (pneumonia)
2. Congestive heart failure (CHF)
3. SLE or rheumatoid arthritis
4. Pancreatitis (sympathetic effusion)
5. Trauma
6. Pulmonary embolism
7. Renal disease
8. Cirrhosis
9. Malignancy (mesothelioma, lymphoma, metastasis)
10. Postpericardiotomy syndrome

What are the symptoms? Dyspnea, pleuritic chest pain

What are the signs? Decreased breath sounds, dullness to percussion, egophony at the upper limit

What are the properties of a transudate?

Specific gravity <1.016
Protein <3 g/dl
Few cells

What are the properties of an exudate?

Specific gravity >1.016
Protein >3 g/dl
Many cells

What is the key diagnostic test? Thoracentesis (needle drainage) with studies including cytology

What is the treatment?

1. Pigtail catheter or thoracostomy (chest tube)
2. Treat underlying condition
3. Consider sclerosis

What is an empyema? Infected pleural effusion; must be drained, usually with chest tube(s)
Decortication may be necessary if the empyema is solid.

What is a decortication? Thoracotomy and removal of an infected fibrous rind from around the lung (think

	of it as taking off a fibrous "cortex" from the lung)

LUNG ABSCESS

What are the signs/ symptoms?	Fever, sputum, sepsis, fatigue
What are the associated diagnostic studies?	CXR: air-fluid level CT scan to define position and to differentiate from an empyema Bronchoscopy (looking for cancer/culture)
What is the treatment?	Antibiotics and bronchoscopy for culture and toilet, with or without surgery
What are the indications for surgery?	Underlying cancer/tumor Refractory to antibiotics
What are the surgical options?	Lobectomy of lobe with abscess Tube drainage

HEMOPTYSIS

What is it?	Bleeding into the bronchial tree
What are the causes?	1. Bronchitis (50%) 2. Tumor mass (20%) 3. TB (8%) Other causes: bronchiectasis, pulmonary catheters, trauma
Define MASSIVE hemoptysis.	More than 600 cc/24 hours
What comprises the workup?	CXR Bronchoscopy Bronchial A-gram
What is the treatment if massive?	Bronchoscopy, intubation of unaffected side, Fogarty catheter, occlusion of bleeding bronchus, bronchial A-gram with or without embolization, surgical resection of involved lung
What is the treatment of moderate to mild bleeding?	Laser coagulation

SPONTANEOUS PNEUMOTHORAX

What is it?
Atraumatic spontaneous development of a pneumothorax

What are the causes?
Idiopathic (primary), bleb disease-emphysema, etc. (secondary)

What body habitus is associated with spontaneous pneumothorax?
Thin and tall

How is the diagnosis made?
CXR

What is the treatment?
Chest tube

What are the options if refractory, recurrent, or bilateral?
Pleurodesis: scar the lung to the parietal pleura with a sclerosant (talc) via chest tube/thoracoscopy or by thoracotomy and mechanical abrasion

Who might also need a pleurodesis after the first episode?
Those whose lifestyles place them at increased risk for pneumothorax (e.g., pilots, skin divers)

MESOTHELIOMA

Malignant Mesothelioma

What is it?
A primary pleural neoplasm

What are the two types?
1. Localized (benign or malignant)
2. Diffuse (highly malignant)

What are the risk factors?
Exposure to asbestos
Smoking

What are the symptoms?
Localized: pleuritic pain, joint pain and swelling, dyspnea
Diffuse: chest pain, malaise, weight loss, cough

What are the signs?
Pleural effusion (present in only 10% to 15% of patients with local disease, almost always in diffuse disease [>75%])

What are the associated radiographic tests?
X-ray may reveal a peripheral mass, often forming an obtuse angle with the chest wall; **CT is also performed.**

How is the diagnosis made? Pleural biopsy, pleural fluid cytology

What is the treatment if localized? Surgical excision

What is the treatment if diffuse? Early stages may be resected, followed by radiation (brachytherapy); for more advanced stages, radiation, chemotherapy, or both are done.

What is the prognosis? Localized: poor if tumor is malignant
Diffuse: **dismal** (average life span after diagnosis is about 1 year)

Benign Mesothelioma

What is it? Benign pleural mesothelioma

What pleura is usually involved? Visceral pleura

What is the gross appearance? Pedunculated "broccoli or cauliflower" tumor on a stalk coming off of the lung

What is the treatment? Surgical resection with at least 1 cm clear margin

What is the prognosis? In contrast to malignant mesothelioma, the benign mesothelioma has an excellent prognosis with cure in the vast majority of cases (possibility of transformation into a malignant mesothelioma if inadequate resection).

DISEASES OF THE LUNGS

BRONCHOGENIC CARCINOMA

What is the annual incidence of lung cancer in the United States? 150,000 new cases

What is the number of annual deaths from lung cancer? 100,000 (increasing in women); most common cancer death in the United States

What is the number one risk factor? Smoking (surprise!)

Does asbestos exposure increase the risk in patients who smoke?

Yes

What type of lung cancer arises in nonsmoking ?

Adenocarcinoma

What are the signs/ symptoms?

Change in a chronic cough
Hemoptysis, chest pain, dyspnea
Pleural effusion (suggests chest wall involvement)
Hoarseness (recurrent laryngeal nerve involvement)
Superior vena cava syndrome
Diaphragmatic paralysis (phrenic nerve involvement)
Symptoms of metastasis/paraneoplastic syndrome
Finger clubbing

What is Pancoast's tumor?

Tumor at the apex of the lung or superior sulcus that may involve the brachial plexus, sympathetic ganglia, and vertebral bodies, leading to pain, upper extremity weakness, and Horner's syndrome

What is Horner's syndrome?

Injury to the cervical sympathetic chain:
1. Miosis (small pupil)
2. Ptosis
3. Enophthalmos
4. Decreased sweating on affected side

What are the four most common sites of extra-thoracic metastases?

1. Bone
2. Liver
3. Adrenals
4. Kidney

What are paraneoplastic syndromes?

Syndromes that are associated with tumors but may affect distant parts of the body; they may be caused by hormones released from endocrinologically active tumors or may be of uncertain etiology

Name five general types of paraneoplastic syndromes.

1. Metabolic: Cushing's, SIADH, hypercalcemia
2. Neuromuscular: Eaton-Lambert, cerebellar ataxia

3. Skeletal: hypertrophic osteoarthropathy
4. Dermatologic: acanthosis nigricans
5. Vascular: thrombophlebitis

What are the associated radiographic tests?

CXR and CT scan

How is the tumor diagnosed?

1. Sputum cytology
2. Needle biopsy (CT or fluoro guidance)
3. Bronchoscopy with brushings, biopsies, or both
4. With or without mediastinoscopy, mediastinotomy, scalene node biopsy, or open lung biopsy for definitive diagnosis

For each tumor listed, recall its usual site in the lung and its natural course:

Squamous cell?

Two-thirds occur centrally in lung hilus; may also be a Pancoast's tumor; slow growth, late metastasis; associated with smoking (think: **S**quamous = **S**entral)

Adenocarcinoma?

Peripheral, rapid growth with hematogenous/nodal metastasis, associated with lung scarring

Small (oat) cell?

Central, highly malignant, usually not operable

Large cell?

Usually peripheral, very malignant

What are the stages of NON-small cell carcinoma of the lungs:

Stage Ia?

Tumor <3 cm, no nodes, no metastases (T1NoMo)

Stage Ib?

Tumor >3 cm, but no nodes and no metastases (T2NoMo)

Stage IIa?

Tumor <3 cm **and** positive nodes to lung or ipsilateral hilum; **no** metastases (T1N1Mo)

Stage IIb?

1. Tumor >3 cm and positive nodes in lung or ipsilateral hilum (T2N1Mo)
2. Tumor that invades chest wall,

diaphragm, mediastinal pleura, or pericardial sac (**no** mediastinal structures) and no nodes and **no** metastases (T3NoMo)

Stage IIIa?

1. Tumor invades chest wall, diaphragm, or mediastinal pleura or pericardial sac **and** positive nodes in lung or ipsilateral hilum with **no** metastases (T3N1Mo).
2. Lymph node metastases to ipsilateral, mediastinal, or subcarinal nodes with **no** metastases and **no** mediastinal tumor invasion (T1N2Mo, T2N2Mo, T3N2Mo)

Stage IIIb?

No distant metastases but mediastinal invasion or lymph node metastases to contralateral hilum or mediastinum Supraclavicular/scalene nodes

Stage IV?

Distant metastasis

What are the surgical contraindications by stage for NON-small cell carcinoma?

Stage IV, Stage IIIb

What is the treatment by stage for NON-small cell lung carcinoma:

Stage I?

Surgical resection

Stage II?

Surgical resection

Stage IIIa?

Surgical resection if early IIIa, chemotherapy with or without XRT

Stage IIIb?

Chemotherapy and XRT

Stage IV?

Chemotherapy +/− XRT

Treatment of isolated brain metastasis?

Surgical resection

What is the approximate prognosis (5-year survival) after treatment of NON-small cell lung carcinoma by stage:

Stage Ia? 65%

Stage Ib? 55%

Stage IIa? 40%

Stage IIb? 35%

Stage IIIa? Approximately 20%

Stage IV? Basically 0%

How is small cell carcinoma treated? Chemotherapy with or without x-ray therapy

What are the six contraindications to surgery for lung cancer? Acronym **STOP IT:**

1. **S**uperior vena cava syndrome, **S**upraclavicular node metastasis, **S**calene node metastasis
2. **T**racheal carina involvement
3. **O**at cell carcinoma (treat with chemotherapy with or without radiation)
4. **P**ulmonary function tests shows FEV1 < 1
5. Myocardial **I**nfarction (or cardiac cripple)
6. **T**umor elsewhere (metastatic disease)

What postoperative FEV1 must you have? FEV1 $>$ 800 cc; thus, a preoperative FEV1 $>$ 2 is usually needed for a pneumonectomy

If FEV1 is $<$ 2, a ventilation perfusion scan should be performed.

What is hypertrophic pulmonary osteoarthropathy? Periosteal proliferation and new bone formation at the end of long bones and in the bones of the hand (seen in 10% of patients with lung cancer)

SOLITARY PULMONARY NODULES (COIN LESIONS)

What are they? Peripheral circumscribed pulmonary lesions

What is the differential diagnosis? Granulomatous disease, benign neoplasms, malignancy

What percentage are malignant?
Overall, 5% to 10% (but >50% are malignant in smokers older than 50 years)

Is there a gender risk?
Yes; the incidence of coin lesions is 3 to 9 times higher and malignancy is nearly twice as common in men as in women.

What are the symptoms?
Usually asymptomatic with solitary nodules, but may include coughing, weight loss, chest pain, and hemoptysis

What are the signs?
Physical findings are uncommon; clubbing is rare; hypertrophic osteoarthropathy implies more than an 80% chance of malignancy.

How is the diagnosis made?
CXR, chest CT

What is the significance of "popcorn" calcification?
Most likely benign (i.e., hamartoma)

What are the risk factors for malignancy?
1. Size: lesions > 1 cm have a significant chance of malignancy, and those > 4 cm are very likely to be malignant.
2. Indistinct margins (corona radiata)
3. Documented growth on follow-up x-ray (if no change in 2 years, most likely benign)
4. Increasing age

What are the associated lab tests?
1. TB skin tests, etc.
2. Sputum cultures
3. Sputum cytology is diagnostic in 5% to 20% of cases.

Which method of tissue diagnosis is used?
Chest CT with needle biopsy, bronchoscopy (+/− transtracheal biopsy), excisional biopsy (open or thoracoscopic)

What is the treatment?
Surgical excision is the mainstay of treatment.
Excisional biopsy is therapeutic for benign lesions, solitary metastasis, and for primary cancer in patients who are poor risks for more extensive surgery.
Lobectomy for centrally placed lesions
Lobectomy with node dissection for primary cancer (if resectable by preop evaluations)

Which solitary nodule can be followed without a tissue diagnosis?
Popcorn calcifications
Mass unchanged for 2 years on previous CXR

What is the prognosis?
For malignant coin lesions <2 cm, 5-year survival is approximately 70%.

What if the patient has an SPN and pulmonary hypertrophic osteoarthropathy?
The patient has more than a 75% chance of having a carcinoma.

What is hypertrophic pulmonary osteoarthropathy?
Periosteal proliferation and new bone formation at the end of long bones and in bones of the hand

What is its incidence?
About 7% of patients with lung cancer (2% to 12%)

What are the signs?
Associated with clubbing of the fingers; diagnosed by x-ray of long bones, revealing periosteal bone hypertrophy

CARCINOID TUMOR

What is it?
An APUD (amine-precursor uptake and decarboxylation) cell tumor of the bronchus

What is its natural course in the lung?
Slow growing (but may be malignant)

What are the primary local findings?
Wheezing and atelectasis caused by bronchial obstruction/stenosis

What condition may it be confused with?
Asthma

How is the diagnosis made?
Bronchoscopy reveals round red-yellow-purple mass covered by epithelium that protrudes into bronchial lumen.

What is the treatment?
Surgical resection (lobectomy with lymph node dissection)
Sleeve resection is also an option for proximal bronchial lesions.

What is a sleeve resection?
Resection of a ring segment of bronchus (with tumor inside) and then end to end

anastomosis of the remaining ends, allowing salvage of lower lobe

What is the prognosis (5-year survival) after complete surgical resection of carcinoid:

Negative nodes? More than 90% are alive at 5 years.

Positive nodes? Two-thirds are alive at 5 years.

What is the most common benign lung tumor? Hamartoma (normal cells in a weird configuration)

PULMONARY SEQUESTRATION

What is it? Abnormal benign lung tissue with separate blood supply that **DOES NOT** communicate with the normal tracheobronchial airway

Define the following terms:

Interlobar Sequestration in normal lung tissue covered by normal visceral pleura

Extralobar Sequestration not in normal lung covered by its own pleura

What are the signs/symptoms? Asymptomatic, recurrent pneumonia

How is the diagnosis made? CXR, chest CT, A-gram, U/S with Doppler flow to ascertain blood supply

What is the treatment in the following cases:

Extralobar? Surgical resection

Intralobar? Lobectomy

What is the major danger during surgery for sequestration? Anomalous blood supply from below the diaphragm (these can be cut and retract into the abdomen and result in exsanguination!)
Always document blood supply by A-gram or U/S with Doppler flow.

DISEASES OF THE MEDIASTINUM

MEDIASTINAL ANATOMY

What structures lie in the following locations:

Superior mediastinum?
Aortic arch, great vessels, upper trachea, esophagus

Anterior mediastinum?
Thymus, ascending aorta, lymph nodes

Middle mediastinum?
Heart, lower trachea and bifurcation, lung hila, phrenic nerves, lymph nodes

Posterior mediastinum?
Esophagus, descending aorta, thoracic duct, vagus and intercostal nerves, sympathetic trunks, azygous and hemizygous veins, lymph nodes

What is the major differential diagnosis for tumors of t he mediastinum:

Anterior mediastinum?
The classic **"four Ts": T**hyroid tumor, **T**hymoma, **T**errible lymphoma, **T**eratoma; also parathyroid tumor, lipoma, vascular aneurysms

Middle mediastinum?
Lymphadenopathy (e.g., lymphoma, sarcoid), teratoma, fat pad, cysts, hernias, extension of esophageal mass, bronchogenic cancer

Posterior mediastinum?
Neurogenic tumors, lymphoma, aortic aneurysm, vertebral lesions, hernias

What is the differential diagnosis for a neurogenic tumor?
Schwannoma (A.K.A. neurolemmoma), neurofibroma, neuroblastoma, ganglioneuroma, ganglioneuroblastoma, pheochromocytoma

PRIMARY MEDIASTINAL TUMORS

Thymoma

Where are they found in the mediastinum?
Anterior

How is the diagnosis made?
CT

What is the treatment?
All thymomas should be surgically resected via midline sternotomy and, if malignant, treated with postoperative radiation therapy (33% 10-year survival rate for malignant thymoma treated with surgery and radiation).

What percentage of thymomas are malignant?
Approximately 25%

How is a malignant thymoma diagnosed?
At surgery with invasion into surrounding structures (not by histology!)

What is myasthenia gravis?
Autoimmune disease with antibodies against the muscle acetylcholine receptors

What percentage of patients with myasthenia gravis have a thymoma?
Approximately 15%

What percentage of patients with thymoma have or will have myasthenia gravis?
Approximately 75%!

Teratomas

What are they?
Tumors of branchial cleft cells; the tumors contain ectoderm, endoderm, and mesoderm

What is a dermoid cyst?
A teratoma made up of ectodermal derivatives (e.g., teeth, skin, hair)

Which age-group is affected?
Usually adolescents, but can occur at any age

Where in the mediastinum do they occur?
Anterior

What are the characteristic x-ray findings?
Calcifications or teeth; tumors may be cystic

What percentage are malignant?
Approximately 15%

What is the treatment of benign dermoid cysts?
Surgical excision

What is the treatment of malignant teratoma?

Preoperative chemotherapy until tumor markers are normal, then surgical resection

Which tumor markers are associated with malignant teratomas?

AFP, CEA

Neurogenic Tumors

What is the incidence?

Most common mediastinal tumors in all age groups

Where in the mediastinum do they occur?

Posterior, in the paravertebral gutters

What percentage are malignant?

50% in children
10% in adults

What are the histologic types (5)? (Note cells of origin and whether benign or malignant)

1. Neurilemmoma or schwannoma (benign)—arise from Schwann cell sheaths of intercostal nerves
2. Neurofibroma (benign)—arise from intercostal nerves; can degenerate into:
3. Neurosarcoma (malignant)
4. Ganglioneuroma (benign)—from sympathetic chain
5. Neuroblastoma (malignant)—also from sympathetic chain

LYMPHOMA

Where in the mediastinum do they occur?

Anywhere, but most often in the anterosuperior mediastinum or hilum in the middle mediastinum

What percentage of lymphomas involve mediastinal nodes?

Approximately 50%

What are the symptoms?

Cough, fever, chest pain, weight loss, SVC syndrome, chylothorax

How is the diagnosis made?

1. CXR, CT
2. Mediastinoscopy or mediastinotomy with node biopsy

What is the treatment?	Nonsurgical (chemotherapy, radiation, or both)

MEDIASTINITIS

Acute Mediastinitis

What is it?	Acute suppurative mediastinal infection
Name the six etiologies:	1. Esophageal perforation (Boerhaave's syndrome) 2. Postoperative wound infection 3. Head and neck infections 4. Lung or pleural infections 5. Rib or vertebral osteomyelitis 6. Distant infections
What are the clinical features?	Fever, chest pain, dysphagia (especially with esophageal perforation), respiratory distress, leukocytosis
What is the treatment?	1. **A**irway, **B**reathing, and **C**irculation (always first!) 2. Wide drainage 3. Treatment of primary cause 4. Antibiotics

Chronic Mediastinitis

What is it?	Mediastinal fibrosis secondary to *chronic* granulomatous infection
What is the most common etiology?	Histoplasma capsulatum
What are the clinical features?	50% are asymptomatic; symptoms are related to compression of adjacent structures: SVC syndrome, bronchial and esophageal strictures, constrictive pericarditis.
How is the diagnosis made?	CXR or CT may be helpful, but surgery/biopsy often makes the diagnosis.
What is the treatment?	Antibiotics; surgical removal of the granulomas is rarely helpful

SUPERIOR VENA CAVA SYNDROME

What is it?	Obstruction of the superior vena cava, usually by extrinsic compression

What is the number one cause? — Malignant tumors cause approximately 90% of cases; lung cancer is by far the most common; other tumors include thymoma, lymphoma, and Hodgkin's disease.

What are the clinical manifestations?

1. Blue discoloration and puffiness of the face, arms, and shoulders
2. CNS manifestations may include headache, nausea, vomiting, visual distortion, stupor, and convulsions.
3. Cough, hoarseness, and dyspnea

What is the treatment?

1. Diuretics and fluid restriction
2. Prompt radiation therapy with or without chemotherapy for any causative cancer

What is the prognosis? — SVC obstruction itself is fatal in less than 5% of cases; mean survival time in patients with malignant obstruction is about 7 months.

DISEASES OF THE ESOPHAGUS

ANATOMIC CONSIDERATIONS

What is the primary function of the UES? — Swallowing

What is the primary function of the LES? — Prevention of reflux

The esophageal venous plexus drains inferiorly into the gastric veins. Why is this important? — The gastric veins are part of the portal venous system; portal hypertension can thus be referred to the esophageal veins, leading to varices.

Identify the esophageal muscle type:

Proximal third — Skeletal muscle

Middle third — Smooth muscle > skeletal muscle

Distal third? — Smooth muscle

What is the length of the esophagus? — Approximately 25 cm in the adult (40 cm from teeth to LES)

Why is the esophagus notorious for anastomotic leaks?
The esophagus has no serosa (same as the distal rectum).

What nerve runs with the esophagus?
The vagus nerve

OROPHARYNGEAL DYSPHAGIA

What is it?
Improper relaxation of the UES

Describe the pathophysiology and the resulting complication.
Incoordination between relaxation of the UES and contraction of the pharynx leads to eventual formation of **Zenker's diverticulum,** which is a false diverticulum (mucosa only) above the cricopharyngeus muscle.

What are the symptoms?
Dysphagia, reflux of undigested food, left-sided neck mass, halitosis

What are the diagnostic tests?
History and physical examination; endoscopy to rule out other esophageal disorders (must be taken with caution as not to rupture through the diverticulum)

What is the treatment?
1. Myotomy of cricopharyngeus muscle
2. Excision of diverticulum

What muscle is involved with a Zenker's diverticulum?
Cricopharyngeus muscle

ACHALASIA

What is it?
1. Failure of the LES to relax during swallowing
2. Loss of esophageal **peristalsis**

What are the proposed etiologies?
1. Neurologic (ganglionic degeneration of Auerbach's plexus, vagus nerve, or both); possibly infectious in nature
2. Chagas' disease in South America

What are the associated long-term conditions?
Esophageal carcinoma secondary to Barrett's esophagus from food stasis

What are the symptoms?
Dysphagia for both solids and liquids, followed by regurgitation; dysphagia for liquids is worse

What are the diagnostic findings?

Radiographic contrast studies reveal dilated esophageal body with narrowing inferiorly.
Manometry: motility studies reveal increased pressure in the LES and failure of the LES to relax during swallowing

What is the treatment?

1. Balloon dilation of the LES
2. Medical treatment of reflux versus Belsey Mark IV 270° fundoplication (do not perform 360° Nissen)
3. Myotomy of the lower esophagus and LES

DIFFUSE ESOPHAGEAL SPASM

What is it?

Strong, nonperistaltic contractions of the esophageal body; sphincter function is usually normal

What is the associated condition?

Gastroesophageal reflux

What are the symptoms?

Spontaneous chest pain that radiates to the back, ears, neck, jaw, or arms

What is the differential diagnosis?

Angina pectoris
Psychoneurosis
Nutcracker esophagus

What are the associated diagnostic tests?

Esophageal manometry: Motility studies reveal repetitive, high-amplitude contractions with normal sphincter response
Upper GI may be normal, but 50% show segmented spasms or corkscrew esophagus
Endoscopy

What is the classic finding on esophageal contrast study (UGI)?

"Corkscrew esophagus"

What is the treatment?

Medical (antireflux measures, Ca channel blockers, nitrates)
Long esophagomyotomy in refractory cases

NUTCRACKER ESOPHAGUS

What is it also known as?

Hypertensive peristalsis

What is it?

Very strong peristaltic waves

What are the symptoms?

Spontaneous chest pain that radiates to the back, ears, neck, jaw, or arms

What is the differential diagnosis?

Angina pectoris
Psychoneurosis
Diffuse esophageal spasm

What are the associated diagnostic tests?

1. Esophageal manometry: motility studies reveal repetitive, high-amplitude contractions with normal sphincter response
2. Results of UGI may be normal (rule out mass)
3. Endoscopy

What is the treatment?

Medical (antireflux measures, Ca channel blockers, nitrates)
Long esophagomyotomy in refractory cases

ESOPHAGEAL REFLUX

What is it?

Reflux of gastric contents into the lower esophagus resulting from the decreased function of the LES

What are the causes?

1. Decreased LES tone
2. Decreased esophageal motility
3. Hiatal hernia
4. Gastric outlet obstruction
5. NGT

Name four associated conditions/factors.

1. Sliding hiatal hernia
2. Tobacco and alcohol
3. Scleroderma
4. Decreased endogenous gastrin production

What are the symptoms?

Substernal pain, heartburn, regurgitation; symptoms are worse when patient is supine and after meals

How is the diagnosis made?

1. pH probe in the lower esophagus reveals acid reflux.
2. EGD shows esophagitis.
3. Manometry reveals decreased LES pressure.
4. Barium swallow

What is the treatment?

Initially medical: H_2 blockers, antacids, metoclopramide, omeprazole
Elevation of the head of the bed; small, multiple meals

Which four complications require surgery?

1. Failure of medical therapy
2. Esophageal strictures
3. Progressive pulmonary insufficiency secondary to documented nocturnal aspiration
4. Barrett's esophagus

Describe each of the following types of surgery:

Nissen

360° fundoplication: wrap fundus of stomach all the way around the esophagus

Belsey Mark IV

270° fundoplication: wrap fundus of stomach, but not all the way around

Hill

Tighten arcuate ligament around esophagus and tack stomach to diaphragm

Lap Nissen

Nissen via laparoscope

Lap Toupet?

Lap fundoplication posteriorly with less than 220 to 250° wrap used with decreased esophageal motility; disadvantage is more postoperative reflux

What is Barrett's esophagus?

Replacement of the lower esophageal squamous epithelium with columnar epithelium secondary to reflux

Why is it significant?

This lesion is premalignant.

What is the treatment?

People with significant reflux should be followed with regular EGDs with biopsies, H_2-blockers, and antireflux precautions; many experts believe that patients with severe dysplasia should undergo esophagectomy.

CAUSTIC ESOPHAGEAL STRICTURES

Which agents may cause strictures if ingested?

Lye, oven cleaners, drain cleaners, batteries, sodium hydroxide tablets (Clinitest)

How is the diagnosis made?

History; EGD is clearly indicated early on to assess the extent of damage (< 24 hrs); scope to level of severe injury (deep ulcer) only, water soluble contrast study for deep ulcers to rule out perforation

What is the initial treatment?

1. NPO/IVF/H_2-blocker
2. Do **not** induce emesis.
3. Corticosteroids (controversial—probably best for shallow/moderate ulcers), antibiotics (penicillin/gentamicin) for moderate ulcers
4. Antibiotic for deep ulcers
5. Upper GI at 10 to 14 days

What is the treatment if stricture develops?

Dilation with Maloney dilator/balloon catheter

In severe refractory cases, esophagectomy with colon interposition or gastric pull up

What is the long-term follow-up?

Because of increased risk of esophageal squamous cancer (especially with ulceration), patients need endoscopies every other year.

What is a Maloney dilator?

Mercury-filled rubber dilator

ESOPHAGEAL CARCINOMA

What are the two main types?

1. Squamous cell carcinoma in most of the esophagus
2. Adenocarcinoma at the GE junction

What is the age and gender distribution?

Most common in the sixth decade of life; men predominate

What are the etiologic factors (4)?

1. Tobacco
2. Alcohol

3. GE reflux
4. Barrett's esophagus

What are the symptoms?

Dysphagia, weight loss
Others symptoms include chest pain, back pain, hoarseness, symptoms of metastasis

What comprises the workup?

1. UGI
2. EGD
3. Transesophageal ultrasound (TEU)
4. CT scan of chest/abdomen

What is the differential diagnosis?

Leiomyoma, metastatic tumor, lymphomas, benign stricture, achalasia, diffuse esophageal spasm, GERD

How is the diagnosis made?

1. Upper GI localizes tumor.
2. EGD obtains biopsy and assesses resectability.
3. Full metastatic workup (CXR, bone scan, CT, LFTs)

Describe the stages of esophageal cancer:

Stage I

Tumor: invades **lamina propria** or **submucosa**
Nodes: negative

Stage IIa

Tumor: invades muscularis propria or adventitia
Nodes: negative

Stage IIb

Tumor: **any tumor** that invades up to the muscularis propria
Nodes: positive regional nodes

Stage III

Tumor: invades adventitia
Nodes: positive regional nodes OR
Tumor: invades adjacent structures
Nodes: positive or negative nodes

Stage IV

Distant metastasis

What is the treatment?

Total thoracic esophagectomy with gastric pull-up or colon interposition (± chemotherapy/radiation, usually in a clinical trial)

What is the operative mortality rate?	About 5%
What is the prognosis (5-year survival) by stage:	
I?	80%
II?	33%
III?	15%
IV?	Basically 0%

68 Cardiovascular Surgery

What do the following abbreviations stand for:

AI?	**A**ortic **I**nsufficiency/regurgitation
AS?	**A**ortic **S**tenosis
CABG?	**C**oronary **A**rtery **B**ypass **G**rafting
CAD?	**C**oronary **A**rtery **D**isease
CPB?	**C**ardio**P**ulmonary **B**ypass
IABP?	**I**ntra-**A**ortic **B**alloon **P**ump
LAD?	**L**eft **A**nterior **D**escending coronary artery
IMA?	**I**nternal **M**ammary **A**rtery
MR?	**M**itral **R**egurgitation
PTCA?	**P**ercutaneous **T**ransluminal **C**oronary **A**ngioplasty (balloon angioplasty)
VAD?	**V**entricular **A**ssist **D**evice
VSD?	**V**entricular **S**eptal **D**efect

Define the following terms:

Stroke volume (SV)	ml of blood pumped per heartbeat ($SV = \frac{CO}{HR}$)
Cardiac output (CO)	Amount of blood pumped by the heart each minute: heart rate $\times$ SV
Cardiac Index (CI)	CO/BSA (body surface area)

Ejection fraction	Percentage of blood pumped out of the left ventricle: SV ÷ end diastolic volume (nl 55% to 70%)
Compliance	Change in volume/change in pressure
SVR	**S**ystemic **V**ascular **R**esistance $\frac{\text{MAP} - \text{CVP}}{\text{CO} \times 80}$
Preload	Left ventricular end diastolic pressure or volume
Afterload	Arterial resistance the heart pumps against
PVR	**P**ulmonary **V**ascular **R**esistance $\text{PA}_{(\text{mean})} - \text{PCWP/CO} \times 80$
MAP	**M**ean **A**rterial **P**ressure = Diastolic BP + 1/3 (Systolic BP–Diastolic BP)
What is a normal CO?	4 to 8 L/minute
What is a normal CI?	2.5 to 4 L/minute
What are the ways to increase CO?	1. **Rate**—Increase heart rate 2. **Rhythm**—Normal sinus 3. **Preload**—Increase preload 4. **Afterload**—Decrease afterload 5. **Inotropes**—Increase contractility 6. **Mechanical** assistance (IABP)
When does most of the coronary blood flow take place?	During diastole (66%)
Name the three major coronary arteries.	1. Left anterior descending (LAD) 2. Circumflex 3. Right coronary
What are the three main "cardiac electrolytes"?	1. Calcium (inotropic) 2. Potassium (dysrhythmias) 3. Magnesium (dysrhythmias)

ACQUIRED HEART DISEASE

CORONARY ARTERY DISEASE (CAD)

What is it?

Atherosclerotic occlusive lesions of the coronary arteries; segmental nature makes CABG possible

What is the incidence?

CAD is the #1 killer in the Western world; more than 50% of cases are triple vessel diseases involving the LAD, circumflex, and right coronary arteries.

What are the symptoms?

If ischemia occurs (low flow, vasospasm, thrombus formation, plaque rupture, or a combination), patient may experience chest pain; crushing, substernal shortness of breath; nausea/upper abdominal pain; sudden death; or may be asymptomatic with fatigue.

Who classically get "silent" MIs?

Patients with diabetes (autonomic dysfunction)

What are the risk factors?

HTN
Smoking
High (>240) cholesterol/lipids
Obesity
Diabetes mellitus
Family history

Which diagnostic tests should be performed?

Exercise stress testing (± thallium)
Echocardiography
Localize dyskinetic wall segments
Valvular dysfunction
Estimate ejection fraction
Cardiac catheterization with coronary angiography and left ventriculography (definitive test)

What is the treatment?

Medical therapy (β-blockers, aspirin, nitrates, HTN medications), angioplasty (PTCA), surgical therapy: CABG

CABG

What is it?

Coronary **A**rtery **B**ypass **G**rafting

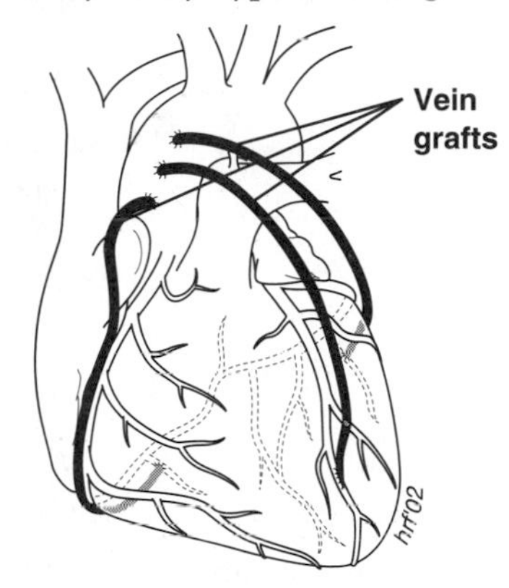

What are the indications?

Left main disease
Three-vessel disease (main arteries—not branches)
Unstable or disabling angina unresponsive to medical therapy
Postinfarct angina
Coronary artery rupture, dissection, thrombosis after PTCA

What procedures are most often used in the treatment?

Coronary arteries grafted (usually 3 to 6): internal mammary pedicle graft and saphenous vein free graft are most often used (IMA 95% 10-year patency vs. 60% to 70% with saphenous); procedure is performed under CPB

What other vessels are occasionally used for grafting?

Gastroepiploic and inferior epigastric veins

What are the possible complications?

MI, dysrhythmias
Infection
Hemorrhage
Graft thrombosis
Sternal dehiscence
Postpericardiotomy syndrome, stroke, tamponade

What is the operative mortality?

Between 1% and 3% for elective CABG (vs. 5% to 10% for acute MI)

What medication should every patient be given after CABG?

Aspirin

POSTPERICARDIOTOMY SYNDROME

What is it?

Pericarditis after pericardiotomy (unknown etiology), occurs weeks to 3 months postoperatively

What are the signs/ symptoms?

Fever
Chest pain, atrial fibrillation
Malaise
Pericardial friction rub
Pericardial effusion/pleural effusion

What is the treatment?

NSAIDs, with or without steroids

What is pericarditis after an MI called?

Dressler's syndrome

CARDIOPULMONARY BYPASS (CPB)

What is it?

Pump and oxygenation apparatus remove blood from SVC and IVC and return it to the aorta, bypassing the heart and lungs and allowing cardiac arrest for open heart procedures, heart transplant, lung transplant, or heart-lung transplant, as well as procedures on the proximal great vessels.

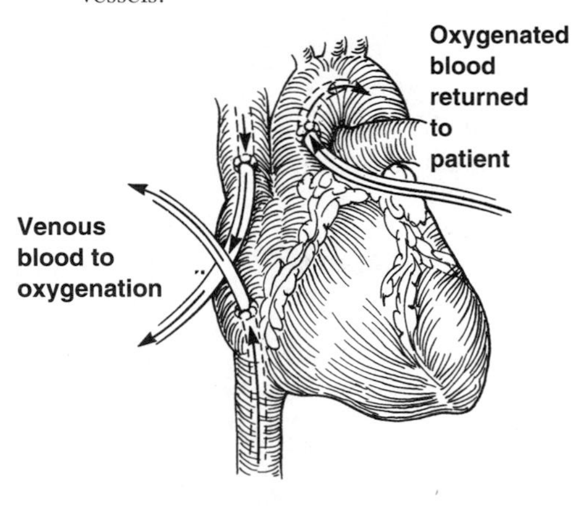

Is anticoagulation necessary?

Yes, just before and during the procedure, with heparin

How is anticoagulation reversed?

Protamine

What are the six ways to manipulate cardiac output after CPB?

Rate, rhythm, afterload, preload, inotropes, mechanical (IABP and VAD)

What mechanical problems can decrease CO after a CPB procedure?

Cardiac tamponade, pneumothorax

What are the possible complications?

Trauma to formed blood elements (especially thrombocytopenia and platelet dysfunction)
Pancreatitis (low flow)
Heparin rebound
CVA
Failure to wean from bypass
Technical complications (operative technique)
MI

What is heparin rebound?

Increased anticoagulation after CPB from increased heparin levels, as increase in peripheral blood flow after CPB returns heparin residual that was in the peripheral tissues

What is the method of lowering SVR after CPB?

Warm the patient, administer sodium nitroprusside (SNP) and dobutamine

What are the options if a patient cannot be weaned from CPB?

Inotropes (e.g., epinephrine)
VAD

What percentage of patients go into AFib after CPB?

Up to 33%

What is the workup of a postoperative patient with AFib?

Rule out PTX (CXR), acidosis (ABG), electrolyte abnormality (chem 10), and ischemia (EKG).

What is a MIDCAB?

Minimally **I**nvasive **D**irect **C**oronary **A**rtery **B**ypass-LIMA to LAD bypass without CPB and through a small thoracotomy

What is TMR?

Trans**myo**cardial laser **Rev**ascularization-laser through groin catheter makes small

	holes (intramyocardial sinusoids) in cardiac muscle to allow blood to nourish the muscle
TMR is modeled after what type of heart?	Reptile and human fetus!

AORTIC STENOSIS (AS)

What is it?	Destruction and calcification of valve leaflets, resulting in obstruction of left ventricular outflow
What are the causes?	Calcification of bicuspid aortic valve Rheumatic fever Acquired calcific AS (7th to 8th decades)
What are the symptoms?	Angina (5 years life expectancy if untreated) Syncope (3 years life expectancy if untreated) CHF (2 years life expectancy if untreated) Often asymptomatic until late Mnemonic: **A**ortic **S**tenosis **C**omplications (**A**ngina **S**yncope **C**HF)—5,3,2
What are the signs?	Murmur: crescendo-decrescendo systolic second right intercostal space with radiation to the carotids Left ventricular heave or lift from left ventricular hypertrophy
What tests should be performed?	CXR, EKG, echocardiography Cardiac catheterization—needed to plan operation
What is the treatment?	Valve replacement with tissue or mechanical prosthesis, if patient is symptomatic or valve cross-sectional area is <0.7 cm^2 (normal 2.5 to 3.5 cm^2) and gradient >50 mm Hg
What are the pros/cons of mechanical valve?	Mechanical valve is more durable, but requires lifetime anticoagulation.
Why is a loud murmur often a good sign?	Implies a high gradient, which indicates preserved LV function

Why might an AS murmur diminish over time?
It may imply a decreasing gradient from a decline in LV function.

AORTIC INSUFFICIENCY (AI)

What is it?
Incompetency of the aortic valve

What are the causes?
Bacterial endocarditis (*Staphylococcus aureus, Streptococcus viridans*)
Rheumatic fever
Annular ectasia from collagen vascular disease (especially Marfan's syndrome)

What are the predisposing conditions?
Bicuspid aortic valve, connective tissue disease

What are the symptoms?
Palpitations from dysrhythmias and dilated left ventricle
Dyspnea/orthopnea from left ventricular failure
Angina from decreased diastolic BP and coronary flow (*Note:* most coronary blood flow occurs during diastole and aorta rebound.)

What are the signs?
Murmur: blowing, decrescendo diastolic at left sternal border
Austin-Flint murmur: reverberation of regurgitant flow
Increased pulse pressure: "pistol shots," "water-hammer" pulse palpated over peripheral arteries

Which diagnostic tests should be performed?
1. CXR: increasing heart size can be used to follow progression
2. Echocardiogram
3. Catheterization (definitive)

What is the treatment?
Aortic valve replacement

What are the indications for surgical treatment?
All symptomatic patients (CHF, PND, etc.), left ventricle dilatation, decreasing LV function, decreasing EF

What is the prognosis?
Low operative risk; surgery gives symptomatic improvement and may improve longevity

MITRAL STENOSIS (MS)

What is it?
Calcific degeneration and narrowing of the mitral valve resulting from rheumatic fever in most cases

What are the symptoms?
1. Dyspnea from increased left atrial pressure, causing pulmonary edema (i.e., CHF)
2. Hemoptysis (rarely life-threatening)
3. Hoarseness from dilated left atrium impinging on the recurrent laryngeal nerve

What are the signs?
Murmur: crescendo diastolic rumble at apex
Irregular pulse from AFib caused by dilated left atrium
Stroke caused by systemic emboli from left atrium (AFib and obstructed valve allow blood to pool in the left atrium and can lead to thrombus formation)

Which diagnostic tests should be performed?
Echocardiogram
Catheterization

What is the treatment?
1. Open commissurotomy: open heart operation with CPB
2. Balloon valvuloplasty: percutaneous; if unsuccessful, surgery is required
3. Valve replacement

What is the prognosis?
More than 80% of patients are well at 10 years with successful operation.

MITRAL REGURGITATION (MR)

What is it?
Incompetence of the mitral valve

What are the causes?
Severe mitral valve prolapse (some prolapse is found in 5% of the population, with women ≥ men)
Rheumatic fever
Post-MI from papillary muscle dysfunction/rupture
Ruptured chordae

What are the most common causes?
Rheumatic fever (#1 worldwide), Ruptured chordae/papillary muscle dysfunction

What are the symptoms? Often insidious and late: dyspnea, palpitations, fatigue

What are the signs? Murmur: holosystolic, apical radiating to the axilla

What are the indications for treatment? Indications for surgery differ from those for MS; in MR, catheter and echocardiogram findings are more revealing than symptoms (e.g., increasing regurgitation, decreasing EF). *Note:* EF first increases in MR; therefore, normal EF may actually indicate decompensation.

What is the treatment?

1. Valve replacement
2. Annuloplasty: suture a prosthetic ring to the dilated valve annulus

What is a normal EF? From 55% to 70%

ARTIFICIAL VALVE PLACEMENT

What is it? Replacement of damaged valves with tissue or mechanical prosthesis

What are the types of valves? **Tissue:** glutaraldehyde-fixed porcine valves deteriorate over time (about 20% require replacement in 10 years); however, they do not require long-term anticoagulation

Contraindicated in children because of calcification

Mechanical: can last for the life of the patient, but require lifelong anticoagulation

Contraindicated in those with bleeding tendency (e.g., PUD, ETOH abuse)

What is the operative mortality? From 1% to 5% in most series

What must patients with an artificial valve receive before dental procedures? Antibiotics

INFECTIOUS ENDOCARDITIS

What is it? Microbial infection of heart valves

What are the predisposing conditions?
Pre-existing valvular lesion, procedures that lead to bacteremia/IV drug use

What are the common causative agents?
S. viridans: associated with abnormal valves
S. aureus: associated with IV drug use
S. epidermidis: associated with prosthetic valves

What are the signs/ symptoms?
Murmur (new or changing)
Petechiae
Splinter hemorrhage (fingernails)
Roth spots (on retina)
Osler nodes (raised, **painful** on soles and palms; **O**sler = **O**uch!)
Janeway lesions (similar to Osler nodes, but flat and **painless**)
(Janeway = pain **away**)

Which diagnostic tests should be performed?
Echocardiogram, TEE
Serial blood cultures (definitive)

What is the treatment?
Prolonged IV therapy with bactericidal antibiotics, to which infecting organisms are sensitive

What is the prognosis?
Infection can progress, requiring valve replacement

CONGENITAL HEART DISEASE

VENTRICULAR SEPTAL DEFECT (VSD)

What is its claim to fame?
Most common congenital heart defect

What is it?
Failure of ventricular septum to completely close; **80% of cases involve the membranous portion of the septum,** resulting in left-to-right shunt, increased pulmonary blood flow, and CHF if pulmonary to systemic flow is >2:1

What is pulmonary vascular obstructive disease?
Pulmonary artery hyperplasia from increased pulmonary pressure caused by a left to right shunt (e.g., VSD)

What is Eisenmenger's syndrome?
Irreversible pulmonary HTN from chronic changes in pulmonary arterioles

and increased right heart pressures; cyanosis develops when the shunt reverses (becomes right to left across the VSD)

What is the treatment of Eisenmenger's syndrome?
The only option is heart-lung transplant; otherwise, the disease is untreatable.

What is the incidence of VSD?
30% of heart defects (most common defect)

PATENT DUCTUS ARTERIOSUS (PDA)

What is it?
Physiologic right-to-left shunt in fetal circulation connecting the pulmonary artery to the aorta bypassing fetal lungs; often, this shunt persists in the neonate

What are the factors preventing closure?
Hypoxia, increased prostaglandins, prematurity

What are the symptoms?
Often asymptomatic
Poor feeding
Respiratory distress
CHF with respiratory infections

What are the signs?
Acyanotic, unless other cardiac lesions are present; continuous "machinery" murmur

Which diagnostic tests should be performed?
Physical examination
Echocardiogram (to rule out associated defects)
Catheter (seldom required)

What is the medical treatment?
Indomethacin is an NSAID: prostaglandin (PG) inhibitor (PG keeps PDA open).

What is the treatment?
Surgical ligation or cardiac catheterization closure at 6 months to 2 years of age

TETRALOGY OF FALLOT (TOF)

What is it?
Malalignment of the infundibular septum in early development, leading to the characteristic tetrad:
1. Pulmonary stenosis/obstruction of right ventricular outflow
2. Overriding aorta
3. Right ventricular hypertrophy
4. VSD

What are the symptoms?
Hypoxic spells (squatting behavior increases SVR and increases pulmonary blood flow)

What are the signs?
Cyanosis
Clubbing
Murmur: SEM at left third intercostal space

Which diagnostic tests should be performed?
CXR: small, "boot-shaped" heart and decreased pulmonary blood flow
Echocardiography

What is the prognosis?
95% survival at specialized centers

IHSS

What is IHSS?
Idiopathic **h**ypertrophic **s**ubaortic **s**tenosis

What is the usual presentation?
Can present with sudden death from:
1. Dysrhythmias
2. Syncope
3. CHF

COARCTATION OF THE AORTA

What is it?
Narrowing of the thoracic aorta, with or without intraluminal "shelf" (infolding of the media); usually found near ductus/ligamentum arteriosum

What are the three types?
1. Preductal (fatal in infancy if untreated)
2. Juxtaductal
3. Postductal

What percentage are associated with other cardiac defects?
60% (bicuspid aortic valve is most common)

What is the major route of collateral circulation?
Subclavian artery to the IMA to the intercostals to the descending aorta

What is the incidence?
From 10% to 15% of defects

What are the symptoms?
Headache
Epistaxis
Lower extremity fatigue → claudication

What are the signs?

Pulses: decreased lower extremity pulses
Murmurs:
1. Systolic—from turbulence across coarctation, often radiating to infrascapular region
2. Continuous—from dilated collaterals

Which diagnostic tests should be performed?

CXR
"3" sign is aortic knob, coarctation, and dilated poststenotic aorta
Rib notching is bony erosion from dilated intercostal collaterals
Echocardiogram
Cardiac catheterization if cardiac defects

What is the treatment?

Surgery
Resection with end-to-end anastomosis
Patch graft (rare)
Subclavian artery flap
Interposition graft
Endovascular repair an option in adults

What are the indications for surgery?

Symptomatic patient
Asymptomatic patient older than 3 to 4 years

What are the possible postoperative complications?

Paraplegia
"Paradoxic" HTN (postoperative)
Mesenteric necrotizing panarteritis (GI bleeding)

What is the prognosis?

Untreated life expectancy: 30 to 40 years

What are the long-term concerns?

Aortic dissection, HTN

TRANSPOSITION OF THE GREAT VESSELS

What is it?

Aorta originates from the right ventricle and the pulmonary artery from the left ventricle; fatal without PDA, ASD, or VSD to allow communication between the left and right circulations

What is the incidence?

From 5% to 8% of defects

What are the signs/symptoms?

Most common lesion that presents with cyanosis and CHF in neonatal period (>90% by day 1)

Which diagnostic tests should be performed?
CXR: "egg-shaped" heart contour
Catheterization (definitive)

What is the treatment?
Arterial switch operation—aorta and pulmonary artery are moved to the correct ventricle and the coronaries are re-implanted

EBSTEIN'S ANOMALY

What is it?
Tricuspid valve is placed abnormally low in the right ventricle, forming a large right atrium and a small right ventricle, leading to tricuspid regurgitation and decreased right ventricular output

What are the risk factors?
400 times the risk if the mother has taken lithium

VASCULAR RINGS

What are they?
Many types; represent an anomalous development of the aorta/pulmonary artery from the embryonic aortic arch that surrounds and obstructs the trachea/esophagus

How are they diagnosed?
Barium swallow, MRI

What are the signs/symptoms?
Most prominent is stridor from tracheal compression

CYANOTIC HEART DISEASE

What are the causes?
The five "Ts" of cyanotic heart disease:
- **T**etralogy of Fallot
- **T**runcus arteriosus
- **T**otally anomalous pulmonary venous return (TAPVR)
- **T**ricuspid atresia
- **T**ransposition of the great vessels

CARDIAC TUMORS

What is the most common benign lesion?
Myxoma in adults, commonly found in the left atrium with pedunculated morphology (60% to 80% of primary cardiac tumors)

What is the most common malignant tumor in children?
Rhabdomyosarcoma

DISEASES OF THE GREAT VESSELS

THORACIC AORTIC ANEURYSM

What is it?
Aneurysm of the thoracic aorta

What is the cause?
Vast majority result from atherosclerosis, connective tissue disease.

What is the major differential diagnosis?
Aortic dissection

What percentage of patients have aneurysms of the aorta at a distant site?
About 33%! (rule out AAA)

What are the signs/ symptoms?
Most are asymptomatic.
Chest pain, stridor, hemoptysis (rare), recurrent laryngeal nerve compression

What is the most common way to diagnose?
Routine CXR

Which diagnostic tests should be performed?
CXR, CT, MRI, aortography

What are the indications for surgical treatment?
>6 cm in diameter
>2.5 times contiguous normal aortic diameter
Symptoms
Rapid increase in diameter
Rupture

What is the treatment?
Replace with graft.

What are the dreaded complications after treatment of a thoracic aortic aneurysm?
Paraplegia (up to 20%)
Anterior spinal syndrome

What is anterior spinal syndrome?
Syndrome characterized by:
Paraplegia
Incontinence (bowel/bladder)
Pain and temperature sensation loss

What is the cause?

Occlusion of the great radicular artery of **Adamkiewicz,** which is one of the intercostal/lumbar arteries from T8 to L4

AORTIC DISSECTION

What is it?

Separation of the walls of the aorta from an intimal tear and disease of the tunica media; a false lumen is formed and a "reentry" tear may occur, resulting in "double-barrel" aorta

What are the aortic dissection classifications?

DeBakey classification
Stanford classification

Define the DeBakey classifications:

DeBakey type I

Involves ascending **and** descending aorta

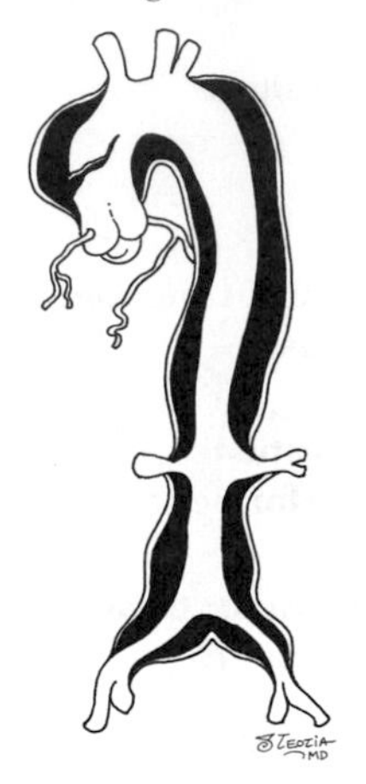

DeBakey type II

Involves ascending aorta only

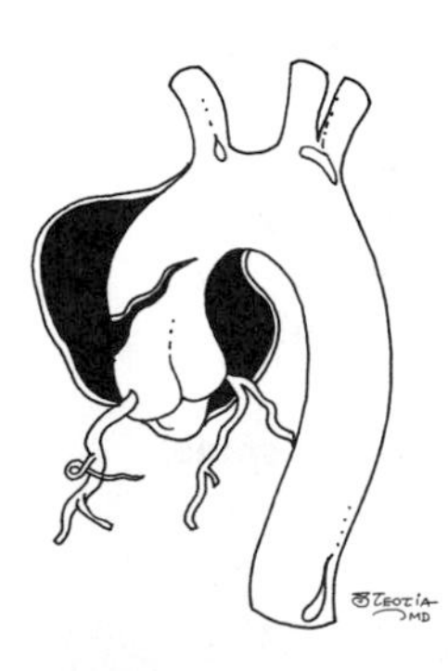

DeBakey type III

Involves descending aorta only

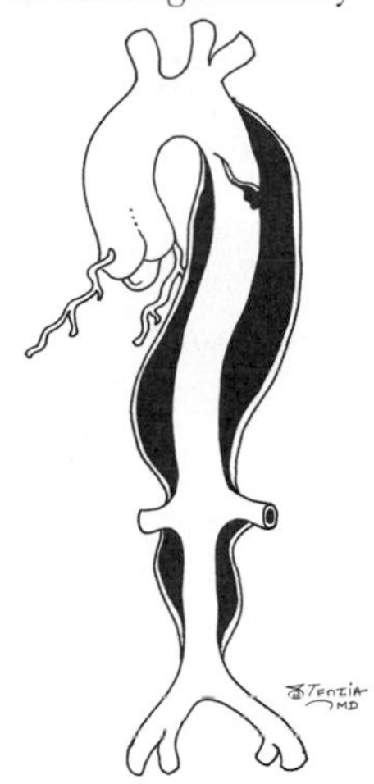

Define the Stanford classifications:

Type A

Ascending aorta (requires surgery) ± Descending aorta (includes DeBakey Types I and II)

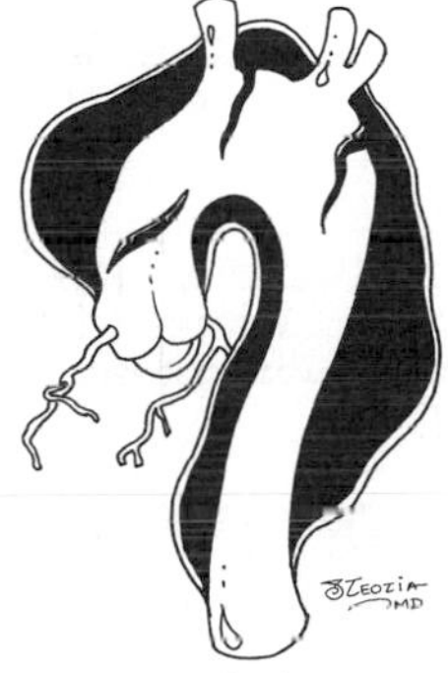

Type B

Descending aorta only (nonoperative, except for complications) (same as DeBakey Type III)

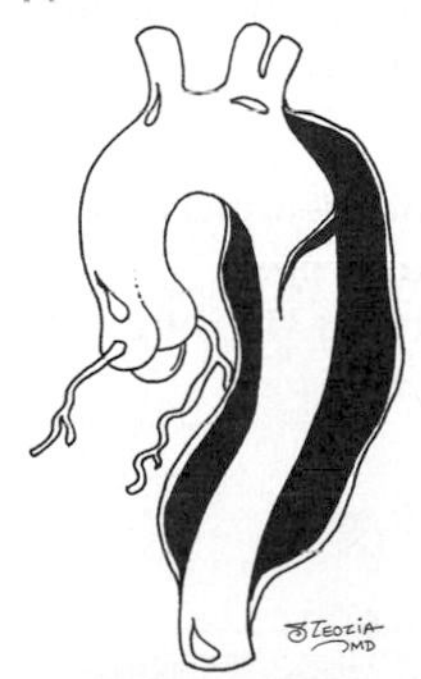

What is the etiology?

HTN (most important)
Marfan's syndrome
Bicuspid aortic valve
Coarctation of the aorta
Cystic medial necrosis
Proximal aortic aneurysm

What are the signs/ symptoms?

Abrupt onset of severe chest pain, most often radiating/tearing to the back; onset is typically more abrupt than that of MI; the pain can migrate as the dissection progresses; patient describes a **"tearing pain"**

Note three other sequelae.

1. Cardiac tamponade; Beck's triad—distant heart sounds, increased CVP with JVD, decreased blood pressure
2. Aortic insufficiency—diastolic murmur
3. Aortic arterial branch occlusion/ shearing, leading to ischemia in the involved circulation (i.e., unequal pulses, CVA, paraplegia, renal insufficiency, bowel ischemia, claudication)

Which diagnostic tests are indicated?

CXR
1. Widened mediastinum
2. Pleural effusion

TEE
CT
Aortography (definitive gold standard but time-consuming!)

What is a dissecting aortic aneurysm?

A misnomer! Not an aneurysm!

What is the treatment of the various types:

Types I and II (Stanford type A)?

Surgical because of risk of:
1. Aortic insufficiency
2. Compromise of cerebral and coronary circulation
3. Tamponade
4. Rupture

Type III (Stanford type B)? Medical (control BP), unless complicated by rupture or significant occlusions

Describe the surgery for an aortic dissection. Open the aorta at the proximal extent of dissection, and then sew—graft to—intimal flap and adventitia circumferentially.

What is the preoperative treatment? Control BP with sodium nitroprusside and β-blockers (e.g., esmolol; β-blockers decrease shear stress).

What is the postoperative treatment? Lifetime control of BP and monitoring of aortic size

What is the possible cause of MI in a patient with aortic dissection? Dissection involves the coronary arteries or underlying LAD.

What are the EKG signs of the following disorders:

Atrial fibrillation? Irregularly irregular

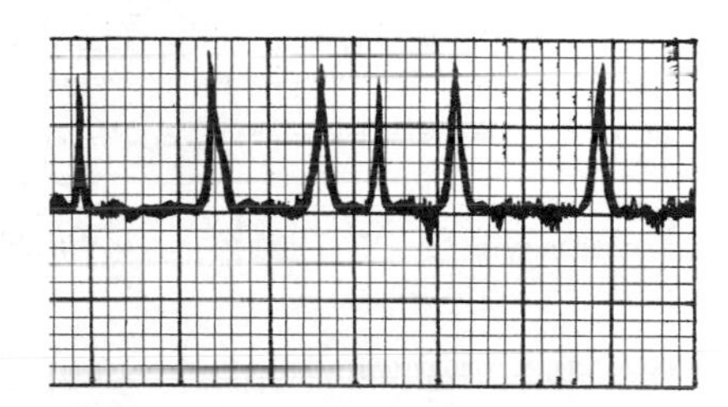

PVC? Premature ventricular complex: Wide QRS

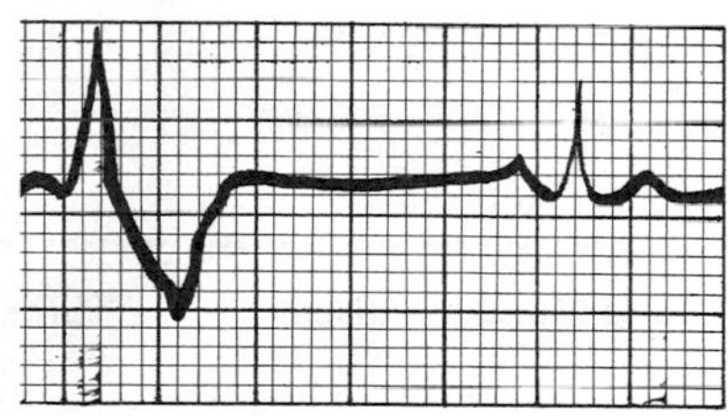

Ventricular aneurysm? ST elevation

Ischemia? ST elevation/ST depression/flipped T waves

Infarction? Q waves

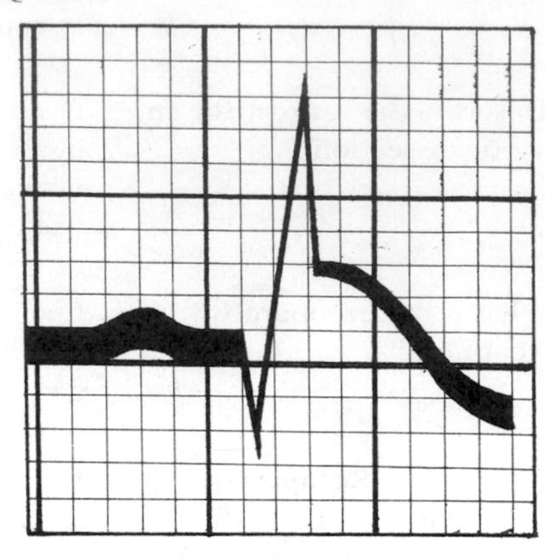

Pericarditis? ST elevation throughout leads

RBBB? **R**ight **b**undle **b**ranch **b**lock: wide QRS and "rabbit ears" or R-R in V1 or V2

LBBB? **L**eft **b**undle **b**ranch **b**lock: wide QRS and "rabbit ears" or R-R in V5 or V6

Wolff-Parkinson-White Delta wave = slurred upswing on QRS

First degree A-V block? Prolonged P-R interval (0.2 second)

Second degree A-V block? Dropped QRS; not all P waves transmit to produce ventricular contraction

Wenckebach phenomenon? Second-degree block with progressive delay in P-R interval prior to dropped beat

Third-degree A-V block? Complete A-V dissociation; random P wave and QRS

MISCELLANEOUS

What is Mondor's disease? Thrombophlebitis of the thoraco-epigastric veins

What is a VAD? **V**entricular **A**ssist **D**evice

How does an IABP work? The **I**ntra-**A**ortic **B**alloon **P**ump has a balloon tip resting in the aorta.

The balloon inflates in diastole, increasing diastolic BP and coronary blood flow. In systole the balloon deflates, creating a negative pressure, lowering afterload, and increasing systolic BP.

What electrolyte must be monitored during diuresis after CPB?

K^+

How is extent/progress of postbypass diuresis followed?

Daily weight, I's and O's, CXR, JVD, edema, etc.

During a CABG, what can be used in place of the saphenous vein?

IMA, inferior epigastric vessels, radial artery, gastroepiploic vessels (*Note:* prosthetic material cannot be used)

What side effect is associated with protamine?

Hypotension

What is an Austin Flint murmur?

Diastolic murmur of AI secondary to regurgitant turbulent flow

Where is the least-oxygenated blood in the body?

Coronary sinus

What is the most common cause of a cardiac tumor?

Metastasis

69 Transplant Surgery

Define the following terms:

Autograft	Same individual is both donor and recipient.
Isograft	Donor and recipient are genetically identical (identical twins).
Allograft	Donor and recipient are genetically dissimilar, but of the same species.
Xenograft	Donor and recipient belong to different species.
Orthotopic	Donor organ is placed in normal anatomic position (liver, heart).
Heterotopic	Donor organ is placed in a different site than the normal anatomic position (kidney, pancreas).
Paratopic	Donor organ is placed close to original organ.

BASIC IMMUNOLOGY

What are histocompatibility antigens?	Distinct (genetically inherited) cell surface proteins of the human leukocyte antigen system (HLA)
Why are they important?	They are targets (class I antigens) and initiators (class II antigens) of immune response to donor tissue (i.e., distinguishing self from nonself).
Which cells have class I antigens?	All nucleated cells (think: class 1 = all cells and thus "one for all")

Which cells have class II antigens?
Macrophages, monocytes, B cells, activated T cells, endothelial cells

What is the MHC called in humans?
HLA (human leukocyte antigen)

What is the location?
Short arm of chromosome 6

What is the code?
Class I, II, and III antigens

CELLS

T CELLS

What is the source?
Thymus

What is the function?
Cell-mediated immunity/rejection

What are the types?
Th (CD4): helper T—help B cells become plasma cells
Ts (CD8): suppressor T—regulate immune response
Tc (CD8): cytotoxic T—kill cell by direct contact

B CELLS

What is the function?
Humoral immunity

What is the cell type that produces antibodies?
B cells differentiate into plasma cells.

MACROPHAGE

What is it?
A monocyte in parenchymal tissue

What is its function?
Processes foreign protein and presents it to lymphocytes

What is it also known as?
Antigen-presenting cell (APC)

Briefly describe the events leading to antibody production.
1. Macrophage engulfs antigen and presents it to Th cells; the macrophage produces IL-1.
2. The Th cells then produce IL-2, and the Th cells proliferate.
3. The Th cells then activate (via IL-4) B cells that differentiate into plasma

cells, which produce antibodies against the antigen presented.

IMMUNOSUPPRESSION

Who needs to be immunosuppressed?
All recipients (except autograft or isograft)

What are the three major drugs used for immunosuppression?
Corticosteroids, azathioprine, cyclosporine

What are the other drugs?
OKT3, ATGAM, FK-506, mycophenolate

What is the advantage of "triple therapy"?
Employs three immunosuppressive drugs; therefore, a lower dose of each can be used, decreasing the toxic side effects of each

CORTICOSTEROIDS

Which is most commonly used in transplants?
Prednisone

How does it function?
Primarily blocks production of IL-1 by macrophage and stabilizes lysosomal membrane of macrophage

What is the associated toxicity?
"Cushingoid," alopecia, striae, HTN, diabetes, pancreatitis, ulcer disease, osteomalacia, aseptic necrosis (especially of the femoral head)

What is the relative potency of the following corticosteroids:

Cortisol?
1

Prednisone?
4

Methylprednisolone?
5

Dexamethasone?
25

AZATHIOPRINE (AZA [IMURAN])

How does it function?
Prodrug that is cleaved into mercaptopurine; inhibits synthesis of DNA and RNA, leading to decreased cellular (T/B cells) production

What is the associated toxicity?	Toxic to bone marrow (leukopenia + thrombocytopenia), hepatotoxic, associated with pancreatitis
When should a lower dose of AZA be administered?	When WBC is <4
What is the associated drug interaction?	Decrease dose if patient is also on allopurinol, because allopurinol inhibits the enzyme xanthine oxidase, which is necessary for the breakdown of azathioprine.

CYCLOSPORINE (CSA)

What is its function?	Inhibits production of IL-2 by Th cells
What is the associated toxicity?	1. Nephrotoxicity (dose-dependent, reversible) 2. Elevated LFTs (50%) 3. Neurotoxic tremor (50%), seizures (5%) 4. HTN 5. Gum hypertrophy 6. Hirsutism 7. Hyperkalemia
What drugs increase CSA levels?	Diltiazem Ketoconazole Erythromycin, fluconazole, **ranitidine**
What drugs decrease CSA levels?	By inducing the p450 system: dilantin, Tegretol, rifampin, isoniazid, barbiturates
What are the drugs of choice for HTN from CSA?	Clonidine, calcium channel blockers

ATGAM/ANTITHYMOCYTE GLOBULIN

How does it function?	An antibody against thymocytes, lymphocytes (cells removed by macrophage phagocytosis)
What is the associated toxicity?	Thrombocytopenia, leukopenia, serum sickness, rigors, fever, anaphylaxis, increased risk of viral infection

OKT3

How does it work?	MONOclonal antibody that binds CD3 receptor (on T cells)

What is a major problem with multiple doses? Blocking antibodies develop, and OKT3 is less effective each time it is used.

FK-506

How does it work? Similar to CSA—blocks IL-2 receptor expression, inhibits T cells

What is its potency compared to CSA? 100 times more potent than CSA

What are its side effects? Nephrotoxicity and CNS toxicity (like CSA)

MYCOPHENOLATE MOFETIL

How does it work? Inhibits T cells and B cells by inhibiting **purine** synthesis

What drug acts at the following sites:

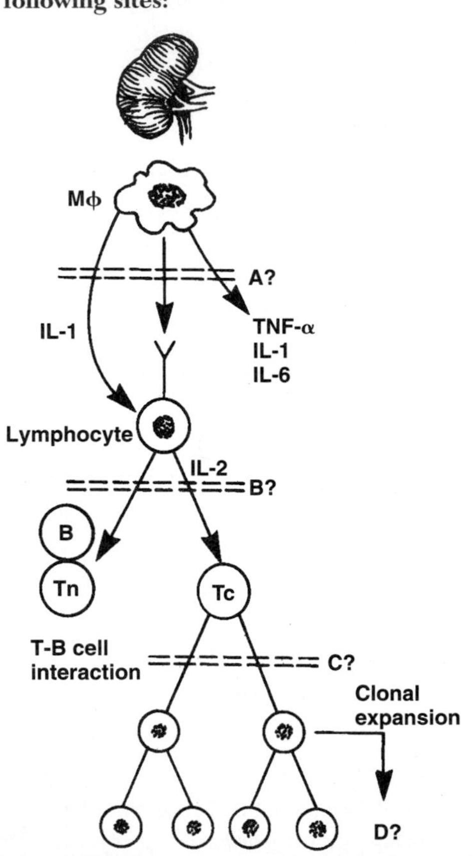

A? Corticosteroids

B? CSA

C? AZA

D? OKT3/ATGAM

MATCHING OF DONOR AND RECIPIENT

How is ABO crossmatching performed? Same procedure as in blood typing

What is the purpose of lymphocytotoxic cross-matching? Tests for HLA antibodies in serum; most important in kidney and pancreas transplants

How is the test performed? Mix recipient serum with donor lymphocyte and rabbit complement.

Is HLA crossmatching important? Yes, for kidney and pancreas transplants

REJECTION

How many methods of rejection are there? Two: humoral and cell-mediated

Name the types of rejection. Hyperacute, accelerated acute, acute, chronic

What are the associated time courses by type?
Hyperacute—immediate in OR
Accelerated acute—7 to 10 days post-transplant
Acute—weeks to months post-transplant
Chronic—months to years post-transplant

What happens in hyperacute rejection? Antigraft antibodies in recipient recognize foreign antigen immediately after blood perfuses transplanted organ.

What happens in acute rejection? T-cell mediated rejection

What type of rejection is responsible for chronic rejection? Cellular, antibody (humoral), or both

What is the treatment of hyperacute rejection? Remove transplanted organ

What is the treatment of acute rejection? High-dose steroids/OKT3

What is the treatment of chronic rejection? Not much (irreversible) or retransplant

ORGAN PRESERVATION

What is the storage temperature of an organ? 4°C—keep on ice in a cooler

Why should it be kept cold? Cold decreases the rate of chemical reactions; decreased energy use minimizes effects of hypoxia and ischemia.

What is U-W solution? University of Wisconsin solution; used to perfuse an organ prior to removal from the donor

What is in it? Potassium phosphate, buffers, starch, steroids, insulin, electrolytes, adenosine

Why should it be used? Lengthens organ preservation time

MAXIMUM TIME BETWEEN HARVEST AND TRANSPLANT OF ORGAN

Heart? 4 hours

Lungs? 6 hours

Pancreas? 24 hours

Liver? 24 hours

Kidney? Up to 48 hours

KIDNEY TRANSPLANT

HISTORY

In what year was the first transplant performed in man? 1954

By whom?

J.E. Murray—1990 Nobel Prize winner in medicine

What are the indications for transplant?

Irreversible renal failure from:

1. Glomerulonephritis (leading cause)
2. Pyelonephritis
3. Polycystic kidney disease
4. Malignant HTN
5. Reflux pyelonephritis
6. Goodpasture's syndrome (antibasement membrane)
7. Congenital renal hyperplasia
8. Fabry's disease
9. Alport's syndrome
10. Renal cortical necrosis
11. Damage caused by type 1 diabetes mellitus

Define renal failure.

GFR < 20% to 25% of normal; as GFR drops to 5% to 10% of normal, uremic symptoms begin (e.g., lethargy, seizures, neuropathy, electrolyte disorders)

What is the most common cause for kidney transplant?

Diabetes (25%)

STATISTICS

What are the sources of donor kidneys?

Cadaveric (70%)
Living related donor (LRD; 30%)

What survival rate is associated with cadaveric source?

85% at 1 year if HLA matched; 80% at 1 year if not HLA matched; 75% graft survival at 3 years

What survival rate is associated with LRD?

Between 90% and 95% patient survival at 3 years; 75% to 85% graft survival at 3 years

What are the tests for compatibility?

ABO, HLA typing

If a choice of left or right donor kidney is available, which is preferred?

Left—longer renal vein allows for easier anastomosis

Should the placement of the kidney be hetero- or orthotopic?

Heterotopic—retroperitoneal in the right lower quadrant or left lower quadrant above the inguinal ligament

Why?

Preserves native kidneys, allows easy access to iliac vessels, places ureter close to the bladder, easy to biopsy kidney

Define anastomoses of a heterotopic kidney transplant.

1. Renal artery to iliac artery
2. Renal vein to iliac vein
3. Ureter to bladder

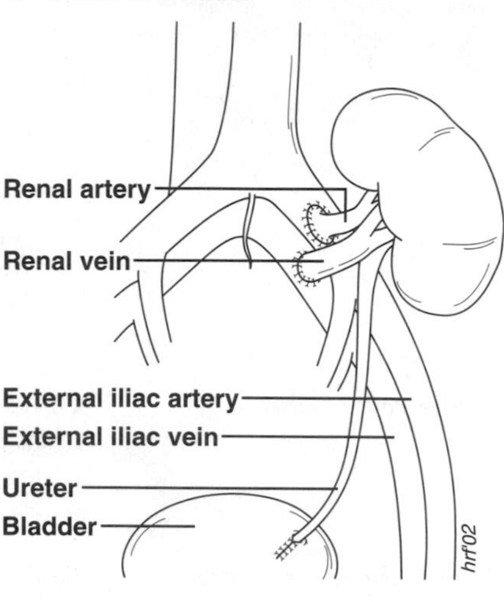

What is the correct placement of the ureter?

Submucosally through the bladder wall—decreases reflux

Why keep native kidneys?

Increased morbidity if they are removed

What is the indication for removal of native kidneys?

Uncontrollable HTN, ongoing renal sepsis

IMMUNOSUPPRESSION

For cadaveric transplant?

CSA, AZA (Imuran), steroids, ATG, OKT3

For LRD transplant?

CSA, AZA (Imuran), steroids

REJECTION

What is the red flag that indicates rejection?

Increasing creatinine

What is the differential diagnosis of increased creatinine?

(Remember: "-**tion**") obstruc**tion,** dehydra**tion,** infec**tion,** intoxica**tion** (CSA); plus lymphocele, ATN

What are the signs/ symptoms?

Fever, malaise, HTN, ipsilateral leg edema, pain at transplant site, oliguria

What is the workup for the following tests:

US/Doppler?

Look for fluid collection around the kidney, hydronephrosis, flow in vessels.

Radionuclide scan?

Look at flow and function.

Biopsy?

Distinguish between rejection and cyclosporine toxicity.

What is the time course for return of normal renal function after transplant?

LRD—3 to 5 days
Cadaveric—7 to 15 days

LIVER TRANSPLANT

What are the indications?

Liver failure from:

1. Cirrhosis (leading indication in adults)
2. Budd-Chiari
3. Biliary atresia (leading indication in children)
4. Neonatal hepatitis
5. Chronic active hepatitis
6. Fulminant hepatitis with drug toxicity—acetaminophen
7. Sclerosing cholangitis
8. Caroli's disease
9. Subacute hepatic necrosis
10. Congenital hepatic fibrosis
11. Inborn errors of metabolism
12. Fibrolamellar hepatocellular carcinoma

Define the following terms:

Liver failure

Stage III or IV encephalopathy in patients with liver disease; also, abnormal synthetic function

Stage III encephalopathy

Deep somnolence, incoherent speech

Stage IV encephalopathy

Coma

What is the test for compatibility?

ABO typing

What is the placement? Orthotopic

What are the options for biliary drainage?
1. Donor common bile to recipient common bile duct end to end
2. Roux-en-Y choledochojejunostomy

What is the correct proportionate size? Donor body weight should be approximately 50% > or 50% < recipient.

Immunosuppression? CSA, AZA (Imuran), steroids

REJECTION

What are the red flags indicating rejection? Decreased bile drainage, increased serum bilirubin, increased LFTs

What is the site of rejection? Rejection involves the biliary epithelium first and later the vascular endothelium.

What is the workup with the following tests:

U/S with Doppler? Look at flow in portal vein, hepatic artery; rule out thrombosis, leaky anastomosis, infection (abscess).

Cholangiogram? Look at bile ducts (easy to do; patients usually have a T-tube if they have first-degree biliary anastomosis).

Biopsy? Especially important 3 to 6 weeks postoperatively, when CMV is of greatest concern

Does hepatorenal syndrome renal function improve after liver transplant? Yes

SURVIVAL STATISTICS

What is the 1-year survival rate? Approximately 80% to 85%

What percentage of patients require retransplant? Approximately 20%

Why? Usually primary graft dysfunction, rejection, infection, vascular thrombosis, or recurrence of primary disease

PANCREAS TRANSPLANT

What are the indications?	Type I (juvenile) diabetes mellitus associated with severe complications (renal failure, blindness, neuropathy) or very poor glucose control
What are the tests for compatibility?	ABO, Dr matching (class II)
What is the placement?	Heterotopic, in iliac fossa or paratopic
Where is anastomosis of the exocrine duct in heterotopic placement?	To the bladder

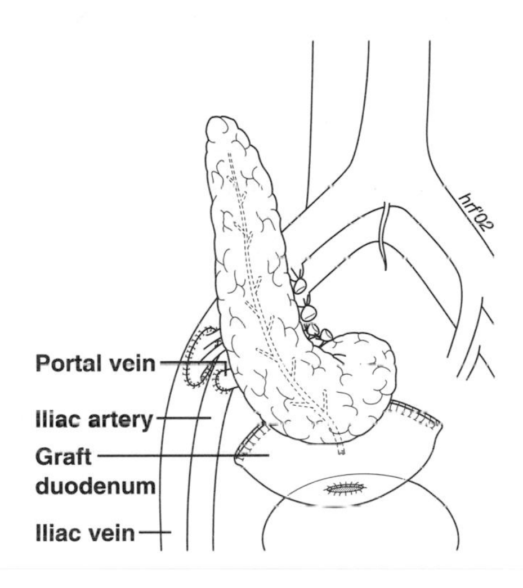

Why?	Measures the amount of amylase in urine, gives an indication of pancreatic function (i.e., high urine amylase indicates good pancreatic function)
What is the associated electrolyte complication?	Loss of bicarbonate
Where is anastomosis of the exocrine duct in paratopic placement?	To the jejunum
Why?	It is close by and physiologic.
What is the advantage of paratopic placement?	Endocrine function drains to the portal vein directly to the liver, and pancreatic

	contents stay within the GI tract (no need to replace bicarbonate).
Immunosuppression?	CSA, AZA (Imuran), steroids
What are the red flags indicating rejection?	Hyperamylasemia, hyperglycemia, hypoamylasuria, graft tenderness
Why should the kidney and pancreas be transplanted together?	Kidney function is a better indicator of rejection; also better survival of graft is associated with kidney-pancreas transplant than pancreas alone.
Why is hyperglycemia not a good indicator for rejection surveillance?	Hyperglycemia appears relatively late with pancreatic rejection

HEART TRANSPLANT

What are the indications?	Age birth to 65 years with terminal acquired heart disease—class IV of New York Heart Association classification (inability to do any physical activity without discomfort = 10% chance of surviving 6 months)
What are the contra-indications?	Older than 65 years of age (variable) Active infection Poor pulmonary function Increased pulmonary artery resistance
What are the tests for compatibility?	ABO, size
What is the placement?	Orthotopic anastomosis of atria, aorta, pulmonary artery
What is used for immuno-suppression?	Cyclosporine, azathioprine (Imuran), steroids
What are the red flags of rejection?	Fever, hypotension or hypertension, increased T4/T8 ratio
What are the tests for rejection?	Endomyocardial biopsy—much more important than clinical signs/symptoms; patient undergoes routine biopsy
What are survival statistics?	Between 85% and 95%

INTESTINAL TRANSPLANTATION

What is it?
Transplantation of the small bowel

What are transplant anastomoses?
Donor SMA to recipient aorta
Donor SMV to recipient portal vein

What are indications?
Short gut syndrome and inability to sustain TPN (liver failure, lack of venous access, etc.)

What percentage of intestinal transplant recipients have an episode of rejection in the first 6 months?
>90%!!!!!!!!!!!

What is a common postoperative problem other than rejection?
GVHD (graft versus host disease) from large lymphoid tissue in transplanted intestines

What is the most common cause of death postoperatively?
Sepsis

How is rejection surveillance conducted?
Endoscopic biopsies

What is graft survival at 1 year?
Approximately 60%

LUNG TRANSPLANT

What are the indications?
Generally, a disease that substantially limits activities of daily living and is likely to result in death within 12 to 18 months:
- Pulmonary fibrosis
- COPD
- Eosinophilic granuloma
- Primary pulmonary HTN
- Eisenmenger's syndrome
- Cystic fibrosis

What are the contraindications?
Current smoking
Active infection

What tests comprise the pretransplant assessment of the recipient?
1. Pulmonary—PFTs, V/Q scan
2. Cardiac—Echo, cath, angiogram
3. Exercise tolerance test

What are the donor requirements?
1. 55 years of age or younger
2. Clear chest film
3. PA oxygen tension of 300 on 100% oxygen and 5 cm PEEP
4. No purulent secretions on bronchoscopy

What are necessary anastomoses?
Bronchi, PA, pulmonary veins
Bronchial artery is not necessary.

What are the red flags of rejection?
Decreased arterial O_2 tension
Fever
Increased fatigability
Infiltrate on x-ray

What are the survival rates associated with the following conditions:

Single lung, 1 year?
Approximately 65%

Double lung, 1 year?
Approximately 70%

TRANSPLANT COMPLICATIONS

Note four major complications.
1. Infection
2. Rejection
3. Post-transplant lymphoproliferative disease
4. Complications of steroids

INFECTION

What are the usual agents?
DNA viruses, especially CMV, HSV, VZV

When should CMV infection be suspected?
More than 21 days post-transplant

What is the time of peak incidence of CMV infections?
4 to 6 weeks post-transplant

What are the signs/ symptoms of CMV?
Fever, neutropenia, signs of rejection of transplant; also can present as viral pneumonitis, hepatitis, colitis

How is CMV diagnosed?
Biopsy of transplant to differentiate rejection, cultures of blood, urine

What is the treatment of CMV?
Ganciclovir, with or without immunoglobin; foscarnet

What are the complications of ganciclovir?	Bone marrow suppression
What are the signs/ symptoms of HSV?	Herpetic lesions, shingles, fever, neutropenia, rejection of transplant
What is the treatment of HSV?	Acyclovir until patient is asymptomatic

MALIGNANCY

What are the most common types?	Skin/lip cancer (40%), B-cell cancer, cervical cancer in women, T-cell lymphoma, Kaposi's sarcoma
Which epithelial cancers are important after transplant?	Skin/lip cancer, especially basal cell and squamous cell
What is post-transplant lymphoma associated with?	Multiple doses of OKT3 EBV Young > elderly
What is the treatment for post-transplant lympho-proliferative disease?	1. Drastically reduce immunosuppression 2. ± Radiation 3. ± Chemotherapy

70 Orthopaedic Surgery

ORTHOPAEDIC TERMS

What do the following abbreviations stand for:

ORIF?	**O**pen **R**eduction **I**nternal **F**ixation
ROM?	**R**ange **O**f **M**otion
FROM?	**F**ull **R**ange **O**f **M**otion
ACL?	**A**nterior **C**ruciate **L**igament
PCL?	**P**osterior **C**ruciate **L**igament
MCL?	**M**edial **C**ollateral **L**igament
PWB?	**P**artial **W**eight **B**earing
FWB?	**F**ull **W**eight **B**earing
WBAT?	**W**eight **B**earing **A**s **T**olerated
THA?	**T**otal **H**ip **A**rthroplasty
TKA?	**T**otal **K**nee **A**rthroplasty
THR?	**T**otal **H**ip **R**eplacement
TKR?	**T**otal **K**nee **R**eplacement

Define the following terms:

Supination	Palm up
Pronation	Palm down
Plantarflexion	Foot down at ankle joint (plant foot in ground)
Foot dorsiflexion	Foot up at ankle joint
Adduction	Movement toward the body (**ADD**uction = **ADD** to the body)

Abduction — Movement away from the body

Inversion — Foot sole faces midline

Eversion — Foot sole faces laterally

Volarflexion — Hand flexes at wrist joint toward flexor tendons

Wrist dorsiflexion — Hand flexes at wrist joint toward extensor tendons

Allograft bone — Bone from human donor other than patient

Reduction — Maneuver to restore proper alignment to fracture or joint

Closed reduction — Reduction done without surgery (e.g., casts, splints)

Open reduction — Surgical reduction

Fixation — Stabilization of a fracture after reduction by means of surgical placement of hardware (e.g., pins, plates, screws); can be external or internal

Unstable fracture or dislocation — Fracture or dislocation in which further deformation will occur if reduction is **not** performed

Varus — Extremity abnormality with apex of defect pointed away from midline (e.g., genu varum = bowlegged; with valgus, this term can also be used to describe fracture displacement)
Think, knees are very **varied** apart

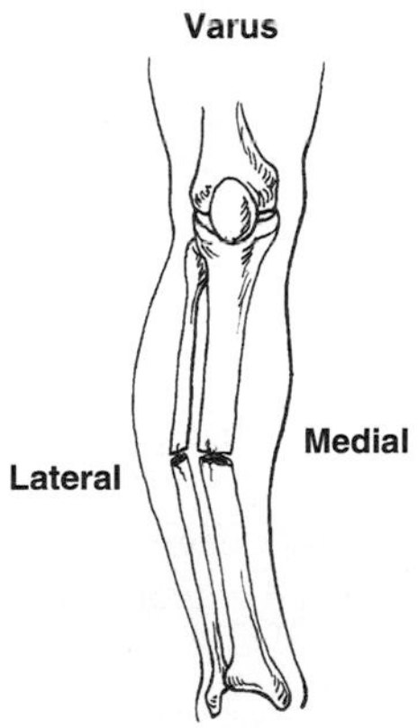

Varus
Lateral
Medial

Valgus — Extremity abnormality with apex of defect pointed toward the midline (e.g., genu valgus = knock-kneed)

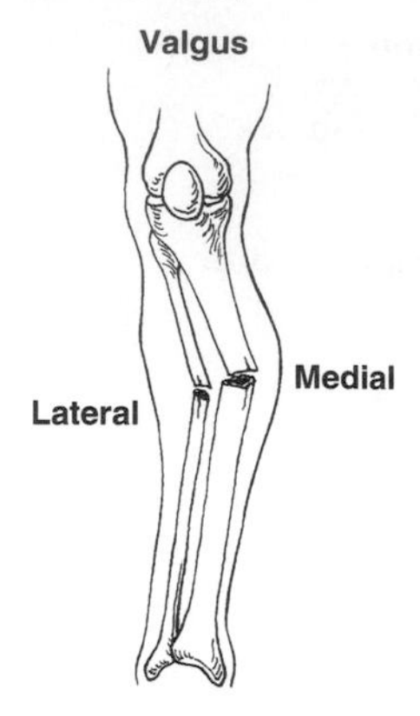

Dislocation — Total loss of congruity and contact between articular surfaces of a joint

Subluxation — Loss of congruity between articular surfaces of a joint; articular contact still remains

Arthroplasty — Total joint replacement (most last 10 to 15 years)

Arthrodesis — Joint fusion with removal of articular surfaces

Osteotomy — Cutting bone (usually wedge resection) to help realigning of joint surfaces

Non-union — Failure of fractured bone ends to fuse

Define each of the following:

Diaphysis — Main shaft of long bone

Metaphysis — Flared end of long bone

Physis — Growth plate, found only in immature bone

TRAUMA GENERAL PRINCIPLES

Define extremity examination in fractured extremities.

1. Observe entire extremity (e.g., open, angulation, joint disruption).
2. Neurologic (sensation, movement)
3. Vascular (e.g., pulses, cap refill)

Which x-rays should be obtained?

Two views (also joint above and below fracture)

How are fractures described?

1. Skin status (open or closed)
2. Bone (by thirds: proximal/middle/distal)
3. Pattern of fracture (e.g., comminuted)
4. Alignment (displacement, angulation, rotation)

How do you define the degree of angulation, displacement, or both?

Define lateral/medial/anterior/posterior displacement and angulation of the distal fragment(s) in relation to the proximal bone.

Identify each numbered structure:

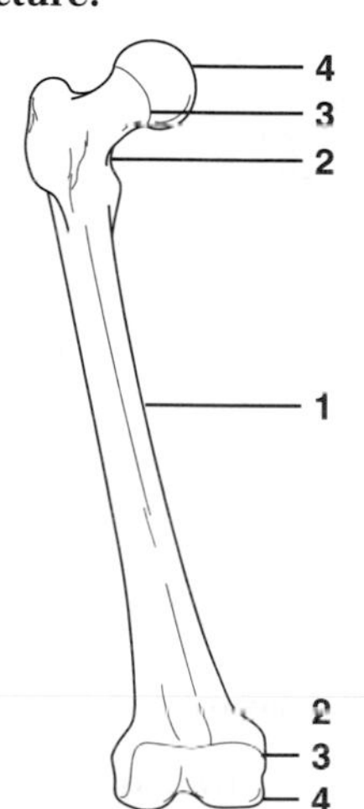

1. Diaphysis
2. Metaphysis
3. Physis
4. Epiphysis

FRACTURES

Define the following patterns of fracture:

Closed fracture

Intact skin over fracture/hematoma

Open fracture

Wound overlying fracture, through which fracture fragments are in continuity with outside environment; high risk of infection
Note: Called compound fracture in the past

Simple fracture

One fracture line, two bone fragments

Comminuted fracture Results in more than two bone fragments; also known as fragmentation

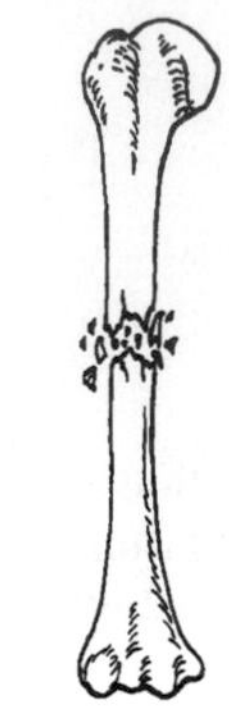

Comminuted fracture

Transverse fracture Fracture line perpendicular to long axis of bone

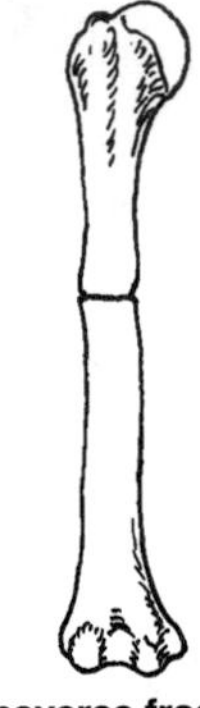

Transverse fracture

Oblique fracture Fracture line creates an oblique angle with long axis of bone

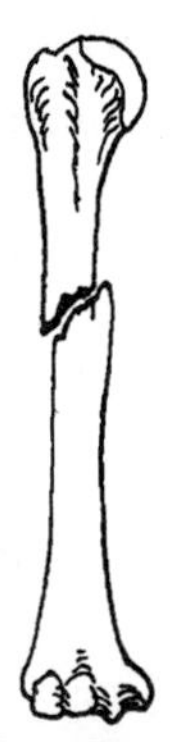

Oblique fracture

Spiral fracture

Severe oblique fracture in which fracture plane rotates along the long axis of bone; caused by a twisting injury

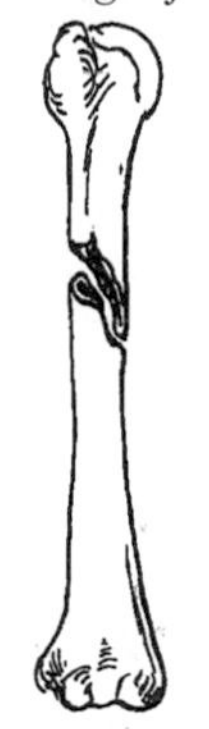

Spiral fracture

Longitudinal fracture

Fracture line parallel to long axis of bone

Impacted fracture

Fracture resulting from compressive force; end of bone is driven into contiguous metaphyseal region without displacement

Pathologic fracture

Fracture through abnormal bone (e.g., tumor-laden or osteoporotic bone)

Stress fracture

Fracture in normal bone from cyclic loading on bone

Greenstick fracture

Incomplete fracture in which cortex on only one side is disrupted; seen in children

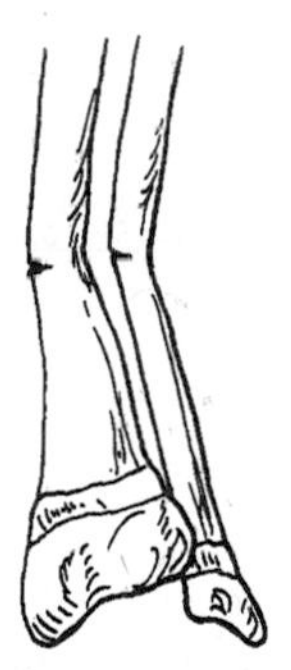

Greenstick fracture

Torus fracture

Impaction injury in children in which cortex is buckled but not disrupted (A.K.A. buckle fracture)

Avulsion fracture — Fracture in which tendon is pulled from bone, carrying with it a bone chip

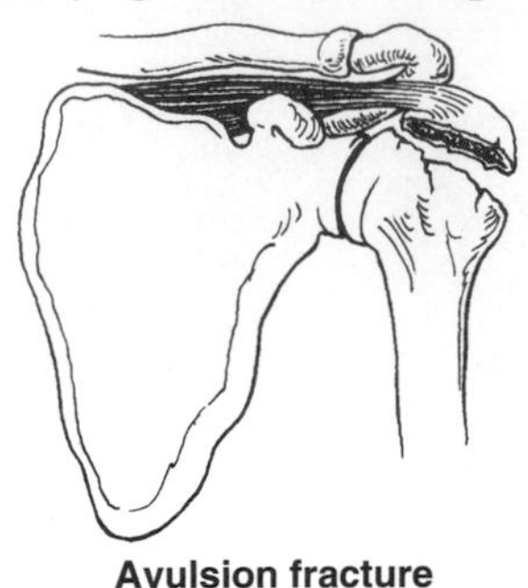

Avulsion fracture

Periarticular fracture — Fracture close to but not involving the joint

Intra-articular fracture — Fracture through the articular surface of a bone (usually requires ORIF)

Define the following specific fractures:

Colles' fracture — Distal radius fracture with dorsal displacement and angulation, usually from falling on an outstretched hand; (a common fracture!)

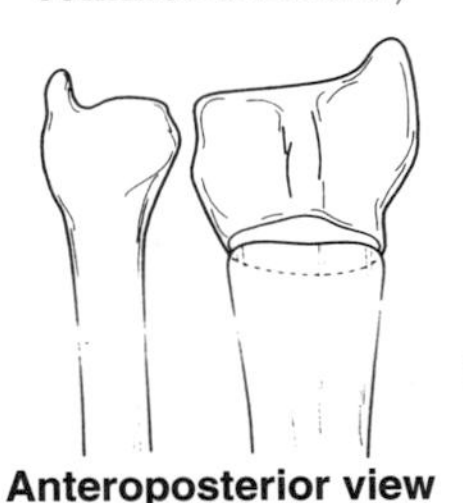

Anteroposterior view

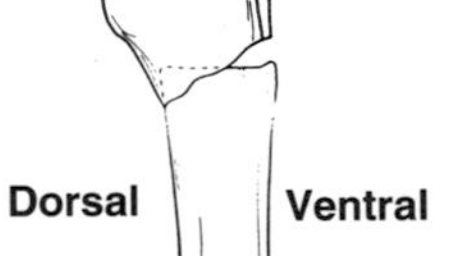

Lateral view

Smith's fracture — "Reverse Colles' fracture"—distal radial fracture with volar displacement and angulation, usually from falling on the **dorsum** of the hand (uncommon)

Jones' fracture — Fracture at the base of the fifth metatarsal diaphysis

Bennett's fracture — Fracture-dislocation of the base of the first metacarpal with disruption of the carpometacarpal joint

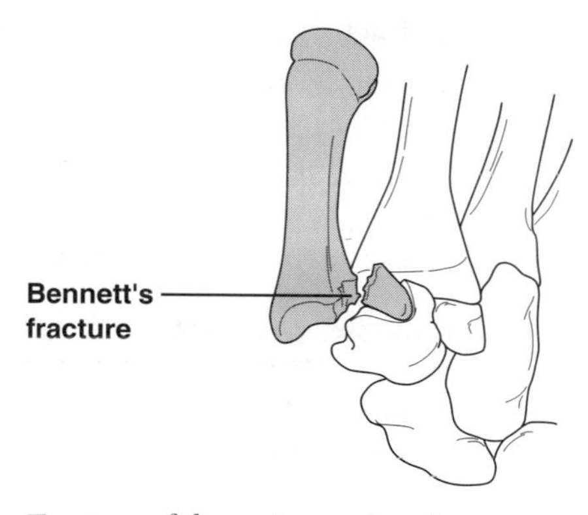

Boxer's fracture	Fracture of the metacarpal neck, "classically" of the small finger

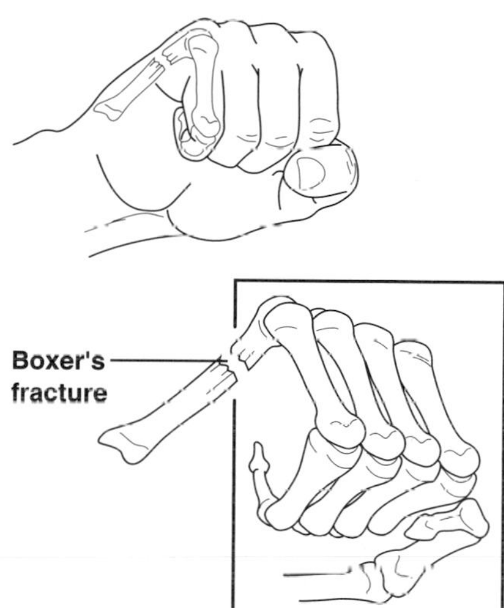

Clay shoveler's avulsion fracture	Fracture of spinous process of C6-C7
Hangman's fracture	Fracture of the pedicles of C2
Transcervical fracture	Fracture through the neck of the femur
Tibial plateau fracture	Intra-articular fracture of the proximal tibia (the plateau is the flared proximal end)
Monteggia fracture	Fracture of the proximal third of the ulna with dislocation of the radial head

Galeazzi fracture	Fracture of the radius at the junction of the middle and distal thirds accompanied by disruption of the distal radioulnar joint
Pott's fracture	Fracture of distal fibula
Pott's disease	Tuberculosis of the spine

ORTHOPAEDIC TRAUMA

What are the major orthopaedic emergencies?

1. Open fractures/dislocations
2. Vascular injuries (e.g., knee dislocation)
3. Compartment syndromes
4. Neural compromise, especially spinal injury
5. Osteomyelitis/septic arthritis; acute, i.e., when aspiration is indicated
6. Hip dislocations—require immediate reduction or patient will develop avascular necrosis; "reduce on the x-ray table"
7. Exsanguinating pelvic fracture (M.A.S.T., external fixator)

What is the main risk when dealing with an open fracture?

Infection

Which fracture has the highest mortality?

Pelvic fracture (up to 50% with open pelvic fractures)

What factors determine the extent of injury?

1. Age: suggests susceptible point in musculoskeletal system:
   Child—growth plate
   Adolescent—ligaments
   Elderly—metaphyseal bone
2. Direction of forces
3. Magnitude of forces

What are indications for open reduction?

1. Intra-articular fractures
2. Extremity function requiring perfect reduction
3. Failed closed reduction
4. Multiple trauma; to allow mobilization at earliest possible date
5. Elderly patients in cases in which a long period without ambulation carries a risk

of compromised cardiopulmonary function
6. Displaced pathologic fractures (not imminently terminal)
7. Major avulsion fractures with important muscle/ligament involvement
8. Selected physeal fractures (e.g., Salter III & IV)
9. Fractures with associated compartment syndrome

What is the acronym for indications for OPEN reduction?

"NO CAST":
N: Nonunion
O: Open fracture
C: Compromise of blood supply
A: Articular surface malalignment
S: Salter Harris grade III, IV, fracture
T: Trauma patients who need early ambulation

How are open fractures classified:

Grade I?

<1-cm laceration

Grade II?

>1-cm and <10-cm laceration

Grade IIIA?:

Open fracture with massive tissue devitalization/loss

Grade IIIB?

Open fracture with massive tissue devitalization/loss and extensive periosteal stripping or extensive gross contamination

Grade IIIC?

Open fracture with massive tissue devitalization/loss and major vascular injury requiring repair

What is the initial treatment of an open fracture?

1. Prophylactic antibiotics to include IV gram-positive ± anaerobic coverage
   Grade I—cefazolin (Ancef)
   Grade II or III—cefoxitin/gentamicin
2. Surgical debridement
3. Inoculation against tetanus
4. Lavage wound <6 hours postincident with high-pressure sterile irrigation
5. Open reduction of fracture and stabilization (e.g., use of external fixation)

What structures are at risk with a humeral fracture?

Radial nerve, brachial artery

What must be done when both forearm bones are broken?

Because precise movements are needed, open reduction and internal fixation are musts.

How have femoral fractures been repaired traditionally?

Traction for 4 to 6 weeks

What is the newer technique?

Intramedullary rod placement

What are the advantages?

Nearly immediate mobility with decreased morbidity/mortality

What is the chief concern following tibial fractures?

Recognition of associated compartment syndrome

What is suggested by pain in the anatomic snuff-box?

Fracture of scaphoid bone (A.K.A. navicular fracture)

What is the most common cause of a "pathologic" fracture in adults?

Osteoporosis

COMPARTMENT SYNDROME

What is acute compartment syndrome?

Increased pressure within an osteofascial compartment that can lead to ischemic necrosis

How is it diagnosed?

Clinically, using intracompartmental pressures is also helpful (especially in unresponsive patients). Fasciotomy is clearly indicated if pressure in the compartment is >40 mm Hg (30 to 40 mm Hg is a gray area).

What are the causes?

Fractures, vascular compromise, reperfusion injury, compressive dressings; can occur after any musculoskeletal injury

What are common causes of forearm compartment syndrome?

Supracondylar humerus fracture, brachial artery injury, radius/ulna fracture, crush injury

What is Volkmann's contracture?

The final sequela of forearm compartment syndrome; **contracture** of the forearm flexors from replacement of dead muscle with fibrous tissue

What is the most common site of compartment syndrome?

Calf (four compartments: anterior, lateral, deep posterior, superficial posterior compartments)

What situations should immediately alert one to be on the lookout for a developing compartment syndrome?

1. Supracondylar elbow fractures in children
2. Proximal/midshaft tibial fractures
3. Electrical burns
4. Arterial/venous disruption

What are the symptoms of compartment syndrome?

Pain, paresthesias, paralysis

What are the signs of compartment syndrome?

Pain on passive movement (out of proportion to injury), cyanosis or pallor, hypoesthesia (decreased sensation, decreased two point discrimination), firm compartment

Can a patient have a compartment syndrome with a palpable or Doppler-detectable distal pulse?

YES!

What are the possible complications of compartment syndrome?

Muscle necrosis, nerve damage, contractures, myoglobinuria

What is the initial treatment of the orthopaedic patient developing compartment syndrome?

Bivalve and split casts, remove constricting clothes/dressings, place extremity at heart level

What is the definitive treatment of compartment syndrome?

Fasciotomy within 4 hours (6 to 8 hours maximum) if at all possible

MISCELLANEOUS TRAUMA INJURIES AND COMPLICATIONS

Name the motor and sensation tests used to assess the following peripheral nerves:

Radial

Wrist extension; dorsal web space between thumb and index finger

Ulnar	Little finger abduction; little finger-distal ulnar aspect
Median	Thumb opposition or thumb pinch; index finger-distal radial aspect
Axillary	Arm abduction; deltoid patch on lateral aspect of upper arm
Musculocutaneous	Elbow (biceps) flexion; lateral forearm

How is a peripheral nerve injury treated?
Controversial, although clean lacerations may be repaired primarily; most injuries are followed for 6 to 8 weeks (EMG)

What fracture is associated with a calcaneus fracture?
L-spine fracture (usually from a fall)

Name the nerves of the brachial plexus.
Think: morning rum or **A.M. RUM** = **A**xillary, **M**edian, then **R**adial, **U**lnar, **M**usculocutaneous nerves

What are the indications for operative exploration with a peripheral nerve injury?
1. Loss of nerve function *after* reduction of fracture
2. No EMG signs of nerve regeneration after 8 weeks (nerve graft)

DISLOCATIONS

SHOULDER

What is the most common type?
95% are anterior (posterior are associated with seizures or electrical shock).

Which structures are at risk?
Axillary nerve and axillary artery

How is it diagnosed?
Indentation of soft tissue beneath acromion

What is the treatment?
1. Reduction via gradual traction
2. Immobilization for 3 weeks in internal rotation
3. ROM exercises

ELBOW

What is the most common type?
Posterior

Which structures are at risk? Brachial artery, ulnar nerve, median nerve

What is the treatment? Reduce and splint for 7 to 10 days.

HIP

When should hip dislocations be reduced? Immediately, to decrease risk of avascular necrosis; "reduce on the x-ray table!"

What is the most common cause of a hip dislocation? High velocity trauma (e.g., MVA)

What is the most common type? Posterior—"dashboard dislocation"—often involves fracture of posterior lip of acetabulum

Which structures are at risk? Sciatic nerve; blood supply to femoral head—avascular necrosis (AVN)

What is the treatment? Closed or open reduction

KNEE

What are the common types? Anterior or posterior

Which structures are at risk? Popliteal artery and vein, peroneal nerve—especially with posterior dislocation, ACL, PCL (Note: need arteriogram)

What is the treatment? Immediate attempt at relocation (do not wait to x-ray), arterial repair, and then ligamentous repair (delayed or primary)

THE KNEE

What are the ligaments of the knee? Anterior cruciate ligament (ACL), posterior cruciate ligament (PCL), medial collateral ligament (MCL), lateral collateral ligament (LCL), patellar ligament

What is the "anterior drawer test" of the knee? Test to ascertain the anterior stability of the knee and integrity of the ACL
Knee is placed in 90° flexion and pulled forward (like opening a drawer). If tibia is

	pulled forward, test is positive and consistent with an ACL tear.
What is the meniscus of the knee?	The cartilage surface of the tibia plateau (lateral and medial meniscus); tears are repaired usually by arthroscopy with removal of torn cartilage fragments
What is the "unhappy triad"?	Lateral knee injury resulting in ACL tear, MCL tear, and a medial meniscus injury

ACHILLES TENDON RUPTURE

What are the signs of an Achilles tendon rupture?	Severe calf pain, also bruised swollen calf, two ends of ruptured tendon may be felt, patient will have weak plantar flexion from great toe flexors that should be intact
Name the test for an intact Achilles tendon.	**Thompson's test:** a squeeze of the gastrocnemius muscle results in plantar flexion of the foot

ROTATOR CUFF

What muscles form the rotator cuff?	1. Supraspinatus (acronym = **"SITS"**) 2. Infraspinatus 3. Teres minor 4. Subscapularis
When do tears usually occur?	Fifth decade
What is the usual history?	Intermittent shoulder pain especially with **overhead** activity, followed by an episode of acute pain corresponding to a tendon tear; weak abduction
What is the treatment?	Most tears: symptomatic pain relief Later: if poor muscular function persists, surgical repair is indicated
What is Volkmann's contracture?	Contracture of forearm flexors secondary to **forearm compartment syndrome**
What is the usual cause of Volkmann's contracture?	Brachial artery injury, **supracondylar humerus fracture,** radius/ulnar fracture, crush injury, etc.

MISCELLANEOUS

Define the following terms:

Dupuytren's contracture — Thickening and contracture of palmar fascia; incidence increases with age

Charcot's joint — Joint arthritis from peripheral neuropathy

Tennis elbow — Tendonitis of the lateral epicondyle of the humerus (classically seen in tennis players)

Turf toe — Hyperextension of the great toe (tear of the tendon of the flexor hallucis brevis); classically seen in football players

Shin splints — Exercise-induced anterior compartment hypertension (compartment syndrome); seen in runners

Heel spur — Plantar fasciitis with abnormal bone growth in the plantar fascia
Classically seen in runners and walkers

What is traumatic myositis? — Abnormal bone deposit in a muscle after blunt trauma deep muscle contusion (benign)

ORTHOPAEDIC INFECTIONS

OSTEOMYELITIS

What is osteomyelitis? — Inflammation/infection of bone marrow and adjacent bone

What are the most likely causative organisms? — Neonates: *Staphylococcus aureus*, gram-negative *streptococcus*
Children: S. *aureus*, *Haemophilus influenzae*, streptococci
Adults: S. *aureus*
Immunocompromised/drug addicts: S. *aureus* gram-negative
Sickle cell: *Salmonella*

What is the most common organism isolated in osteomyelitis in the general adult population? — S. *aureus*

What is the most common isolated organism in patients with sickle cell disease?
Salmonella

What is seen on physical examination?
Tenderness, decreased movement, swelling

What are the diagnostic steps?
History and physical examination, needle aspirate, blood cultures, CBC, ESR, CRP, bone scan

What are the treatment options?
Antibiotics with or without surgical drainage

What is a Marjolin's ulcer?
Squamous cell carcinoma that arises in a chronic sinus from osteomyelitis

SEPTIC ARTHRITIS

What is septic arthritis?
Inflammation of a joint beginning as synovitis and ending with destruction of articular cartilage if left untreated

What are the causative agents?
Same as in osteomyelitis, except that gonococcus is a common agent in the adult population

What are the findings on physical examination?
Joint pain, decreased motion, joint swelling, joint warm to the touch

What are the diagnostic steps?
Needle aspirate (look for pus; culture plus Gram stain), x-ray, blood cultures, ESR

What is the treatment?
Decompression of the joint via needle aspiration and IV antibiotics; hip, shoulder, and spine must be surgically incised, débrided, and drained

ORTHOPAEDIC TUMORS

What is the most common type in adults?
Metastatic!

What are the common sources?
Breast, lung, prostate, kidney, thyroid, and multiple myeloma

What is the usual presentation?
Bone pain or as a pathologic fracture

What is the most common primary malignant bone tumor?

Multiple myeloma (45%)

What is the differential diagnosis of a possible bone tumor?

1. Metastatic disease
2. Primary bone tumors
3. Metabolic disorders (e.g., hyperparathyroidism)
4. Infection

What are the benign bone tumors?

1. Osteochondroma
2. Enchondroma
3. Unicameral/aneurysmal bone cysts
4. Osteoid osteoma
5. Chondroblastoma
6. Fibroxanthoma
7. Fibrous dysplasia
8. Nonossifying fibroma

What are the malignant bone tumors?

1. Multiple myeloma
2. Osteosarcoma
3. Chondrosarcoma
4. Ewing's sarcoma
5. Giant cell tumor (locally malignant)
6. Malignant melanoma
7. Metastatic

Compare benign and malignant bone tumors in terms of:

Size

Benign—small; <1 cm
Malignant— >1 cm

Bone reaction

Benign—sclerotic bone reaction
Malignant—little reaction

Margins

Benign—sharp
Malignant—poorly defined

Invasive

Benign—confined to bone
Malignant—often extends to surrounding tissues

Are most pediatric bone tumors benign or malignant?

80% are benign (most common is osteochondroma).

Are most adult bone tumors benign or malignant?

66% are malignant (most commonly metastatic).

What are the diagnostic steps?
1. PE/lab tests
2. Radiographs
3. CT scan, technetium scan, or both
4. Biopsy

What are radiographic signs of malignant tumors?
Large size
Aggressive bone destruction, poorly defined margins
Ineffective bone reaction to tumor
Extension to soft tissues

What are the radiographic signs of benign tumor?
Small
Well circumscribed, sharp margins
Effective bone reaction to the tumor (sclerotic periostitis)
No extension—confined to bone

What are some specific radiographic findings of the following:

Osteosarcoma?
"Sunburst pattern"

Fibrous dysplasia
Bubbly lytic lesion "ground glass"

Ewing's sarcoma
"Onion skinning"

What is the mainstay of treatment for bone tumors?
Surgery (excision plus debridement) for both malignant and benign lesions; radiation therapy and chemotherapy as adjuvant therapy for many malignant tumors

OSTEOSARCOMA

What is the usual age at presentation?
Between 10 and 20 years

What is the gender distribution?
Men > women

What is the most common location?
Approximately two-thirds in the distal femur, proximal tibia

What is the radiographic sine qua non?
Bone formation somewhere within tumor

What is the treatment?
Resection (limb sparing if possible) plus chemotherapy

What is the 5-year survival rate? Approximately 70%

What is the most common site of metastasis? Lungs

What is the most common benign bone tumor? **Osteochondroma;** it is cartilaginous in origin and may undergo malignant degeneration

What is a chondrosarcoma? Malignant tumor of cartilaginous origin; presents in middle-aged and older patients and is unresponsive to chemotherapy and radiotherapy

EWING'S SARCOMA

What is the usual presentation? Pain, swelling in involved area

What is the most common location? Around the knee (distal femur, proximal tibia)

What is the usual age at presentation? Evenly spread among those younger than 20 years of age

What are the associated radiographic findings? Lytic lesion with periosteal reaction termed "onion skinning," which is calcified layering
Central areas of tumor can undergo liquefaction necrosis, which may be confused with purulent infection (particularly in a child with fever, leukocytosis, and bone pain).

What is the 5-year survival rate? 50%

How can Ewing's sarcoma mimic the appearance of osteomyelitis? Bone cysts

What is a unicameral bone cyst? Fluid-filled cyst most commonly found in the proximal humerus in children 5 to 15 years of age

What is the usual presentation? Asymptomatic until pathologic fracture

What is the treatment? Steroid injections

What is an aneurysmal bone cyst?
A hemorrhagic lesion that is locally destructive by expansile growth, but does not metastasize

What is the usual presentation?
Pain and swelling; pathologic fractures are rare

What is the treatment?
Curettage and bone grafting

ARTHRITIS

Which arthritides are classified as degenerative?
Osteoarthritis
Post-traumatic arthritis

What signs characterize osteoarthritis?
Heberden's nodes/Bouchard's nodes
Symmetric destruction, usually of the hip, knee, or spine

What are Bouchard's nodes?
Enlarged PIP joints of the hand from cartilage/bone growth

What are Heberden's nodes?
Enlarged DIP joints of the hand from cartilage/bone growth

What is post-traumatic arthritis?
Usually involves one joint of past trauma

What are the treatment options for degenerative arthritis?
1. NSAIDS for acute flare-ups, **not** for long-term management
2. Local corticosteroid injections
3. Surgery

What are the characteristics of rheumatoid arthritis?
Autoimmune reaction in which invasive pannus attacks hyaline articular cartilage, rheumatoid factor (anti-IgG/IgM) in 80% of patients, three times more common in women, skin nodules (e.g., rheumatoid nodule)

What is pannus?
Inflammatory exudate overlying synovial cells inside the joint

What are the classic hand findings with rheumatoid arthritis?
Wrist: radial deviation
Fingers: ulnar deviation

What are the surgical management options for joint/bone diseases?
1. Arthroplasty
2. Arthrodesis (fusion)
3. Osteotomy

What is the major difference between gout and pseudogout?
Gout: caused by urate deposition
Pseudogout: caused by calcium pyrophosphate positive birefringent

square crystals (think: **P**ositive **S**quare crystals = **PS**eudogout)

What is a Charcot's joint?

Arthritic joint from peripheral neuropathy

PEDIATRIC ORTHOPAEDICS

What are the major differences between pediatric and adult bones?

Children: increased bone flexibility and bone healing (thus, many fractures are treated closed, whereas an adult would require O.R.I.F.), physis (weak point)

What types of fractures are unique to children?

Greenstick fracture
Torus fracture
Fracture through physis

SALTER CLASSIFICATION

What does it describe?

Fractures in children involving physis

What does it indicate high risk of?

Potential growth arrest

Define the following terms:

Salter I

Through physeal plate only

Salter II

Involves physis and metaphysis

Salter III

Involves physis and epiphysis

Salter IV

Extends from metaphysis through physis, into epiphysis

Salter V

Axial force crushes physeal plate.

Define the following fractures by Salter-Harris grade:

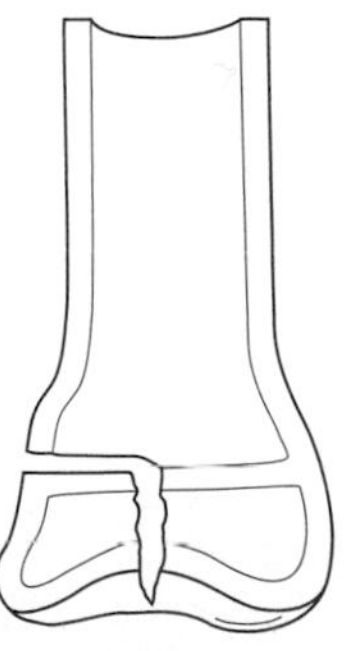

Salter III

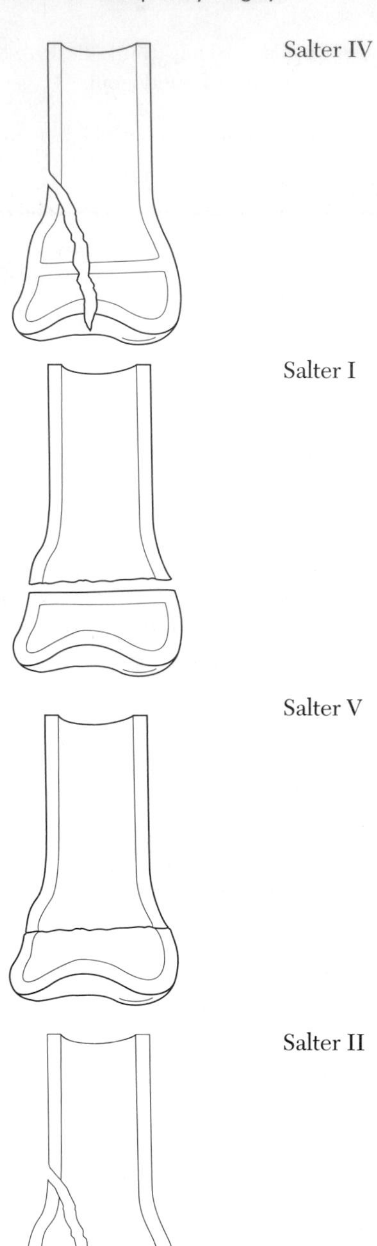

Salter IV

Salter I

Salter V

Salter II

What acronym can help you remember the SALTER classifications?

SALTR:
S = **S**eparated = type I
A = **A**bove = type II

L = **L**ower = type III
T = **T**hrough = type IV
R = **R**uined = type V

Why is the growth plate of concern in childhood fractures?

The growth plate represents the "weak link" in the child's musculoskeletal system. Fractures involving the growth plate of long bones may compromise normal growth, so special attention should be given to them.

What is a chief concern when oblique/spiral fractures of long bones are seen in children?

Child abuse is a possibility; other signs of abuse should be investigated.

What is usually done during reduction of a femoral fracture?

A small amount of overlap is allowed because increased vascularity from injury may make the affected limb longer if overlap is not present. Treatment after reduction is a spica cast.

What is unique about ligamentous injury in children?

Most "ligamentous" injuries are actually fractures involving the growth plate!

What two fractures have a high incidence of associated compartment syndrome?

1. Tibial fractures
2. Supracondylar fractures of humerus (Volkmann's contracture)

CONGENITAL HIP DISLOCATION

What is the epidemiology?

Female > male, firstborn children, breech
Presentation, 1–1000 births

What percentage are bilateral?

10%

How is the diagnosis made?

Barlow's maneuver, Ortolani's sign
Radiographic confirmation is required.

What is Barlow's maneuver?

Detects unstable hip: patient is placed in the supine position and attempt is made to push femurs posteriorly with knees at 90°/hip flexed and hip will dislocate (think: push **B**ack = **B**arlow)

What is Ortolani's sign?
The "clunk" produced by relocation of a dislocated femoral head when the examiner abducts the flexed hip and lifts the greater trochanter anteriorly; detects a dislocated hip (think **O**ut = **O**rtolani's)

What is the treatment?
Pavlik harness—maintains hip reduction with hips flexed at 100° to 110°

SCOLIOSIS

What is the definition?
Lateral curvature of a portion of the spine
Nonstructural: corrects with positional change
Structural: does not correct

What are the treatment options?
1. Observation
2. Braces (Milwaukee brace)
3. Surgery

What are the indications for surgery for scoliosis?
Respiratory compromise
Rapid progressive
Curves more than 40°
Failure of brace

MISCELLANEOUS

Define the following terms:

Legg-Calvé-Perthes disease
Idiopathic avascular necrosis of femoral head in children

Slipped capital femoral epiphysis
Migration of proximal femoral epiphysis on the metaphysis in children. The proximal femoral epiphysis externally rotates and displaces anteriorly from the capital femoral epiphysis, which stays reduced in the acetabulum.
Note: Hip pain in children often presents as knee pain.

Blount's disease
Idiopathic varus bowing of tibia

Osgood-Schlatter's disease
Apophysitis of the tibial tubercle resulting from repeated powerful contractions of the quadriceps; seen in adolescents with an open physis
Treatment of mild cases: activity restriction
Treatment of severe cases: cast

What is the most common pediatric bone tumor?
Osteochondroma (remember, 80% of bone tumors are benign in children)

71 Neurosurgery

HEAD TRAUMA

What is the incidence?

70,000 fatal injuries/year in the United States, 500,000 head injuries per year

What percentage of trauma deaths result from head trauma?

50%

Dermatomes:

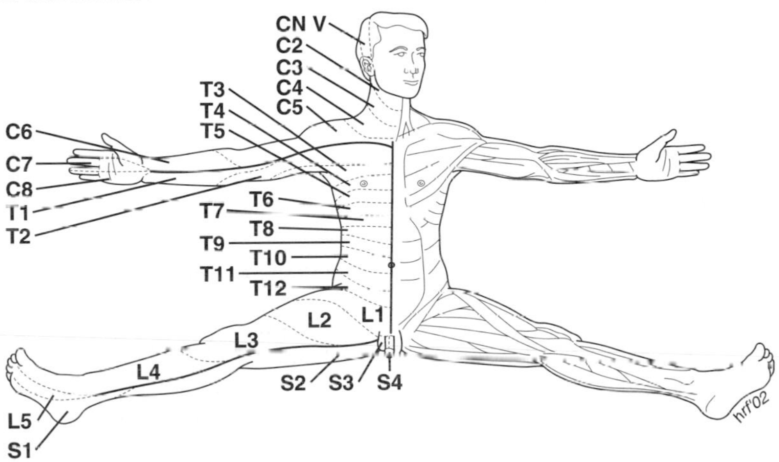

What is the Glasgow Coma Scale (GCS)?

The GCS is an objective assessment of the level of consciousness after trauma.

GCS SCORING SYSTEM

Eyes?

Eye Opening (E)
4—opens spontaneously
3—opens to voice (command)
2—opens to painful stimulus
1—does not open eyes
(Think = "4 eyes")

Motor?

Motor Response (M)
6—obeys commands
5—localizes painful stimulus
4—withdraws from pain
3—decorticate posture
2—decerebrate posture
1—no movement
(Think = 6-cylinder motor)

Verbal?

Verbal Response (V)
5—appropriate and oriented
4—confused
3—inappropriate words
2—incomprehensible sounds
1—no sounds
(**Think =** Jackson 5 = verbal 5)

What indicates coma by GCS score?

<8 (think: "less than eight—it may be too late")

What does unilateral, dilated, nonreactive pupil suggest?

Focal mass lesion with ipsilateral herniation with compression of CN III

What do bilateral fixed and dilated pupils suggest?

Diffusely increased ICP

What are the four signs of basilar skull fracture?

1. **Raccoon eyes**—periorbital ecchymoses
2. **Battle's sign**—postauricular ecchymoses
3. **Hemotympanum**
4. **CSF** rhinorrhea/otorrhea

What is the initial radiographic imaging in trauma?

1. Plain films of C-spine (C1-C7/T1): AP, lateral, odontoid
2. Head CT (if LOC or GCS < 15)
3. T/L spine AP and lateral

Should the trauma head CT be with or without IV contrast?

Without!

What is normal ICP?

Between 5 and 15 mm H_2O

What is the worrisome ICP?

More than 20 mm H_2O

What determines ICP (Monroe-Kelly hypothesis)?

1. Volume of brain
2. Volume of blood
3. Volume of CSF

What is the CPP?

Cerebral **P**erfusion **P**ressure = mean arterial pressure—ICP (normal CPP is >70)

What is Cushing's reflex?

Physiologic response to increased ICP:

1. Hypertension
2. Bradycardia
3. Decreased RR

What are the general indications to monitor ICP after trauma?

1. GCS <9
2. Altered level of consciousness or unconsciousness with multiple system trauma
3. Decreased consciousness with focal neurologic examination abnormality

What is Kocher's point?

Landmark for placement of ICP monitor bolt:

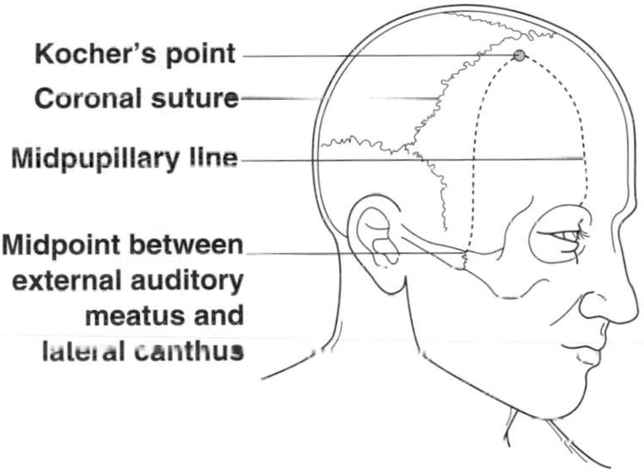

Kocher's point
Coronal suture
Midpupillary line
Midpoint between external auditory meatus and lateral canthus

What nonoperative techniques are used to decrease ICP?

1. **Elevate** head of bed (HOB) 30° (if spine cleared)
2. Diuresis-Mannitol (osmotic diuretic), Lasix, limit fluids
3. Intubation plus hyperventilation (intermittent)
4. Sedation
5. Pharmacologic paralysis
6. Ventriculostomy (CSF drainage)

Why is prolonged hyperventilation dangerous?

May result in severe vasoconstriction and ischemic brain necrosis!
Use only for very brief periods

What is a Kjellberg?

Decompressive bifrontal craniectomy (pronounced "shellberg") with removal of frontal bone placed in freezer for possible later replacement

How does cranial nerve examination localize the injury in a comatose patient?

The CNs proceed caudally in the brain stem as numbered. Presence of corneal reflex (CN 5 + 7) indicates intact pons. Intact gag reflex (CN 9 + 10) shows functioning upper medulla. Be aware that CN 6 palsy is often a false localizing sign.

What is acute treatment of seizures after head trauma?

Benzodiazepines (Ativan)

What is the significance of hyponatremia (low sodium level) after head injury?

S.I.A.D.H. must be ruled out

EPIDURAL HEMATOMA

What is an epidural hematoma?

Collection of blood between the skull and dura

What causes it?

Usually occurs in association with a skull fracture as bone fragments lacerate meningeal arteries

What artery is associated with epidural hematomas?

Middle meningeal artery

What is the most common sign of an epidural hematoma?

More than 50% have ipsilateral blown pupil.

What is the classic history with an epidural hematoma?

LOC followed by a "lucid interval" followed by neurologic deterioration

What are the classic CT findings with an epidural hematoma?

Lenticular-shaped hematoma

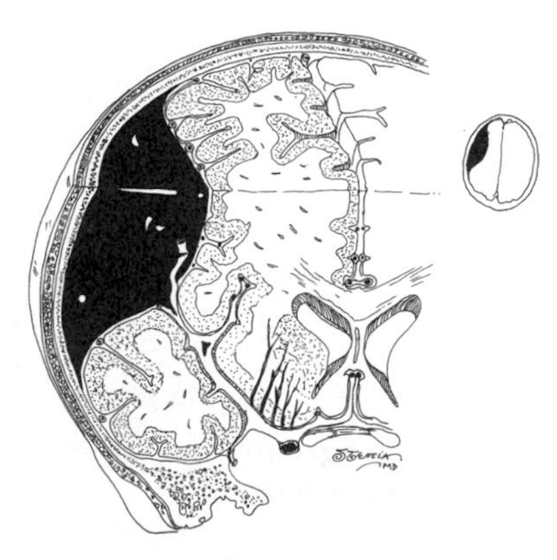

What is the surgical treatment for an epidural hematoma?

Surgical evacuation

What are the indications for surgery with an epidural hematoma?

Any symptomatic epidural hematoma; any epidural hematoma > 1 cm

SUBDURAL HEMATOMA

What is it?

Blood collection under the dura

What causes it?

Tearing of "bridging" veins that pass through the space between the cortical surface and the dural venous sinuses or injury to the brain surface with resultant bleeding from cortical vessels

What are the three types of subdurals?

1. Acute—symptoms within 48 hours of injury
2. Subacute—symptoms within 3 to 14 days
3. Chronic—symptoms after 2 weeks or longer

What is the treatment of epidural and subdural hematomas?

The mass effect (pressure) must be reduced. Craniotomy with clot evacuation is usually required

What classic CT findings appear on head CT for a subdural hematoma?

Crescent-shaped hematoma

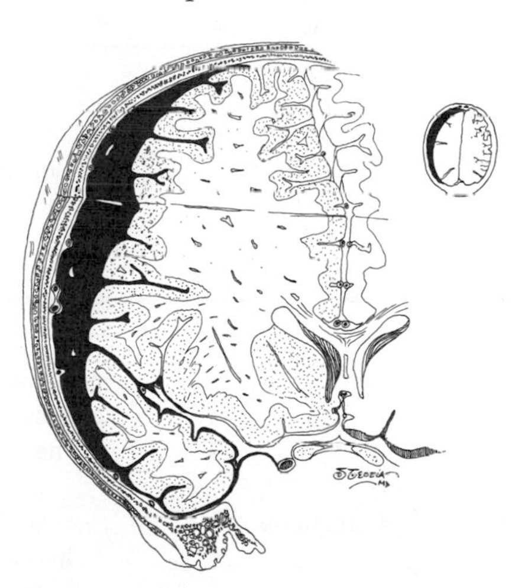

TRAUMATIC SUBARACHNOID HEMORRHAGE

What is it?
Head trauma resulting in blood below the arachnoid membrane and above the pia

What is the treatment?
Anticonvulsants and observation

CEREBRAL CONTUSION

What is it?
Hemorrhagic contusion of brain parenchyma

What is a coup and contrecoup injury?
Coup—injury at the site of impact
Contrecoup—injury at the site opposite the point of impact

What is DAI?
Diffuse **A**xonal **I**njury (shear injury to brain parenchyma) from rapid deceleration injury; 33% mortality; long-term coma

SKULL FRACTURE

What is a depressed skull fracture?
A fracture in which one or more fragments of the skull are forced below the inner table of the skull

What are the indications for surgery?
1. Contaminated wound requiring cleaning and debridement
2. Severe deformity
3. Impingement on cortex
4. Open fracture
5. CSF leak

What is the treatment for open skull fractures?
1. Antibiotics
2. Seizure prophylaxis (phenytoin)
3. Surgical therapy

SPINAL CORD TRAUMA

What are the two general types of injury?
1. Complete—no motor/sensory function below the level of injury
2. Incomplete—residual function below the level of injury

Define "spinal shock."
Loss of all reflexes and motor function, hypotension, bradycardia

Define "sacral sparing."

Sparing of sacral nerve level: anal sphincter intact, toe flexion, perianal sensation

What initial studies/ intervention are important?

1. ABCs obtain airway and ventilate if needed
2. Maintain BP (IVF, pressors if refractory to fluids)
3. NG tube—prevents aspiration
4. Foley
5. High-dose steroids—proven to improve outcome if given <8 hours post injury
6. Complete cervical x-rays and those of lower levels as indicated by examination

What are the diagnostic studies?

Plain films, CT, MRI

What are the indications for emergent surgery with spinal cord injury?

Unstable vertebral fracture
Incomplete injury with extrinsic compression
Spinal epidural or subdural hematoma

What is the indication for IV high-dose steroids with spinal cord injury?

Spinal cord injury with neurologic deficit (methylprednisolone: high-dose bolus [30 mg/kg] followed by continuous infusion [5.4 mg/kg] for 23 hours)

Have steroids been proven to help after PENETRATING spine injury?

No

Describe the following conditions:

Anterior cord syndrome

Affects corticospinal and lateral spinothalamic tracts, paraplegia, loss of pain/temperature sensation, preserved touch/vibration/proprioception

Central cord syndrome

Preservation of some lower extremity motor and sensory ability with upper extremity weakness

Brown-Séquard syndrome

Hemisection of cord resulting in ipsilateral motor weakness and touch/proprioception loss with contralateral pain/temperature loss

Posterior cord syndrome — Injury to posterior spinal cord with loss of proprioception distally

How can the findings associated with Brown-Séquard syndrome be remembered? — Think: Captain Brown-Séquard = **CPT** = **C**ontralateral **P**ain **T**emperature loss

Define the following terms:

Jefferson's fracture — Fracture through **C1** arches from axial loading (unstable fracture)

Hangman's fracture — Fracture through the pedicles of **C2** from hyperextension; usually stable
Think: hangman (C2) is below stature of President T. Jefferson (C1)

Odontoid fracture — Fracture of the odontoid process of C2 (view with open-mouth odontoid x-ray)

Priapism — Penile erection seen with spinal cord injury

Chance fracture — Transverse vertebral fracture

Clay shoveler's fracture — Fracture of spinous process of C7

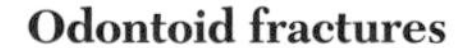

Odontoid fractures — A: Type I—fracture through tip of dens
B: Type II—fracture through base of dens
C: Type III—fracture through body of C2

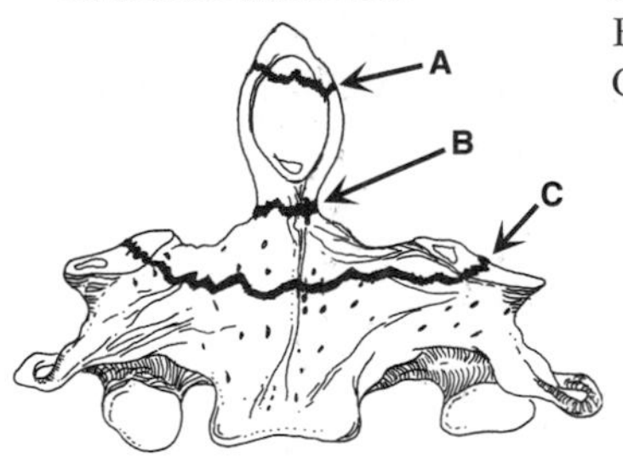

TUMORS

GENERAL

What is the incidence of CNS tumors? — Approximately 1% of all cancers; third leading cause of cancer deaths in people 15 to 34 years of age; second leading cause of cancer deaths in children

What is the usual location of primary tumors in adults/children? — In adults, roughly two-thirds of tumors are supratentorial, one-third are infratentorial; the reverse is true in children.

What is the differential diagnosis of a ring-enhancing brain lesion?

Metastatic carcinoma, abscess, GBM, lymphoma

What are the adverse effects of tumors on the brain?

1. Increased ICP
2. Mass effect on cranial nerves
3. Invasion of brain parenchyma, disrupting nuclei/tracts
4. Seizure foci
5. Hemorrhage into/around tumor mass

What are the signs/symptoms of brain tumors?

1. Neurologic deficit (66%)
2. Headache (50%)
3. Seizures (25%)
4. Vomiting (classically in the morning)

How is the diagnosis made?

CT or MRI is the standard diagnostic study.

What are the surgical indications?

1. Establishing a tissue diagnosis
2. Relief of increased ICP
3. Relief of neurologic dysfunction caused by tissue compression
4. Attempt to cure in the setting of localized tumor

What are the most common intracranial tumors in adults?

Metastatic neoplasms are most common; among primaries, gliomas are number 1 (50%) and meningiomas are number 2 (25%).

What are the most common in children?

1. Medulloblastomas (33%)
2. Astrocytomas (33%)
3. Ependymomas (10%)

GLIOMAS

What is a glioma?

A general name for several tumors of neuroglial origin (e.g., astrocytes, ependymal, oligodendrocytes)

What are the characteristics of a LOW-grade astrocytoma?

Nuclear atypia, high mitotic rate, high signal on T2 weighted images, nonenhancing with contrast CT

What is the most common primary brain tumor in adults?

Glioblastoma multiforme (GBM)
Think GBM = Greatest Brain Malignancy

What are its characteristics? Poorly defined, highly aggressive tumors occurring in the white matter of the cerebral hemispheres; spread extremely rapidly

What is the average age of onset? Fifth decade

What is the treatment? Surgical debulking followed by radiation therapy

What is the prognosis? Without treatment, more than 90% of patients die within 3 months of diagnosis. With treatment, 90% die within 2 years.

MENINGIOMAS

What is the layer of origination? Arachnoid cap cells

What are the associated histologic findings? Psammoma bodies (concentric calcifications), Whorl formations (onion skin pattern)

What is the histologic malignancy determination? Brain parenchymal invasion

What is the peak age of occurrence? Between 40 and 50 years

What is the gender ratio? Females predominate almost 2:1.

What is the clinical presentation? Variable depending on location; lateral cerebral convexity tumors can cause focal deficits or headache; sphenoid tumors can present with seizures; posterior fossa tumors with CN deficits; olfactory groove tumors with anosmia

What is the treatment? Preop embolization and surgical resection

CEREBELLAR ASTROCYTOMAS

What is the peak age of occurrence? Between 5 and 9 years

What is the usual location? Usually in the cerebellar hemispheres; less frequently in the vermis

What are the signs/ symptoms?

Usually lateral cerebellar signs occur: ipsilateral incoordination or dysmetria (patient tends to fall to side of tumor), as well as nystagmus and ataxia; CN deficits are also frequently present, especially in CNs VI and VII.

What are the treatment and prognosis?

Completely resectable in 75% of cases, which usually results in a cure; overall 5-year survival rate exceeds 90%

MEDULLOBLASTOMA

What is the peak age of occurrence?

First decade (3 to 7 years)

What is the cell of origin?

External granular cells of cerebellum

What is the most common location?

Cerebellar vermis in children; cerebellar hemispheres of adolescents and adults

What are the signs/ symptoms?

Headache, vomiting, and other signs of increased ICP; also usually truncal ataxia

What are the treatment and prognosis?

Best current treatment includes surgery to debulk the tumor, cranial and spinal radiation, and chemotherapy; 5-year survival rate is more than 50%.

METASTATIC TUMORS

What are the three main patterns of intracranial metastasis and what are the most common primary tumors involved?

Metastases to

1. Skull/dura: breast, prostate, multiple myeloma
2. Brain parenchyma: lung, breast, skin, kidney, GI tract
3. Meningeal carcinomatosis: lung, leukemia, lymphoma, breast, GI

Where do cerebral metastases occur within the brain?

At the junction of gray and white matter (MCA territory)

What are the signs/ symptoms?

Same as those of primary tumors

What are the treatment and prognosis?

Surgical resection if lesion is solitary and accessible; otherwise, radiation is most frequently used

Chemotherapy has been used with some success for lung, breast, and testicular primaries.
Average survival is approximately 6 months.

What are the signs/ symptoms of meningeal carcinomatosis?

Headache, backache, mental status changes, radiculopathy, and CN palsies are common.

How is the diagnosis of meningeal carcinomatosis made?

Head CT is usually normal, but may show a diffuse enhancement of the meninges. A demonstration of malignant cells in the CSF is required for diagnosis.

What are the treatment and prognosis?

Intrathecal chemotherapy and radiation; mean survival is about 6 months

VASCULAR NEUROSURGERY

SUBARACHNOID HEMORRHAGE (SAH)

What are the usual causes?

Most cases are due to **trauma;** of nontraumatic SAH, the leading cause is ruptured **berry aneurysm,** followed by arteriovenous malformations

What is a berry aneurysm?

Saccular outpouching of vessels in the circle of Willis, usually at bifurcations

What is the usual location of a berry aneurysm?

Anterior communicating artery is number one (30%), followed by posterior communicating artery and middle cerebral artery.

What medical disease increases the risk of berry aneurysms?

Polycystic kidney disease and connective tissue disorders (e.g., Marfan's syndrome)

What is an AVM?

A congenital abnormality of the vasculature with connections between the **arterial** and **venous** circulations without interposed capillary network

Where do they occur?

More than 75% are supratentorial.

What are the signs/ symptoms of SAH?

Classic symptom is **"the worst headache of my life."** Meningismus is documented by neck pain and positive Kernig's and Brudzinski's signs. Occasionally LOC, vomiting, and CN deficits occur.

What comprises the workup of SAH?

If SAH is suspected, head CT should be the first test ordered to look for subarachnoid blood. LP may show xanthochromic CSF, but is not necessary if CT is definitive. This test should be followed by arteriogram to look for aneurysms or AVMs.

What are the possible complications of SAH?

1. Brain edema leading to increased ICP
2. Rebleeding (most common in the first 24 to 48 hours posthemorrhage)
3. **Vasospasm** (most common cause of morbidity and mortality)

What is the treatment for vasospasm?

Nimodipine (calcium channel blocker)

What is the treatment of aneurysm?

Surgical treatment by placing a metal clip on the aneurysm is the mainstay of therapy. Alternatives include balloon occlusion or coil embolization.

What is the treatment of AVM?

Many are on the brain surface and accessible operatively. Preoperative embolization can reduce the size of the AVM. For surgically inaccessible lesions, radiosurgery (gamma knife) has been effective in treating AVMs less than 3 cm in diameter.

INTRACEREBRAL HEMORRHAGE

What is it?

Bleeding into the brain parenchyma

What is the etiology?

Number one is hypertensive/atherosclerotic disease giving rise to Charcot-Bouchard aneurysms (small tubular aneurysms along smaller terminal arteries); other causes include coagulopathies, AVMs, amyloid angiopathy, bleeding into a tumor, and trauma.

Where does it occur?

Two-thirds occur in the basal ganglia; putamen is the structure most commonly affected.

How often does blood spread to the ventricular system?
Two-thirds of cases

What is the usual presentation?
Two-thirds present with coma; large putamen bleeding classically presents with contralateral hemiplegia and hemisensory deficits, lateral gaze preference, aphasia, and homonymous hemianopsia.

What is the associated diagnostic study?
CT

What are the surgical indications?
CN III palsy, progressive alteration of consciousness

What is the prognosis?
Poor, especially with ventricular or diencephalons involvement

SPINE

LUMBAR DISC HERNIATION

What is it?
Extrusion of the inner portion of the intervertebral disc (nucleus pulposus) through the outer annulus fibrosis, causing impingement on nerve roots exiting the spinal canal

Which nerve is affected?
The nerve exiting at the level below (e.g., an L4-L5 disc impinges on the L5 nerve exiting between L5-S1)

Who is affected?
Middle-aged and older individuals

What is the usual cause?
Loss of elasticity of the posterior longitudinal ligaments and annulus fibrosis as a result of aging

What are the most common sites?
L5-S1 (45%)
L4-L5 (40%)

What is the usual presenting symptom?
Low back pain

What are the signs:

L5-S1?
Decreased ankle jerk reflex
Weakness of plantar flexors in foot

	Pain in back/midgluteal region to posterior calf to lateral foot Ipsilateral radiculopathy on straight leg raise
L4-L5?	Decreased biceps femoris reflex Weak extensors of foot
L3-L4?	Decrease or absence of knee jerks, weakness of the quadriceps femoris, pain in lower back/buttock, pain in lateral thigh and anterior thigh Pain in hip/groin region to posterolateral thigh, lateral leg, and medial toes
What is cauda equina syndrome?	Herniated disc compressing multiple S1, S2, S3, S4 nerve roots, resulting in bowel/bladder incontinence, "saddle anesthesia" over buttocks/perineum, low back pain, sciatica
What is "sciatica"?	Radicular or nerve root pain
How is the diagnosis made?	CT, CT myelogram, or MRI
What is the treatment?	Conservative—bed rest and analgesics Surgical—partial hemilaminectomy and discectomy (removal of herniated disc)
What are the indications for emergent surgery?	1. Cauda equina syndrome 2. Progressive motor deficits

CERVICAL DISC DISEASE

What is it?	Basically the same pathology as previously described, except in the cervical region; the disc impinges on the nerve exiting the canal at the same level of the disease (e.g., a C6-C7 disc impinges on the C7 nerve root exiting at the C6-C7 foramen)
What are the most common sites?	C6-C7 (70%) C5-C6 (20%) C7-T1 (10%)
What are the signs/symptoms:	
C7?	Decreased triceps reflex/strength, weakness of forearm extension

Pain from neck, through triceps and into index and middle finger

C6?

Decreased biceps and brachioradialis reflex
Weakness in forearm flexion
Pain in neck, radial forearm, and thumb

C8?

Weakness in intrinsic hand muscles, pain in fourth/fifth fingers

What is Spurling's sign?

Reproduction of radicular pain by having the patient turn his head to the affected side and applying axial pressure to the top of the head

How is the diagnosis made?

CT or MRI

What is the treatment?

Anterior or posterior discectomy with fusion PRN

What are the symptoms of central cervical cord compression from disc fragments?

Myelopathic syndrome with LMN signs at level of compression and UMN signs distally; e.g., C7 compression may cause bilateral loss of triceps reflex and bilateral hyperreflexia, clonus, and Babinski signs in lower extremities

SPINAL EPIDURAL ABSCESS

What is the etiology?

Hematogenous spread from skin infections is most common; also, distant abscesses/infections, UTIs, postoperative infections, and LPS, spine surgery

What is the commonly associated medical condition?

Diabetes mellitus

What are the most common sites?

1. Thoracic
2. Lumbar
3. Cervical

What is the most common organism?

Staphylococcus aureus

What are the signs/symptoms?

Fever; severe pain over affected area and with flexion/extension of spine; weakness can develop, ultimately leading to paraplegia; 15% of patients have a back furuncle

How is the diagnosis made?
MRI is test of choice.

Which test is contraindicated?
LP, because of the risk of seeding CSF with bacteria, causing meningitis

What is the treatment?
Surgical drainage and appropriate antibiotic coverage

What is the prognosis?
Depends on preop condition; severe neurologic deficits (e.g., paraplegia) show little recovery; 15% to 20% of cases are fatal

PEDIATRIC NEUROSURGERY

HYDROCEPHALUS

What is it?
Abnormal condition consisting of an increased volume of CSF along with distension of CSF spaces

What are the three general causes?
1. Increased production of CSF
2. Decreased absorption of CSF
3. Obstruction of normal flow of CSF (90% of cases)

What is the normal daily CSF production?
Approximately 500 ml

What is the normal volume of CSF?
Approximately 150 ml in the average adult

Define "communicating" versus "noncommunicating" hydrocephalus.
Communicating—unimpaired connection of CSF pathway from lateral ventricle to subarachnoid space
Noncommunicating—complete or incomplete obstruction of CSF flow within or at the exit of the ventricular system

What are the specific causes of hydrocephalus?
1. Congenital malformation
   Aqueductal stenosis
   Myelomeningocele
2. Tumors obstructing CSF flow

3. Inflammation causing impaired absorption of fluid
   Subarachnoid hemorrhage
   Meningitis
4. Choroid plexus papilloma causing increased production of CSF

What are the signs/ symptoms?

Signs of increased ICP: HA, nausea, vomiting, ataxia, increasing head circumference exceeding norms for age

How is the diagnosis made?

CT, MRI, measurement of head circumference

What is the treatment?

1. Remove obvious offenders.
2. Perform bypass obstruction with ventriculoperitoneal shunt or ventriculoatrial shunt.

What is the prognosis if untreated?

50% mortality; survivors show decreased IQ (mean = 69); neurologic sequelae: ataxia, paraparesis, visual deficits

What are the possible complications of treatment?

1. Blockage/shunt malfunction
2. Infection

What is hydrocephalus ex vacuo?

Increased volume of CSF spaces from brain atrophy, not from any pathology in the amount of CSF absorbed or produced

What is a "shunt series"?

A series of x-rays covering the entire shunt length—looking for shunt disruption/ kinking to explain malfunction of shunt

SPINAL DYSRAPHISM/NEURAL TUBE DEFECTS

What is the incidence?

Approximately 1/1000 live births in the United States

What are the race/gender demographics?

More common in white patients and female patients

Define spina bifida occulta.

Defect in the development of the posterior portion of the vertebrae

What are the signs/ symptoms?

Usually asymptomatic, though it may be associated with other spinal abnormalities; usually found incidentally on x-rays

What is the most common clinically significant defect?

Myelomeningocele: herniation of nerve roots and spinal cord through a defect in the posterior elements of the vertebra(e); the sac surrounding the neural tissue may be intact, but more commonly is ruptured and therefore exposes the CNS to the external environment

What are the most common anatomic sites?

#1 lumbar region; #2 lower thoracic region; #3 upper sacral region

What are the signs/symptoms?

Variable from mild skeletal deformities to a complete motor/sensory loss; bowel/bladder function is difficult to evaluate, but often is affected and can adversely affect survival

What is the treatment?

With open myelomeningoceles, patients are operated on immediately to prevent infection.

What is the prognosis?

Approximately 95% survival for the first 2 years, compared with 25% in patients not undergoing surgical procedures

Which vitamin is thought to lower the rate of neural tube defects in utero?

Folic acid

CRANIOSYNOSTOSIS

What is it?

Premature closure of one or more of the sutures between the skull plates

What is the incidence?

1/200 live births in the United States

What are the types?

Named for the suture that is fused (e.g., sagittal, coronal, lambdoid); sagittal craniosynostosis accounts for more than 50% of all cases; more than one suture can be fused, and all or part of a suture may be affected

How is the diagnosis made?

Physical examination can reveal ridges along fused sutures and lessened suture mobility. Plain x-rays can show a lack of lucency along the fused suture, but are rarely required.

What are the indications for surgery?

Most often the reasons are cosmetic, as the cranial vault will continue to deform with growth. Occasionally, a child will present with increased ICP secondary to restricted brain growth.

What is the timing of surgery?

Usually 3 to 4 months of age; earlier surgery increases the risk of anesthesia; later surgeries are more difficult because of the worsening deformities and decreasing malleability of the skull

What is the operative mortality?

Less than 1%

MISCELLANEOUS

Which IV anesthetic increases ICP?

Ketamine; consequently, this medication should be avoided in head trauma patients

What is the most common bacteria causing post-neurosurgery meningitis?

Staphylococcus aureus (skin flora)

What classically presents as the "worst headache of my life"?

Spontaneous subarachnoid hemorrhage

What classically has a "lucid interval"?

Epidural hemorrhage

What is the most common location of a hypertensive intracerebral hemorrhage?

Putamen

What is Horner's syndrome?

Cervical sympathetic chain lesion: M.A.P.:

1. **M**iosis
2. **A**nhydrosis of ipsilateral face
3. **P**tosis

What is a third-nerve palsy?

Think: the third nerve does three things:

1. Diplopia
2. Ptosis
3. Mydriasis

What is Millard-Gubler syndrome?

Pons infarction:
1. VI nerve palsy
2. VII nerve palsy
3. Contralateral hemiplegia

What is syringomyelia?

Central pathologic cavitations of the spinal cord

72 Urology

Define the following terms:

Cystogram	Contrast study of the bladder
Ureteral stents	Plastic tubes placed via cystoscope into the ureters for stenting, identification, etc.
Cystoscope	Scope placed into the urethra and into the bladder to visualize the bladder
Perc nephrostomy	Catheter placed through the skin into the kidney pelvis to drain urine with distal obstruction, etc.
Retrograde pyelogram	Dye injected into the ureter up into the kidney and films taken
RUG	**R**etrograde **U**rethro**G**ram (dye injected into the urethra and films taken; rules out urethral injury, usually in trauma patients)
Gomco clamp	Clamp used for circumcision; protects penis glans
Bell clapper's deformity	Condition of congenital absence of gubernaculum attachment to scrotum
Fournier's gangrene	Extensive tissue necrosis/infection of the perineum in patients with diabetes
Coudé catheter	Basically, a Foley catheter with hook on the end to get around a large prostate
Foley catheter	Straight bladder catheter placed through the urethra
Suprapubic catheter	Bladder catheter placed through the skin above the pubic symphysis into the bladder

Posthitis	Foreskin infection
Hydrocele	Clear fluid in the processus vaginalis membrane
Communicating hydrocele	Hydrocele that communicates with peritoneal cavity and, thus, gets smaller and larger as fluid drains and then reaccumulates
Noncommunicating hydrocele	Hydrocele that does not communicate with the peritoneal cavity; hydrocele remains the same size
Varicocele	Abnormal dilation of the pampiniform plexus to the spermatic vein in the spermatic cord; described as a "bag of worms"
Spermatocele	Dilatation of epididymis or vas deferens
Epididymitis	Infection of the epididymis
Prehn's sign	Elevation of the painful testicle that reduces the pain of epididymitis
TRUS	**T**rans **R**ectal **U**ltra**S**ound
DRE	**D**igital **R**ectal **E**xamination
Orchitis	Inflammation/infection of the testicle
Pseudohermaphroditism	Genetically **one** sex; partial or complete opposite-sex genitalia
Urgency	Overwhelming sensation to void immediately
Dysuria	Painful urination (usually burning sensation)
Frequency	Urination more times than usual
Polyuria	Urination in larger amounts than usual
Nocturia	Awakening to urinate
Hesitancy	Delay in urination

Pneumaturia	Air passed with urine via the urethra
Pyuria	WBC in urine; usually >10 WBC/HPF
Cryptorchidism	Undescended testicle
IVP	**I**ntra**V**enous **P**yelogram (dye is injected into the vein, collects in the renal collecting system, and an x-ray is taken)
Hematuria	RBCs in urine
Space of Retzius	Anatomic extraperitoneal space in front of the bladder
Enuresis	Involuntary urination while asleep
Incontinence	Involuntary urination
TURP	**T**rans**U**rethral **R**esection of the **P**rostate
PVR	**P**ost**V**oid **R**esidual
Priapism	Prolonged, painful erection
Paraphimosis	Foreskin held (stuck) in the retracted position
Phimosis	Inability to retract the foreskin
Balanitis	Inflammation/infection of the glans penis
Balanoposthitis	Inflammation/infection of the glans and prepuce of the penis
UTI	**U**rinary **T**ract **I**nfection
Peyronie's disease	Abnormal fibrosis of the penis shaft, resulting in a bend upon erection
BPH	**B**enign **P**rostatic **H**yperplasia
Epispadias	Abnormal urethral opening on the dorsal surface of the penis
Hypospadiasis	Abnormal urethral opening on the ventral surface of the penis

Impotence	Inability to achieve an erection
Sterility	Inability to reproduce
Appendix testis	Common redundant testicular tissue
VUR	**V**esico**U**reteral **R**eflux

UROLOGIC DIFFERENTIAL DIAGNOSIS

What is the differential diagnosis of scrotal mass?	Cancer, torsion, epididymitis, hydrocele, spermatocele, varicocele, inguinal hernia, testicular appendage, swollen testicle after trauma, nontesticular tumor (paratesticular tumor: e.g., rhabdomyosarcoma, leiomyosarcoma, liposarcoma)
What are the causes of hematuria?	Bladder cancer, trauma, UTI, cystitis from chemotherapy or radiation, stones, kidney lesion, BPH
What is the most common cause of severe gross hematuria without trauma or chemotherapy/radiation?	Bladder cancer
What is the differential diagnosis for bladder outlet obstruction?	BPH, stone, foreign body, urethral stricture, urethral valve
What is the differential diagnosis for ureteral obstruction?	Stone, tumor, iatrogenic (suture), stricture, gravid uterus, radiation injury, retroperitoneal fibrosis
What is the differential diagnosis for kidney tumor?	Renal cell carcinoma, sarcoma, adenoma, angiomyolipoma, hemangiopericytoma, oncocytoma

RENAL CELL CARCINOMA

What is it?	Most common solid renal tumor (90%); originates from proximal renal tubular epithelium
What is the epidemiology?	Primarily a tumor of adults 40 to 60 years of age with a 2:1 male:female ratio; makes up less than 5% of cancers in adults; equal incidence in white and African-American patients

What percentage of the tumors are bilateral?

1%

What are the symptoms?

Pain (40%), hematuria (35%), weight loss (35%), flank mass (25%), HTN (20%)

What is the classic TRIAD of renal cell carcinoma?

1. Flank pain
2. Hematuria
3. Palpable mass (**triad** occurs in only 10% to 15% of cases)

How are most cases diagnosed these days?

Found incidentally on an imaging study (CT, MRI, U/S) for another reason

What radiologic tests are performed?

1. IVP
2. Abdominal CT with contrast

Define the stages (AJCC):

I

Tumor <2.5 cm, no nodes, no metastases

II

Tumor >2.5 cm limited to kidney, no nodes, no metastases

III

Tumor extends into IVC or main renal vein; positive regional lymph nodes but <2 cm in diameter and no metastases

IV

Distant metastasis or positive lymph node >2 cm in diameter or tumor extends past Gerota's fascia

What is the metastatic workup?

CXR, IVP, CT, LFTs, calcium

What gland is removed with a radical nephrectomy?

Adrenal gland

What are the sites of metastases?

Lung, liver, brain, bone; tumor thrombus entering renal vein or IVC is not uncommon

What is the unique route of spread?

Tumor thrombus into **IVC lumen**

What is the treatment?

Radical nephrectomy (excision of the kidney and adrenal, including Gerota's fascia) for stages I through IV

What is the unique treatment for metastatic spread?	Interleukin-2 (IL-2) and alpha-interferon (IFN-a)

BLADDER CANCER

What is the incidence?	Second most common urologic malignancy Male:female ratio of 3:1 White patients are more commonly affected than are African-American patients.
What is the histology?	Transitional cell carcinoma (TCC)—90%; remaining cases are squamous or adenocarcinomas
What are the risk factors?	Smoking, industrial carcinogens (aromatic amines), schistosomiasis, truck drivers, petroleum workers
What are the symptoms?	**Hematuria,** with or without irritative symptoms (e.g., dysuria)
What is the classic presentation of bladder cancer?	"Painless hematuria"
What tests are included in the workup?	Urinalysis and culture, IVP, cystoscopy with cytology and biopsy
Define the stages (according to the Jewett/Marshall system):	
O	Superficial, limited to mucosa; also known as carcinoma in situ (CIS)
A	Involves lamina propria
B	Muscle invasion
C	Extends to perivesicular fat
D	Abdominal organ metastasis (contiguous), lymph node metastasis, distant metastasis
What is the treatment according to stage:	
Stage O?	Bladder chemotherapy (intravesical chemotherapy)

Stage A?	TURB
Stages B and C?	Radical cystectomy, lymph node dissection, removal of prostate/uterus/ovaries/anterior vaginal wall, and urinary diversion (e.g., ileal conduit)
Stage D?	+/− Cystectomy and **systemic chemotherapy**
What is TURB?	**T**rans-**U**rethral **R**esection of the **B**ladder

PROSTATE CANCER

What is the incidence?	Number one GU cancer (>100,000 new cases per year in the United States); most common carcinoma in men in the United States; second most common cause of death in men in the United States
What is the epidemiology?	"A disease of elderly men" present in one-third of men 70 to 79 years of age and in two-thirds of men 80 to 89 years of age at autopsy; African-American patients have a 50% higher incidence than do white patients.
What is the histology?	Adenocarcinoma (95%)
What are the symptoms?	Often asymptomatic; usually presents as a nodule found on routine rectal examination; in 70% of cases, cancer begins in the periphery of the gland and moves centrally; thus, obstructive symptoms occur late; 40% of patients have metastatic disease at presentation, with symptoms of bone pain and weight loss
What are the common sites of metastasis?	Osteoblastic bony lesions, lung, liver, adrenal
What provides lymphatic drainage?	Obturator and hypogastric nodes
What is the significance of Batson's plexus?	Spinal cord venous plexus; route of isolated skull/brain metastasis

What are the steps in early detection and surveillance?

1. Prostate-specific antigen (PSA)—most sensitive and specific marker
2. Acid phosphatase—often elevated in metastatic prostate cancer; used mostly to detect recurrences
3. Rectal examination

How is the diagnosis made?

Transrectal biopsy

What are the indications for transrectal biopsy with normal rectal examination?

PSA >10 or abnormal transrectal ultrasound

Staging (AJCC):

Stage I?

Clinically inapparent tumor, no nodes, no metastases

Stage II?

Tumor within prostate, no nodes, no metastases

Stage III?

Tumor through prostate capsule, no nodes, no metastases

Stage IV?

Tumor extends into adjacent structures or + nodes or + metastases.

What are the treatment options according to stage:

Stage I

Radical prostatectomy +/− external beam radiation

Stage II?

Radical prostatectomy +/− radiation

Stage III?

Radiation therapy

Stage IV?

Hormonal treatment

What is the role of chemotherapy for prostate cancer?

None

What is the hormonal treatment?

Deprive androgens/testosterone:

Hormonal therapy (palliative); androgen blockade with estrogen diethylstilbestrol (DES) or

Luteinizing hormone-releasing hormone (LHRH) agonists

Surgical castration (orchiectomy)

BENIGN PROSTATIC HYPERPLASIA

What is it also known as?
BPH

What is it?
Disease of elderly men (average age is 60 to 65 years); prostate gradually enlarges, creating symptoms of urinary outflow obstruction

What is the size of a normal prostate?
Between 20 and 25 gm

Where does BPH occur?
Periurethrally (note: prostate cancer occurs in the periphery of the gland)

What are the symptoms?
Obstructive-type symptoms: hesitancy, weak stream, nocturia, intermittency, UTI, urinary retention

How is the diagnosis made?
History, DRE, elevated postvoid residual (PVR), urinalysis, cystoscopy, U/S

What lab tests should be performed?
Urinalysis, PSA, BUN, CR

What is the differential diagnosis?
Prostate cancer (e.g., nodular)—biopsy
Neurogenic bladder—history of neurologic disease
Acute prostatitis—hot, tender gland
Urethral stricture—RUG, history of STD
Stone
UTI

What are the treatment options?
Pharmacologic—α-1 blockade
Hormonal—antiandrogens
Surgical—TURP, TUIP, open prostate resection
Transurethral balloon dilation

What is Proscar?
Finasteride: 5-α-reductase inhibitor; blocks transformation of testosterone to dihydrotestosterone; may shrink and slow progression of BPH

What is Hytrin?
Terazosin: α-blocker; may increase urine outflow by relaxing prostatic smooth muscles

What are the indications for surgery?	Due to obstruction: Urinary retention Hydronephrosis UTIs Severe symptoms
What is "TURP"?	**T**rans**U**rethral **R**esection of **P**rostate: resection of prostate tissue via a scope
What is "TUIP"?	**T**rans**U**rethral **I**ncision of **P**rostate
What percentage of tissue removed for BPH will have malignant tissue on histology?	Up to 10%!
What are the possible complications of TURP?	Immediate: Failure to void Bleeding Clot retention UTI Incontinence

TESTICULAR CANCER

What is the incidence?	Rare; 2 to 3 new cases per 100,000 men per year in the United States
What is its claim to fame?	Most common solid tumor of young adult men (20 to 40 years)
What are the risk factors?	Cryptorchidism (6% of testicular tumors develop in patients with a history of cryptorchidism)
What is cryptorchidism?	Failure of the testicle to descend into the scrotum
Does orchiopexy as an adult remove the risk of testicular cancer?	NO
What are the symptoms?	Most patients present with a painless lump, swelling, or firmness of the testicle; they often notice it after incidental trauma to the groin.
What percentage of patients present with an acute hydrocele?	10%

What percentage present with symptoms of metastatic disease (back pain, anorexia)?
Approximately 10%

What are the classifications?
Germ cell tumors (95%):
- Seminomatous (35%)
- Nonseminomatous (65%)
- Embryonal cell carcinoma
- Teratoma
- Mixed cell
- Choriocarcinoma

Nongerminal (5%)
- Leydig cell
- Sertoli cell
- Gonadoblastoma

What is the major classification based on therapy?
Seminomas and nonseminoma tumors

What are the tumor markers for testicular tumors?
1. Human chorionic gonadotropin (HCG)
2. Alpha-fetoprotein (AFP)

What are the tumor markers by tumor type?
HCG—increased in choriocarcinoma (100%), embryonal carcinoma (50%), and rarely in pure seminomas (10%); (half of nonseminomatous tumors)
AFP—increased in embryonal carcinoma and yolk sac tumors (half of nonseminomatous tumors)

Which tumors almost never have an elevated AFP?
Choriocarcinoma and seminoma

In which tumor is HCG almost always found elevated?
Choriocarcinoma

How often is HCG elevated in patients with pure seminoma?
Only about 10% of the time!

What other tumor markers may be elevated and useful for recurrence surveillance?
LDH, CEA, human chorionic somatomammotropic (HCS), gamma-glutamyl transpeptidase (GGT), placental alkaline phosphate (PLAP)

What are the steps in workup?
PE, scrotal U/S, check tumor markers, CXR, CT (chest/pelvis/abd)

Define the stages according to TMN staging (AJCC):

Stage I — Confined to testis, into tunica albuginea or epididymis, no nodes, no metastases

Stage II? — **Positive** nodes, no metastases, any tumor

Stage III? — Distant metastases (any nodal status, any size tumor)

What is the initial treatment for all testicular tumors? — **Inguinal** orchiectomy (removal of testicle through a groin incision)

What is the treatment of seminoma at the various stages:

Stage I and IIA and B? — Inguinal orchiectomy and radiation to retroperitoneal nodal basins

Stages IIC and III? — Orchiectomy and chemotherapy

What is the treatment of nonseminomatous disease at the various stages:

Stage I? — Orchiectomy and retroperitoneal lymph node dissection versus close follow-up for retroperitoneal nodal involvement

Stages II and III? — Orchiectomy and chemotherapy (platinum based) +/− retroperitoneal lymph node dissection

What percentage of stage I seminomas are cured after treatment? — 95%

Which type is most radiosensitive? — Seminoma (think **S**eminoma = **S**ensitive to radiation)

Why not remove testis with cancer through a scrotal incision? — It could result in tumor seeding of the scrotum.

What is the major side effect of retroperitoneal lymph node dissection? — Impotence

TESTICULAR TORSION

What is it?
Torsion (twist) of the spermatic cord, resulting in venous outflow obstruction, and subsequent arterial occlusion → infarction of the testicle

What is the classic history?
Acute onset of scrotal pain usually after vigorous activity or minor trauma

What is a "bell clapper" deformity?
Bilateral nonattachment of the testicles by the gubernaculum to the scrotum (free like the clappers of a bell)

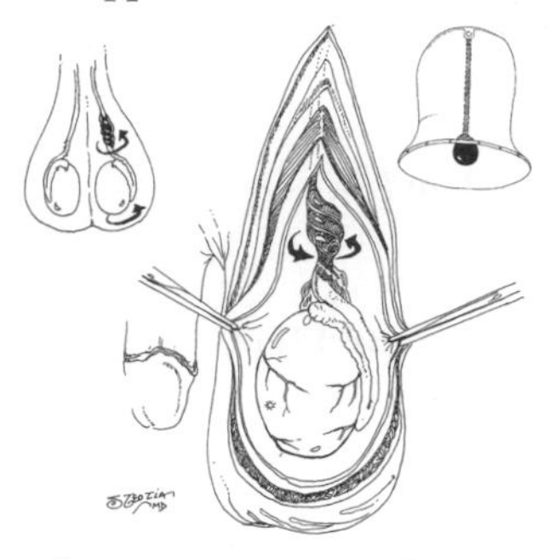

What are the symptoms?
Pain in the scrotum, suprapubic pain

What are the signs?
Very tender, swollen, elevated testicle; nonillumination; absence of cremasteric reflex

What is the differential diagnosis?
Testicular trauma, inguinal hernia, epididymitis, appendage torsion

How is the diagnosis made?
Surgical exploration, U/S (solid mass) and Doppler flow study, cold Tc-99m scan (nuclear study)

What is the treatment?
Surgical detorsion and bilateral orchiopexy to the scrotum

How much time is available from the onset of symptoms to detorse the testicle?
Less than 6 hours will bring about the best results; >90% salvage rate

What are the chances of testicle salvage after 24 hours?
<10%

EPIDIDYMITIS

What is it?
Infection of the epididymis

What are the signs/ symptoms?
Swollen, tender testicle; dysuria; scrotal ache/pain; fever; chills; scrotal mass

What is the cause?
Bacteria from the urethra

What are the common bugs in the following types of patients:

Elderly patients/children?
Escherichia coli

Young men?
STD bacteria: Gonorrhea, Chlamydia

What is the major differential diagnosis
Testicular torsion

What is the work up?
U/A, urine culture, swab if STD suspected, +/− U/S with Doppler or nuclear study to rule out torsion

What is the treatment?
Antibiotics

PRIAPISM

What is priapism?
Persistent penile erection

What are its causes?
Low flow: leukemia, drugs (e.g., prazosin), sickle-cell disease, impotence treatment gone wrong,
High flow; pudendal artery fistula, usually from trauma

What is first-line treatment?
1. Aspiration of blood from corporus cavernosum
2. Alpha-adrenergic agent

IMPOTENCE

What is it?
Inability to achieve an erection

What are the six major causes?
1. **Vascular:** decreased blood flow or leak of blood from the corpus cavernosus (most common cause)
2. **Endocrine:** low testosterone
3. **Anatomic:** structural abnormality of the erectile apparatus (e.g., Peyronie's disease)

4. **Neurologic:** damage to nerves (e.g., postoperative, IDDM)
5. **Medications** (e.g., clonidine)
6. **Psychologic:** performance anxiety, etc. (very rare)

What lab tests should be performed?

Fasting GLC (rule out diabetes and thus diabetic neuropathy)
Serum testosterone
Serum prolactin

What test evaluates for vascular causation of impotence?

Intracavernous vasoactive injection: injection of papaverine or PGE1 into the cavernous cavity of the penis; a full erection subsequently rules out a vascular cause of the impotence

What other diagnostic tests are often useful?

U/S with Doppler flow studies, cavernous pressures, arteriography (pudendal), penile monitoring for erection

What is the treatment?

Depends on the cause: vacuum pump, penile prosthesis, vasoactive injections (inject PGE1, papaverine, sildenafil, phentolamine), psychologic therapy, testosterone injections, Viagra

CALCULUS DISEASE

What is the incidence?

One in ten people will have stones.

What are the risk factors?

Poor fluid intake, IBD, hypercalcemia ("CHIMPANZEES"), renal tubular acidosis, small bowel bypass

What are the types of stones?

1. Calcium oxalate/calcium PO4 (75%)—secondary to hypercalciuria (increased intestinal absorption, decreased renal reabsorption, increased bone reabsorption)
2. Struvite (MgAmPh)(15%)—infection stones; E more than M; seen in UTI with urea-splitting bacteria (Proteus); may cause staghorn calculi; high urine pH
3. Uric acid (7%)—stones are radiolucent (think: **u**ric = **u**nseen); seen in gout,

Lesch-Nyhan, chronic diarrhea, cancer; low urine pH
4. Cystine (1%)—genetic predisposition

What type of stones are not seen on AXR?

Uric acid (Think: **U**ric = **U**nseen)

What stone is associated with UTIs?

Struvite stones (Think: **S**truvite = **S**epsis)

What stones are seen in IBD/bowel bypass?

Calcium oxalate

What are the symptoms?

Severe pain; patient cannot sit still: renal colic (typically pain in the kidney/ureter that radiates to the testis or penis), hematuria (remember, patients with peritoneal signs are motionless)

What are the classic findings/symptoms?

Flank pain, stone on AXR, hematuria

Diagnosis?

KUB (90% radiopaque), IVP, urinalysis and culture, BUN/Cr, CBC

What is the significance of hematuria and pyuria?

Stone with concomitant infection

Treatment?

Narcotics for pain, vigorous hydration, observation
Further options: ESWL (lithotripsy), ureteroscopy, percutaneous lithotripsy, open surgery; metabolic workup for recurrence

What are the indications for intervention?

Urinary tract obstruction
Persistent infection
Impaired renal function

What are the contra-indications of outpatient treatment?

Pregnancy, diabetes, obstruction, severe dehydration, severe pain, urosepsis/fever, pyelonephritis, previous urologic surgery/ one functioning kidney

What are the three common sites of obstruction?

1. Ureteropelvic junction (UPJ)
2. Ureterovesicular junction (UVJ)
3. Intersection of the ureter and the iliac vessels

INCONTINENCE

What are the common types of incontinence?	Stress incontinence, overflow incontinence, urge incontinence
Define the following terms:	
Stress incontinence	Loss of urine associated with coughing, lifting, exercise, etc.; seen most often in women, secondary to relaxation of pelvic floor following multiple deliveries
Overflow incontinence	Failure of the bladder to empty properly; may be caused by bladder outlet obstruction (BPH or stricture) or detrusor hypotonicity
Urge incontinence	Loss of urine secondary to detrusor instability in patients with stroke, dementia, Parkinson's disease, etc.
Enuresis	Bedwetting in children
How is the diagnosis made?	History (including meds), physical examination (including pelvic/rectal examination), urinalysis, postvoid residual (PR), urodynamics, cystoscopy/vesicocystourethrogram (VCUG) may be necessary
What is the "Marshall test"?	Woman with urinary stress incontinence placed in the lithotomy position with a full bladder leaks urine when asked to cough.
What is the treatment of the following disorders:	
Stress incontinence?	Bladder neck suspension
Urge incontinence?	Pharmacotherapy (anticholinergics, α-agonists)
Overflow incontinence?	Self-catheterization, surgical relief of obstruction, alpha blockers

UTI

What is it?	Urinary tract infection

What is the etiology?

Ascending infection, instrumentation, sex in females

What are the common organisms?

1. *E. coli* (90%)
2. *Proteus*
3. *Klebsiella, Pseudomonas*

What are the predisposing factors?

Stones, obstruction, reflux, diabetes mellitus, pregnancy, indwelling catheter/stent

What are the symptoms?

Lower UTI—frequency, urgency, dysuria, nocturia
Upper UTI—back/flank pain, fever, chills

How is the diagnosis made?

Symptoms, urinalysis (>10 WBCs/HPF, >105 CFU grown from clean-catch urine)

When should workup be performed?

After first infection in male patients (unless Foley is in place)
After first pyelonephritis in prepubescent female patients

What is the treatment?

Lower: 1 to 4 days of oral antibiotics
Upper: 3 to 7 days of IV antibiotics

WARD QUESTIONS

Why should orchiopexy be performed?

Decreases the susceptibility to blunt trauma
Increases the ease of follow-up examinations

In which area of the prostate does BPH arise?

Periurethral

In which area of the prostate does prostate cancer arise?

Periphery

What type of bony lesions are seen in metastatic prostate cancer?

Osteoblastic (radiopaque)

What percentage of renal cell carcinoma shows evidence of metastatic disease at presentation?

Approximately 33%

What is the most common site of distant metastasis in renal cell carcinoma?

Lung

What is the most common solid renal tumor of childhood?

Wilms' tumor

What type of renal stone is radiolucent?

Uric acid (Think: **U**ric = **U**nseen)

What are posterior urethral valves?

The most common obstructive urethral lesion in infants and newborns; occurs only in males; found at the distal prostatic urethra

What is the most common intraoperative bladder tumor?

A Foley catheter—don't fall victim!

What provides drainage of the left gonadal (e.g., testicular) vein?

Left renal vein

What provides drainage of the right gonadal vein?

IVC

What are the signs of urethral injury in the trauma patient?

"High-riding, ballottable" prostate, blood at the urethral meatus, severe pelvic fracture, ecchymosis of scrotum

What is the evaluation for urethral injury in the trauma patient?

RUG (**R**etrograde **U**rethro**G**ram)

What is the evaluation for a transected ureter intra-operatively?

IV indigo carmine and then look for leak of blue urine in the operative field

What aid is used to help identify the ureters in a previously radiated retroperitoneum?

Ureteral stents

How should a small traumatic PREperitoneal bladder rupture be treated?

Foley catheter

How should a traumatic INTRAperitoneal bladder rupture be treated?	Operative repair
What percentage of patients with an injured ureter will have no blood on urinalysis?	33%

73 Ophthalmology

Define the following terms:

Astigmatism	Asymmetric cornea
Esotropia	Eyes inward
Exotropia	Eyes outward
Hypertropia	Eyes upward
Hypotropia	Eyes downward
Hyperopia	Farsightedness
Diplopia	Double vision
Strabismus	Eye malalignment
Hyphema	Blood in anterior chamber of eye
Chemosis	Edema of the conjunctiva
Endophthalmitis	Intraocular infection
Ptosis	Eyelid droop
Anisocoria	Asymmetric pupil diameter
Nystagmus	Back and forth jerky movement of the eyes
Dacryocystitis	Lacrimal sac infection
Mydriasis	Pupil dilation (Think: my**D**riasis = **D**ilation)
Miosis	Pupil constriction
Myopia	Nearsightedness

PHACO	Phacoemulsification
PRK	**P**hoto**R**efractive **K**eratectomy
LASIK	**LAS**er **I**n situ **K**eratomileusis
AK	**A**stigmatic **K**eratotomy

OCULAR TRAUMA

What are the signs/symptoms of corneal abrasions?	Pain! History of ocular trauma
How are corneal abrasions diagnosed?	Fluorescein test
With a laceration of the eyebrow, should the eyebrow be shaved prior to suturing closed?	NO; 20% of the time the eyebrow will not grow back!
What is a retinal detachment?	A **separation** of the neurosensory retina from the pigment epithelium and its supportive choroid, resulting in retinal infarction
What causes retinal detachment?	**Trauma,** ocular surgery, diabetes, spontaneous—small rent in retina allows fluid to insinuate itself in the subretinal space, causing a retinal detachment
What are the signs/ symptoms of a retinal detachment?	Floaters, blind spots, flashing lights
What is the treatment for a retinal detachment?	Surgery—sclera buckling therapy
What is the major symptom of a lens detachment?	Blurred vision
What is the common ocular physical finding after a sinus fracture?	Conjunctivae emphysema
How are acid and alkali chemical eye burns treated?	Copious eye irrigation for both

What is sympathetic ophthalmia?	Autoimmune destruction of the contralateral **good eye** after penetrating injury causing blindness to ipsilateral eye; remove blind eye within 2 weeks following penetrating injury to avoid this condition
Should a penetrating eye object be removed?	NO! Call the ophthalmologist and do not remove.
What are the symptoms of BLOWOUT fracture?	Double vision
What is a concern if post-traumatic PROPTOSIS develops?	Retrobulbar hematoma (if severe treat with lateral canthotomy)
What is an eye finding with electrocution?	Cataracts
Refractive Surgery	
What is it?	Surgery to correct vision by reshaping the cornea
What are types?	PRK, AK, LASIK
What is PRK?	Photorefractive keratotomy—shaping of the cornea with a **laser only**
What is AK?	Astigmatic keratotomy—curved incisions are made into the cornea to smooth the asymmetric areas
What is LASIK?	Laser in situ keratotomy—the cutting of the cornea with a scalpel blade **and** then using a laser to modify the shape of the cornea

THE RED EYE

Give the classic signs/ symptoms of the following conditions:	
Bacterial conjunctivitis	Conjunctival redness with purulent discharge
Viral conjunctivitis	Conjunctival redness with serous discharge

Allergic conjunctivitis	Clear conjunctival discharge
Acute narrow angle glaucoma (congenital glaucoma)	Acute pain, cloudy cornea, perilimbal redness, blurred vision
Iritis	Perilimbal redness, irregular pupil, pain, decreased vision
Corneal ulcer	Epithelial defect with infiltrate, pain
Corneal abrasion	Epithelial defect, no infiltrate, pain
Orbital cellulitis	Periocular swelling, erythematous ocular surface, decreased vision

OPHTHALMOLOGY QUESTIONS

What is a cataract?	Opacification of the lens (treated by surgical removal)
What is strabismus?	Misalignment of the eyes
Why is it important to correct strabismus?	To allow proper development of visual acuity and binocular vision
What is a pterygium?	A plaque-like extension of fibrovascular tissue onto the cornea
In what cases should a blind eye be removed?	Blind and painful, malignancy, blind traumatized eye, diagnostic purposes
What is Horner's syndrome?	Sympathetic nerve lesion of the neck resulting in: 1. Miotic pupil 2. Ptosis 3. Decreased facial diaphoresis
What is a PHACO?	Phacoemulsification: cataract is removed with ultrasonic dissector/aspirator
What prophylactic antibiotics are given for eye surgery?	Gentamicin or tobramycin eye drops

Figure Credit Lines

Chapter 9 (carotid endarterectomy)
Lawrence PF, Bell RM, Dayton MT: ESSENTIALS OF GENERAL SURGERY, 3rd edition. Philadelphia, Lippincott Williams & Wilkins, 2000. p. 545

Chapter 27 (craniocaudal view and MLO view mammograms)
Gay SB, Woodcock RJ, Jr: RADIOLOGY RECALL. Philadelphia, Lippincott Williams & Wilkins, 2000. p. 522

Chapter 35 (anatomy of the larynx)
Doherty GM, Meko JB, Olson JA, et al: THE WASHINGTON MANUAL OF SURGERY, 2nd edition. Philadelphia, Lippincott Williams & Wilkins, 1999. p. 635, Fig 42-6

Chapter 37 (Sengstaken-Blakemore balloon)
Lawrence PF, Bell, RM, Dayton MT: ESSENTIALS OF GENERAL SURGERY, 3rd edition. Philadelphia, Lippincott Williams & Wilkins, 2000. p. 353, Fig 18-8

Chapter 53 (rectus abdominis flap reconstruction)
Greenfield LJ, Mulholland M, Oldham KT, Zelenock GB, Lillemoe KD: SURGERY: SCIENTIFIC PRINCIPLES AND PRACTICES, 2nd edition. Philadelphia, Lippincott-Raven Publishers, 1997. p. 2283, Fig 114-4

Chapter 54 (gastrinoma triangle)
Greenfield LJ, Mulholland M, Oldham KT, Zelenock GB, Lillemoe, KD: SURGERY: SCIENTIFIC PRINCIPLES AND PRACTICES, 2nd edition. Philadelphia, Lippincott-Raven Publishers, 1997. p. 924, Fig 34-8

Chapter 70-9B (Colles' fracture)
McKenney MG, Mangonon PC, Moylan JA: UNDERSTANDING SURGICAL DISEASE: THE MIAMI MANUAL OF SURGERY. Philadelphia, Lippincott-Raven Publishers, 1998. p. 355, Fig 4

Chapter 71-2 (Kocher's point)
Spector SA: CLINICAL COMPANION IN SURGERY. Philadelphia, Lippincott Williams & Wilkins, 1999. p. 430, Fig 33-1

Index

Page numbers in *italics* denote figures; those followed by a t denote tables.